Behavior Analysis and Substance Dependence

Simone Martin Oliani • Richard Alecsander Reichert • Roberto Alves Banaco
Editors

Behavior Analysis and Substance Dependence

Theory, Research and Intervention

Springer

Editors
Simone Martin Oliani
Centro Integrado de Neuropsiquiatria e Psicologia Comportamental (CINP)
Londrina, PR, Brazil

Roberto Alves Banaco
Paradigma - Centro de Ciências e Tecnologia do Comportamento
São Paulo, SP, Brazil

Richard Alecsander Reichert
Department of Psychobiology
Universidade Federal de São Paulo (UNIFESP)
São Paulo, SP, Brazil

ISBN 978-3-030-75960-5 ISBN 978-3-030-75961-2 (eBook)
https://doi.org/10.1007/978-3-030-75961-2

This Springer imprint is published by the registered company Springer Nature Switzerland AG
The registered company address is: Gewerbestrasse 11, 6330 Cham, Switzerland

Foreword

The book *Behavior Analysis and Substance Dependence: Theory, Research and Intervention*, organized by Simone Oliani, Richard Reichert and Roberto Banaco, is another example of the breadth of the field explored by Behavior Analysis. I have already written about this amplitude when talking about *Aplysia*, in one extreme, and the analysis of the Brazilian Constitution, in the other.[1] Focusing on the theme of behavioral analysis of drug dependence, its effects and possibilities of intervention by the psychologist, the chapters deal with diagnostic criteria, basic concepts of behavioral pharmacology, functional analysis of the use and dependence on psychoactive substances, establishing and abiding contingencies of the use of these substances, and various behavioral methods and techniques to address the problem; and among the authors are the greatest Brazilian specialists in the study and treatment of substance use disorders.

Association for Behavior Analysis International (ABAI),
Universidade de Brasília
João Claudio Todorov,

Brasília, Brazil
January 2021

[1] Todorov, J. (2004). From Aplysia to the Constitution: Evolution of Concepts in Behavior Analysis. *Psicologia: Reflexão e Crítica*, *17*(2), 151–156. https://doi.org/10.1590/S0102-79722004000200003

Preface

There is a certain comfort in being a Darwinist. The belief in continuity between species allows us to look elsewhere for the causes of problematic human behavior rather than within ourselves. Many human behaviors seem to insist on going in the opposite direction of survival and reproduction, in the saga of living in a hostile environment, as if seeking to eliminate individuals so that they disappear in the times to come. When we pursue the species' hesitant steps in this direction, or even against such fate, at first, we go after that which would be illogical for the species to remain on the face of the Earth. And we call the behaviors found in this collision course with human destruction itself as bizarre, inadequate, unsuitable or pathological. We then proceed in search of what we supposedly know: solving problems of Creation – be it attributed to a god, be it attributed to nature.

This is what happens with drug addiction. Although the beginning of its use may have had some pleasant and reinforcing effects, the subsequent observation of the harmful effects of its abuse should be enough for the other members to try to avoid them. But it is not.

A refusal to the laws of Natural Selection was also created. Rather than, like in other species, allowing it to act on the weakest and most maladaptive individuals, sweeping them out of existence, we have followed a different path. We've tried to avoid with all our strength that our peers say farewell to life, even when their own behavior directs them towards it.

Perhaps we can find the explanation for the interference with other people's lives in the physically fragile origin of the human species in relation to other species (the felines, for example), at the time when culture was beginning to develop. At that time, living in a pack was good, because it was important for us to have behaviors that could protect one another. The phylogenetic contingency prayed that the more numerous we were within a group, the better it would be for everyone. And the stronger we were, the better. Therefore, continuing our assumption, caring for each other was a selected behavior in our species. Making a weak individual become strong, a sick person getting healthy, started bringing benefits to everyone, making the group and culture survive (Marcuse & Pear, 1979). Making the individual produce behaviors that left one strengthened and healthy also became a value towards the direction in which culture has walked. And perhaps medical therapies and later psychological therapies started there. Therapies are nothing more than attempts to make individuals who would be wiped out of existence by their behaviors stay here a little longer.

One of the problematic behaviors that appeared, and that seemed to destroy the existence of Humans was the adhesion of some individuals to the excessive use of substances that altered the states of consciousness. In addition to putting the organism at risk, this behavior sometimes created problems for group living. And the group is now more organized, trying to solve the problems caused by the individual who was abusing drug use.

Many conceptions started to explain and to try solving the problem from that explanation. They are described in Table 2.1 of Chap. 2, and I will not dwell on them now. But the Darwinian conception, once again, was to look for traces of the problem in phylogenesis. And it was found that so many other species also sought to change their behavior when they consumed certain vegetables or their products. For example, legend has it that coffee was discovered for human use in this way: an Ethiopian shepherd who noticed that his sheep were excited when they ate the fruits of the coffee tree. From that observation, many cultural practices have evolved, making coffee today the second most consumed beverage in the world, second only to tea.

But other species have been found that also seek to alter their states of balance and behavior. Ronald Siegel (1979) mentions some of those: elephants look for alcohol from fermented marula fruits or the drink already made from the fermentation of these fruits. For this reason, they illustrate the "Amarula"® liquor label. But monkeys, ostriches, wildebeest, wild boar, giraffes and birds have already been registered that look for this fruit and have drunken effects.[1] And they look for it again. Cats – and other felines – are also fascinated by a hallucinogenic herb called Nepeta cataria, which has, as an effect on their behavior, playing with "imaginary butterflies". The "pet" market sells it under the name "catnip", and it is possible to watch on YouTube some videos about the hallucinogenic effects and the high caused by the drug in animals.[2] Pigeons and other birds, in turn, look for cannabis seeds and experience behavioral changes. So much that they end up inadvertently identifying and denouncing plantations.[3] And, as it is in the public domain, koalas look for eucalyptus that appears to have narcotic effects on them when consumed.[4]

The fact is that drugs end up becoming reinforcers acquired by their behavioral and pharmacological effects (Garcia-Mijares & Silva, 2006) and some of them interfere with responding processes, which in turn determine the operant behavior of looking for the drug (Banaco & Montan, 2018). According to Cunningham (1998), these responding processes are due to aversive sensations produced by the

[1] An illustration can be seen in https://youtu.be/Aq9xx3hD-K0

[2] https://youtu.be/cmkNtrno2Ek

[3] https://www.youtube.com/watch?v=DN5HOMgZL-U

[4] https://www.youtube.com/watch?v=DYFBsAG3VQs

opposite effect to that of the drug (which we usually call “craving”), elicited by the antecedent stimuli conditioned to the drug use. For this reason, the drug is also considered an unconditioned stimulus, since its administration and its effects are also controlled by the “cues” which precede them, turning these cues into conditioned stimuli (Cunningham, 1998). Thus, the use of the drug would be negatively reinforced by the temporary relief experienced in the “craving” state in which the organism is when it comes in contact with the cues, which predict the relapse from time to time, even after long periods without using the drug. Having contact with any significant level of the stimulus conditioned to the use would already be enough for the active search for the drug to begin, since in the past it has brought relief to the discomfort caused by such stimulus.

Solutions to this problem which plagues society are sought, both by those who try to “get people out” of substance dependence, and those who find themselves “trapped” by it. In addition to several kinds of therapies already tried, several experimental models, mostly with animals, seek to extract relevant variables to be manipulated in the treatments. Hartnoll (1991), making a constructive criticism for this search, without intending to discourage, points out some aspects that must be taken into account in relation to the use of experimental models to search for solutions to the problem.

The first one is that the classification of what would be considered a drug of abuse is directly linked to the culture and the historical moment that is determining the criterion from which the use will be considered abusive. For example, Hartnoll points out that, from the legal point of view, at the time the author wrote the article, the use and sale of marijuana, amphetamine, psychotropic drugs, cocaine and heroin was considered illegal in the West, while in the East, especially in Arab countries, alcohol use was very poorly evaluated. Today, in the West, marijuana has gradually found a greater acceptance, both in recreational and medical use, given some of its components. Nowadays, there is also a gradual increase in the acceptance of psychotropic drugs, especially in psychotherapeutic processes.[5] These types of substances, which were already widely used recreationally and religiously in the 60s and 70s, have gone through a severe ban in the West in the 80s and onwards.

If the behavioral control agency is Health and General Medicine, then they consider drugs of abuse to be those that are most likely to cause harmful consequences to one’s health. In this case, the worst use will be considered by professionals, in the following order of importance: tobacco, alcohol, tranquilizers, opiates and stimulants. From the point of view of Epidemiology (frequency of use in the population), by far the biggest drug of abuse is caffeine (found in coffee, teas, soft drinks). Then alcohol, tobacco, marijuana, tranquilizers, and far behind, amphetamines, psychotropics, cocaine and opiates. If the assessment is made by the criterion of self-administration, that is, drugs that produce a greater craving, the sequence, in order of damage relevance is: cocaine and amphetamines, opiates, barbiturates,

[5] https://icpr2020.net/tc-events/icpr-2020-online/

dissociative anesthetics, alcohol, nicotine, caffeine and benzodiazepines, and finally, with a low level of physical dependence, marijuana (Hartnoll, 1991).

As for drug abuse and self-administration, experimental models reveal that drugs widely used by man are not self-administered in the laboratory (tobacco, marijuana, caffeine) or are not easily self-administered (alcohol, benzodiazepines, psychotropics). Other drugs that are easily self-administered in the laboratory in animals are not widely used by men (especially opioids and some stimulants). To get an idea of the difficulty in making an experimental model to study self-administration, Elsmore, Fletcher, Conrad and Sodetz (1980) subjected baboons to choices between food and heroin by attempts, increasing the cost of the choice response, simply by gradually increasing the interval between attempts. The monkeys kept their number of choices for food stable in each successive phase of increasing the cost of the response, and decreased their choice of heroin, proportionally to the cost. The data obtained were analyzed by Green and Freed (1998) representing, in Behavioral Economics, as food being an inelastic asset (its high importance was maintained, despite successive increases in the response cost), while heroin proved to be an elastic asset (its choice decreased as the "price" to be paid increased). In humans, we see some users who stop eating to use drugs. But it is far from the majority. Most cocaine users, for example, are occasional and do not become addicted. Of those who have become addicted, most return to moderate use. And it is known that users who require treatment already suffered from other problems before cocaine addiction (Cunningham, 1998).

When taken to the laboratory, cocaine has a high potential for abuse. Under conditions of unlimited access to the drug, monkeys and rats can self-administer it until they reach the point of having seizures and, in some cases, causing their death. Cunningham recalls, however, that the animals used in the laboratory live in isolation, kept in small cages. Self-administration takes place through an implanted catheter, with few responses available in the experimental environment, other than to press the bar to release the drug. Men in isolation (prisons, for example) can do the same thing, if the drug is available, since functionally the environment for them is very similar: cells with little space for good coexistence, few activities, and at the same time with the drug being available. Self-administration studies in isolated animals, therefore, have a doubtful validity about how humans behave in their social and natural environments.

In addition, it is known that rats and monkeys are social animals and, therefore, to mimic the human problem in the laboratory, one should use social models with availability of drug use, but these are difficult to craft. Perhaps this type of model would bring relevant knowledge, at least, about the first times individuals use drugs. In humans, usually, the first experiences with drugs are situations of social conformity (teenagers starting to smoke, for example), some social rituals (drinking coffee in pairs or groups in the morning), situations of reinforcement for "being part of the group" (for example, the use of alcohol since one's childhood, in a family that takes pride in drinking a lot[6]). There are also cases in which people start using drugs in search of a meaning for life (psychotropic to increase awareness: *Santo Daime* in religious rituals, psilocybin and other psychedelic drugs in psychotherapies[7]).

Even with these difficulties in transposing animal models to humans and vice versa, some ways of dealing with the problem end up being extracted from this literature. According to Cunningham (1998) there are several:

One is the effort to remove stimuli associated with the drug, or to remove the individual from the environment associated with it. This is extremely difficult, but there are strong indications that this removal is beneficial: of the total number of substance dependent people who returned from the Vietnam war and went to a rehabilitation service, it was observed that 54% of those who went to new homes remained abstinent, while only 12% remained abstinent when they returned to their original homes. But, obviously, this change to new environments after detoxification is practically impossible.

Another procedure extracted from these models is to make the respondent extinction by unpairing the stimuli that are triggers for craving responses from drug use. The major difficulty lies in identifying which aspects of the environment the drug was paired with.

A good clue that we can use is found in the Latent Inhibition literature. For example, Lubow and Moore (1959) exposed sheep to a sun picture several times, without any event following that exposure. This made "sun" a known stimulus, not paired with anything. Then, they made a Pavlovian pairing between that same picture with light shocks released on the animal's hind leg, which produced responsive flexing, up to the point that the sun picture, now assuming the function of conditioned stimulus after training, produced the leg flexing before the shock release.

They proceeded in the same way with a cloud picture, which was a new stimulus for the sheep. The data showed that the cloud picture has acquired the property of conditioned stimulus much earlier than the sun picture. This means that more common stimuli in one's life take longer to have the property of producing the conditioned response. One way, therefore, of being able to find the relevant stimuli for relapses, would be to probe with the drug dependent individual which stimuli were new when the substance use started. These stimuli are likely to elicit craving responses.

One can also try the contextual control of extinction that is set by exposing the individual to the complete context of pairing with drugs, obviously without allowing its use. The limitation of this proposal is clearly "convincing" the context (especially the social one) to take part in it.

Another possibility is called "conditioned inhibition", a procedure in which the presentation of a stimulus that was previously paired with "non-drug" must inhibit the conditioned response when presented with the drug-paired stimulus. The

[6] "In my house everyone is groovy, everyone drinks, everyone dances" – Martinho da Vila (Brazilian singer). https://www.youtube.com/watch?v=Wht3Ab8DJ6w

[7] https://www.uol.com.br/ecoa/reportagens-especiais/terapias-psicodelicas-podem-virar-o-jogo-no-tratamento-de-doencas-mentais/#page33

obstacle to this procedure is the same as above: finding out what is the conditioned stimulus that produces craving responses.

The difficulties do not end there. There are also other respondent properties that hinder the management of antecedent stimuli. Many of the CSs for CRs can be interoceptive (e.g., mood states). When this is identified, it becomes much more difficult to program the extinction of the pairing, since the control of mood states depends on events in the outside world. Sometimes due to aversive situations, which would not be ethical or possible to be manipulated (for example, the depression caused by the abandonment caused by a significant other). Another difficulty, disinhibition of the already extinct pairing can also occur when a new and intense stimulus restores the conditioned response to a conditioned stimulus after the extinction of the pairing has been completed (Cunningham, 1998).

In conclusion, the challenge is huge, relevant and important to be faced. More and more humans are dependent on substances either to achieve well-being, or to live the lifestyle which was promised in a capitalist system. It is not uncommon to see people who are dependent on sleep inducers or anxiolytics in order to be able to sleep. And a good percentage of those same people, need to take stimulating drugs in order to be able to do their jobs or acquire a desired level of concentration the next day. We are at a time when we are encouraged not to feel a minute of suffering. And we are presented, as one of the possibilities of not feeling, the use of substances that have the property of "erasing" such feelings, keeping us in the contingency that produces them. In any case, it is necessary for behavior analysts who deal with substance dependence to take into account respondent processes with the same importance as they deal with operant processes and verbal operants. The control of nature is still far from being achieved. Let us keep studying it in every possible way.

From the eighth month of reclusion during the COVID-19 pandemic

Londrina, Paraná, Brazil Roberto Alves Banaco

References

Banaco, R., & Montan, R. (2018). Teoria analítico-comportamental. In N. Zanelatto & R. Laranjeira (Eds.), *O tratamento da dependência química e as terapias cognitivo-comportamentais: um guia para terapeutas* (2nd ed., pp. 115–132). Artmed.

Cunningham, C.L. (1998) Drug Conditioning and drug-seeking behavior. In W. O´Donohue (Ed.) *Learning and behavior therapy* (pp. 518–544). Allyn & Bacon.

Elsmore, T. F., Fletcher, G. V., Conrad, D. G. & Sodetz, F. J. (1980). Reduction of heroine intake in baboons by an economic constraint. *Pharmacology, Biochemistry & Behavior 38*, 715–721. https://doi.org/10.1016/0091-3057(80)90018-0

Garcia-Mijares, M., & Silva, M. T. A. (2006). Dependência de drogas. *Psicologia USP, 17*(4). https://doi.org/10.1590/S0103-65642006000400012

Green, L., & Freed, D.E. (1998). Behavioral Economics. In W. O´Donohue (Ed.) *Learning and behavior therapy* (pp. 274–300). Allyn & Bacon.

Hartnoll, R. (1991). The relevance of behavioural models of drug abuse and dependence liabilities to the understanding of drug misuse in humans. In P. Willner (Ed.), *Behavioural models in psychopharmacology: theoretical, industrial and clinical perspectives* (503–519). Cambridge University Press.

Lubow, R. E., & Moore, A. U. (1959). Latent inhibition: The effect of nonreinforced pre-exposure to the conditional stimulus. *Journal of Comparative and Physiological Psychology* *52*(4), 415–419. https://doi.org/10.1037/h0046700

Marcuse, F. L., & Pear, J. J. (1979). Ethics and animal experimentation: personal views. In J.D. Keehn (Ed.), *Psychopathology in animals: research and clinical implications* (pp. 305–329). Academic Press.

Siegel, R. K. (1979). Natural animal addictions: an ethological perspective. In J.D. Keehn (Ed.), *Psychopathology in animals: research and clinical implications* (pp. 29–60). Academic Press.

Contents

About the Contributors

Eduardo Coelho Abreu Master in Social Psychology from the Post-Graduate Program in Psychology of the Federal University of Espírito Santo (UFES) and graduated in Psychology from the Faculdade Brasileira.

Alan Souza Aranha PhD student in the Department of Clinical Psychology of the University of São Paulo (USP). Specialist in Behavioral Therapy from the Institute of Therapy by Contingencies of Reinforcement (ITCR-Campinas).

Fábio Henrique Baia Master and Doctor in Behavioral Sciences from the Universidade de Brasília (UnB); and Bachelor in Psychology from the Pontifícia Universidade Católica de Minas Gerais (PUC-Minas). He is currently a Full Professor at the School of Psychology of the Universidade de Rio Verdade (UniRV) and a post-doctoral fellow in Experimental Psychology at the Universidade de São Paulo (USP).

Roberto Alves Banaco Master and PhD in Experimental Psychology from the Universidade de São Paulo (USP); and graduated in Psychology from the Pontifícia Universidade Católica de São Paulo (PUC-SP). He is academic director and professor of the Paradigma – Centro de Ciências e Tecnologia do Comportamento (Center for Behavior Sciences and Technology); Member of the Brazilian Society of Psychology (Sociedade Brasileira de Psicologia – SBP); Member of the Board of the Brazilian Association of Psychology and Behavior Medicine (Associação Brasileira de Psicologia e Medicina Comportamental – ABPMC); and Behavior Analyst accredited by the ABPMC. He has experience in Psychology, with emphasis on Psychological Treatment and Prevention, acting mainly in the following themes: behavior analysis, experimental behavior analysis, behavior analytic therapy, radical behaviorism and applied behavior analysis.

Elizeu Borloti PhD in Psychology from the Pontifical Catholic University of São Paulo (PUC-SP); Master in Psychology from the Federal University of Espírito Santo (UFES); and Specialist in Chemical Dependency from UFES. He is a

Behavioral Therapist, professor and researcher of the Post-Graduation Program in Psychology at UFES. He has experience in Psychology, with emphasis on Experimental Behavior Analysis and Psychological Prevention and Treatment, acting mainly on the following themes: verbal behavior, psychological disorders, stress, culture behavioral analysis, behavior and health and substance dependence.

André Amaral Bravin Master and Doctor in Behavior Sciences from the Universidade de Brasília (UnB); Expert in Clinical Psychology (Clinical Behavioral Analysis) from the Brasiliense Behavior Analysis Institute (Instituto Brasiliense de Análise do Comportamento – IBAC); and Bachelor in Psychology from the Universidade Católica de Brasília (UCB). He is currently a Full Professor at the School of Psychology of the Universidade Federal de Jataí (UFJ).

Fernanda Calixto She holds a Ph.D. in Psychology, and a post-doctoral degree from the Federal University of São Carlos (UFSCAR) and the Paradigm Center for Behavioral Sciences and Technology; a Master's degree in Behavioral Analysis from the State University of Londrina (UEL); and a degree in Psychology from the Federal University of Mato Grosso do Sul (UFMS). She develops research, interventions, and supervision related to the following themes: self-control, impulsiveness, gaming and internet addiction, aggressiveness, compulsion, substance dependence, decision making, and personality disorders.

Carlos Eduardo Costa Graduated in Psychology at the Universidade Estadual de Londrina (UEL); Master and PhD in Experimental Psychology at the Universidade de São Paulo (USP). He did a post-doctoral internship with the Programa de Mestrado Profissional em Análise do Comportamento Aplicada no Paradigma: centro de ciências e tecnologia do comportamento (Professional Master's Program in Applied Behavior Analysis at Paradigma – Behavioral Sciences and Technology Center. He is an Associate Professor at the Universidade Estadual de Londrina (UEL); Permanent Professor of the Programa de Pós-Graduação em Análise do Comportamento – UEL (Graduate Program in Behavior Analysis at UEL); General Editor of the journal Acta Comportamentalia and Associate Editor of the periodicals Revista Brasileira de Análise do Comportamento (REBAC) and Perspectivas em Análise do Comportamento; Member of REDETAC (www.redetac.org).

Débora Barbosa de Deus Master in Psychology from Universidade Estadual de Maringá (UEM); Specialist in Behavioral Psychotherapy from UEM; Specialist in Psychological Evaluation from Centro Universitário Integrado de Campo Mourão (INTEGRADO); and graduated in Psychology from UEM.

Célio Roberto Estanislau holds a degree in Psychology and a Masters in Neurosciences from the Universidade Federal de Santa Catarina (UFSC) and a PhD in Psychobiology from the Universidade de São Paulo (USP). He did postdoctoral studies at the Universitat Autònoma de Barcelona. He is a Professor at the

Universidade Estadual de Londrina (UEL). He has experience in Psychology, with emphasis on Psychobiology and Behavioral Neuroscience.

Jaqueline R. de Q. Vago Ferrari Master and PhD student in Psychology from the Universidade Federal do Espírito Santo (UFES); Specialist in Epidemiology from the UFES; Specialist in Cognitive-Behavioral Therapy from the Centro Universitário Amparense (UNIFIA); and graduated in Psychology from the UFES. She has experience in Psychology with emphasis on Mental Health, Substance Dependency and Clinical Psychology, working mainly with the following themes: welcoming and humanization in the treatment of substance dependence, love relationship in substance dependence and prevention of substance use for children and adolescents.

Fábio Leyser Gonçalves Is graduated in Psychology and got a Master's and Ph.D. in Neuroscience and Behavior at the University of São Paulo (USP), where he also served as post-doc. Currently, he is Professor in the Department of Psychology of the School of Sciences at São Paulo State University (UNESP) and on the Graduate Program in Neuroscience and Behavior of the Institute of Psychology – USP. He has experience in Psychology and Behavior Analysis, with emphasis in Electric and Drug Stimulation, acting mainly in the following themes: impulsivity, delay discounting, depression, drug abuse and sensitivity to reinforcement.

Edson Massayuki Huziwara PhD in Experimental Psychology from the Universidade de São Paulo (USP); Master in Special Education and graduated in Psychology from the Universidade Federal de São Carlos (UFSCar). He is an Adjunct Professor of the Department of Psychology and of the Post-Graduate Program in Psychology: Cognition and Behavior at the Universidade Federal de Minas Gerais (UFMG). He has experience in Psychology, with emphasis on Experimental Psychology, acting mainly in the following themes: stimulus equivalence, stimulus control and conditional discrimination with human participants and non-human subjects.

Dan Josua holds a bachelor's degree in Psychology from PUC-SP, specialization in Cognitive-Behavior Therapy from USP, training in Dialectical Behavioral Therapy by Behavioral Tech, and a master's degree in Clinical Psychology from PUC-SP. He is currently the coordinator of Evidence-Based Psychotherapy Training at InPBE – Institute for Evidence-Based Psychology, in addition to acting as a clinical psychologist.

Eduardo José Legal Master and PhD in Experimental Psychology from the Universidade de São Paulo (USP); and Bachelor in Psychology from the Universidade Federal de Santa Catarina (UFSC). He is currently a professor in undergraduate and master's courses in Psychology at the Universidade do Vale do Itajaí (UNIVALI). His research addresses the topics: neuropsychology of executive functions, resilience and well being.

Jan Luiz Leonardi holds a bachelor's degree in Psychology from PUC-SP, specialization in Behavioral Therapy from Paradigma, training in Dialectical Behavioral Therapy by Behavioral Tech, a master's degree in Experimental Psychology: Behavior Analysis from PUC-SP, and a PhD in Clinical Psychology from Universidade de São Paulo (USP). He was the academic coordinator of Paradigma's advanced qualification program in Behavioral Therapy between 2014 and 2020 and vice-president of the Brazilian Association for Behavioral Psychology and Medicine (ABPMC) in the 2015-2016 term. He is currently the coordinator of Evidence-Based Psychotherapy Training at InPBE – Institute for Evidence-Based Psychology and professor at Paradigma, in addition to acting as a clinical psychologist.

Fernanda Machado Lopes Psychologist, Specialist in Psychotherapy of Integrated Techniques and Certified Therapist by the Federação Brasileira de Terapias Cognitivas (Brazilian Federation of Cognitive Therapies). Master and PhD in Developmental Psychology from the Universidade Federal do Rio Grande do Sul (UFRGS), linked to the Laboratory of Experimental Psychology, Neuroscience and Behavior (LPNeC-UFRGS) and Post-Doctorate in Neuroscience, linked to the Laboratory of Psychobiology and Neurocomputation (LPBNC-UFRGS). Experience as an Organizational Psychologist with an emphasis on Human Resources Management and Traffic Psychology; as a Clinical Psychologist with an emphasis on Cognitive-Behavioral Therapy and as a Teacher. Currently works as an Adjunct Professor in the Department of Psychology at the Universidade Federal de Santa Catarina (UFSC) and coordinates the Laboratory of Basic and Applied Cognitive Psychology (LPCOG). Research Areas of Interest: Cognitive and Neuropsychological Processes, Cognitive-behavioral Therapy, Drugs, Depression and Anxiety.

André Luiz PhD student in Behavior Analysis at Universidade Estadual de Londrina (UEL); Master in Behavior Analysis at UEL; Graduated in Psychology at Universidade Positivo (Curitiba). He is an Adjunct Professor at Universidade Positivo (Londrina) and Behavior Analyst at Núcleo Evoluir (Londrina). He develops research on behavioral resistance to change and response-cost.

Wilson Benício Martins Bachelor in Psychology at the Universidade de Rio Verde (UniRV).

Denise De Micheli Graduated in Psychology from Universidade Paulista (UNIP), with a PhD in Psychobiology and a Post-Doctorate in Science from Universidade Federal de São Paulo (UNIFESP). Associate Professor of Medicine and Sociology of Drug Abuse (DIMESAD) at the Department of Psychobiology of UNIFESP. Coordinator of the Interdisciplinary Center for Studies in Neuroscience and Behavior in Childhood and Adolescence (CIENCIA-UNIFESP). Member of the Association for Medical Education and Research in Substance Abuse (AMERSA) and the Brazilian Multidisciplinary Association of Drug Studies (Associação Brasileira Multidisciplinar de Estudos sobre Drogas – ABRAMD).

André Q. C. Miguel Obtained his Doctoral degree at the Department of Psychiatry of the Universidade Federal de São Paulo (UNIFESP); completed his Master in Pathological Dependencies at the University of Pisa (Italy); and graduated in Psychology by the Pontifícia Universidade Católica de São Paulo (PUC-SP). He has a Post-Doctorate from the Department of Psychiatry of Yale University and the Department of Psychiatry of UNIFESP and is currently an Assistant Professor at the Elson S. Floyd College of Medicine at Washington State University.

Rodrigo Noia Mattos Montan Master Student in Applied Behavior Analysis at the Associação Paradigma – Centro de Ciências e Tecnologia do Comportamento (in english Paradigma Association – Center for Sciences and Technology of Behavior); Specialist in Chemical Dependency at the Medical School of Universidade de São Paulo (FMUSP); and a graduate in Psychology from Universidade Presbiteriana Mackenzie. He was a member of the Interdisciplinary Group for the Study of Alcohol and Drugs of the Institute of Psychiatry of the Clinical Hospital of the Universidade de São Paulo (GREA - IPq/HC-FMUSP), and worked in Centers of Psychosocial Attention Alcohol and other Drugs (CAPS ad). He develops studies with cue exposure therapy and virtual reality for crack users. He volunteers as a Clinical Supervisor at CAPS for cases of drug abuse among teenagers. Coordinator and teacher of the Extension Course in Intervention in Cases of Chemical and Behavioral Dependence at the Associação Paradigma – Centro de Ciências e Tecnologia do Comportamento.

Luciana Pellizzaro Naine Specialist in Behavioral Therapy from the Institute of Contingencies of Reinforcement (ITCR-Campinas). Clinical Psychologist in private practice and supervisor of the Behavioral Therapy Specialization course at ITCR-Campinas.

Rafael R. de Q. Balbi Neto Master and PhD in Psychology from the Universidade Federal do Espírito Santo (UFES); and graduated in Psychology from UFES. He has experience in the area of Clinical Psychology, with emphasis on Psychological Assessment, Psychotherapy, Severe Mental Disorder and Substance Dependence. He works mainly in the following themes: Behavior Analysis, Behavior Therapy, Cognitive-Behavior Therapy and Substance Dependence.

Simone Martin Oliani Graduation in Psychology from Centro de Estudos Superiores de Londrina (CESULON). Specialization in Psychotherapy in Behavior Analysis and Master in Behavior Analysis from the Universidade Estadual de Londrina (UEL). Affiliate of ABPMC (Brazilian Association of Medicine and Behavioral Psychology), regional coordinator of the ABPMC Community project. She is also affiliated to ABEAD (Brazilian Association for the Study of Alcohol and Other Drugs) and ACBS (Association for Contextual Behavioral Science). Experience in Psychology, with an emphasis on Clinical Psychology, acting mainly on the following themes: behavior analysis, substance dependence, prevention / intervention and health psychology.

César Silva Rodrigues Oliveira Master in Development Neuropsychology from the Universidade Federal Minas Gerais (UFMG); Specialist in Substance Dependence from the Universidade Federal de São Paulo (UNIFESP); and graduated in Psychology from UFMG. He has experience in the Psychology area, with emphasis on Behavior Analysis, acting mainly in the following themes: clinical psychology, behavior analysis, psychiatric disorders, substance dependence and group therapy.

Claudia Kami Bastos Oshiro PhD from the Department of Clinical Psychology of the University of São Paulo (USP); Bachelor and Master in Special Education from the Federal University of São Carlos (UFSCar). Specialist in Behavioral and Cognitive Therapy from USP. Professor in the Department of Clinical Psychology of USP.

Richard Alecsander Reichert PhD student in Psychobiology at the Universidade Federal de São Paulo (UNIFESP); Researcher in the area of Medicine and Sociology of Drug Abuse; Bachelors in Psychology at the Universidade do Vale do Itajaí (UNIVALI); Member of the Interdisciplinary Center for Studies in Neuroscience and Behavior in Childhood and Adolescence (CIENCIA-UNIFESP); Collaborator of the Laboratory of Basic and Applied Cognitive Psychology (LPCOG) of the Universidade Federal de Santa Catarina (UFSC); and associate member of the Brazilian Multidisciplinary Association of Studies on Drugs (Associação Brasileira Multidisciplinar de Estudos sobre Drogas – ABRAMD), International Society of Substance Use Professionals, Brazilian Society for Neuroscience and Behavior (Sociedade Brasileira de Neurociências e Comportamento, SBNeC), Brazilian Network for Science and Education on Alcohol and other Drugs (Rede Brasileira de Ciência e Educação sobre Álcool e outras Drogas), and International Network on Brief Interventions for Alcohol & Other Drugs (INEBRIA).

Vânia Lúcia Pestana Sant'Ana PhD in Clinical Psychology from the Universidade de São Paulo (USP); Master in Psychology from the Pontíficia Universidade Católica de São Paulo (PUC-SP); Specialist in Psychology from the Centro de Estudos Superiores de Londrina (CESULON); and graduated in Psychology from the Universidade do Sagrado Coração (USC). She has experience in Psychology, with emphasis on Sexuality and Learning, acting mainly in the following themes: treatment, prevention, psychological intervention, radical behaviorism and human sexuality.

Rogério Guaita dos Santos Baia Bachelor in Nursing from the Universidade de Rio Verde (UniRV). He is a member of the Behavioral Analysis Research Group and acts as a researcher in the Behavioral Medicine area.

Kallinca Merillen Silveira Graduated in Psychology at the Universidade Federal de Santa Catarina (UFSC). Research Areas of Interest: Cognitive-behavioral Therapy and Drugs.

Viviane Simões Has a Master's degree in Substance Use Disorder obtained at the Universidade Federal de São Paulo (UNIFESP); Graduated in Nursing and in Psychology at in Universidade Nove de Julho (UNINOVE).

Myenne Mieko Ayres Tsutsumi PhD student in Behavior Analysis at Universidade Estadual de Londrina (UEL); Master in Neurosciences and Behavior at Universidade Federal do Pará (UFPA); Specialist in Neurosciences at the UEL; and Bachelor in Psychology at the UFPA. She is an Assistent Professor at Pontifícia Universidade Católica do Paraná (Londrina) and an Adjunct Professor at Universidade Positivo (Londrina). She develops research on aversive control and Autistic Spectrum Disorder.

Elliot Cozzens Wallace Research Coordinator in the Department of Psychology and The Department of Psychiatry and Behavioral Sciences at the University of Washington. Bachelor's of Science in Psychology from the University of Washington. Bachelor's of Arts in Spanish Literature and Language from the University of Washington.

Rodolfo Yamauchi Has a Master's degree in Substance Use Disorder obtained at the Universidade Federal de São Paulo (UNIFESP) and in Neuropsychology from the Conselho Federal de Psicologia (CFP); and graduated in Psychology at the Universidade Metodista de São Paulo (UMESP).

Denis Roberto Zamignani PhD in Clinical Psychology from the Universidade de São Paulo (USP); and Master in Experimental Psychology: Behavior Analysis from the Pontifícia Universidade Católica de São Paulo (PUC-SP). Behavior Analyst accredited by the Brazilian Association of Psychology and Behavioral Medicine (Associação Brasileira de Psicologia e Medicina Comportamental – ABPMC); Academic Coordinator and Professor of Paradigma – Centro de Ciências e Tecnologia do Comportamento; Member of the Editorial Board of Perspectives on Behavior Analysis and the Brazilian Journal of Behavioral and Cognitive Therapy, published by ABPMC; Member of the Brazilian Society of Psychology and Society for Psychotherapy Research. Coordinator of the Process-Based Studies Laboratory in Analytical-Behavioral Therapy (TACn1) at the Paradigma – Centro de Ciências e Tecnologia do Comportamento. He has experience in the Psychology area, with emphasis on therapeutic intervention, psychotherapy research and professional training for psychologists.

Part I
Introductory Aspects and Main Concepts

Chapter 1
Drug Abuse: Classifications, Effects and Risks

Richard Alecsander Reichert, Kallinca Merillen Silveira, Fernanda Machado Lopes, and Denise De Micheli

Introduction

Drugs use is an ancient habit in human history. Over time, different substances have been used in order to obtain pleasurable sensations, to mitigate or to eliminate aversive feelings and to comply with several social, religious, and cultural purposes. Psychoactive drugs, due to their action in the central nervous system (CNS), are capable of generating modifications in the functioning of the organism, be it in behaviors, in consciousness, in perceptions, or in emotion. Psychoactive drugs, in addition to these modifications, usually, can also cause dependence. From a neuropsychological perspective, the continuous drug use behavior can be understood as a learning process, in which the substance use is sustained due to the production of a positive or negative reinforcing effect to the user. The issue of sustained use and abuse of drugs is a complex one, and is related to biological, psychological, and

This text is an adapted translation of a chapter entitled: "Do consumo de álcool às drogas sintéticas: efeitos e riscos do uso abusivo", which is part of the book "Drogas, ciências e políticas públicas: discussões interdisciplinares e práticas de saúde", organized by Zaluar and colleagues (2019) and published in Brazil.

R. A. Reichert (✉) · D. De Micheli
Department of Psychobiology, Universidade Federal de São Paulo (UNIFESP), São Paulo, SP, Brazil
e-mail: reichert@unifesp.br

K. M. Silveira
Universidade Federal de Santa Catarina (UFSC), Florianópolis, SC, Brazil

F. M. Lopes
Department of Psychology, Universidade Federal de Santa Catarina (UFSC), Florianópolis, SC, Brazil

S. M. Oliani et al. (eds.), *Behavior Analysis and Substance Dependence*,
https://doi.org/10.1007/978-3-030-75961-2_1

Table 1.1 Classification of psychoactive substances

Depressants	Stimulants	Hallucinogens
They reduce or inhibit the activity of the CNS (alcohol, solvents, inhalants, anxiolytics, among others).	They accelerate the activity of the CNS (amphetamines, cocaine, nicotine, caffeine, among others).	They alter the functioning of the CNS in a qualitative and quantitative way, and may cause hallucinations and delirium (marijuana, ecstasy, LSD, among others).

sociocultural factors (Bedendo et al., 2017; Cho et al., 2019; Masur & Carlini, 2004; Uhl et al., 2019) (Table 1.1).

The associated risks of the use of each of these substances are related to their indiscriminate or abusive use (i.e. in inappropriate contexts and at inappropriate times, when there is a higher probability of harm to yourself or others; in a high frequency; or in a high quantity). Under the effect of psychoactive substances, several negative consequences can occur, such as traffic accidents, unprotected sexual activity (and, consequently, sexually transmitted diseases or unplanned pregnancy), involvement in violent situations, difficulties in academic and professional life, among others (De Micheli et al., 2015; UNODC, 2019; Whitesell et al., 2013; WHO, 2009). In addition to these possible risks to the general population, the World Health Organization (WHO, 2018), in one of the topics of its report on global alcohol use, discusses substance use specifically in adolescents; and warns of impacts on the brain and neurocognitive development of adolescents, such as changes in learning processes, memory, and attention, which can lead to physical and emotional health problems in adult life. Moreover, it is important to highlight the possible social harm to the lives of adolescents who use substances, such as harm to their social, family, and other interpersonal relationships.

Epidemiological Data

In Brazil, drug consumption has been increasing in the last 20 years and it has also been associated with the occurrence of several social problems such as violence, accidents, and diseases that can lead to death (Carlini et al., 2010). Data has also been showing that drug abuse has been associated with the occurrence of serious disorders that affect all areas of a person's life, harming the individual's integral health (Oliveira & Argimon, 2015; Rangé & Marlatt, 2008). In addition, the fact that the age group of drug consumption is becoming increasingly younger is also a matter of concern, especially because the earlier the use, the greater the chances of developing patterns of drug dependency. All these elements make the abuse of psychotropic substances a major public health issue.

Epidemiological data from the VI National Survey on Drug Use among Brazilian Elementary and High School Students (Carlini et al., 2010) showed that drug experimentation between youngsters in Brazil usually begins with licit drugs, about 13 years old for alcohol (predominantly in the family environment) and tobacco. Later, between 14 and 15 years old, tends to occur the experimentation of illicit drugs, such as marijuana (about 14.6 years) and cocaine/crack (about 14.9 and 14.8 years, respectively).

Regarding last year's consumption, licit drugs were the most cited (alcohol, 42.4%; tobacco, 9.6%), followed by inhalants (5.2%), marijuana (3.7%), anxiolytics (2.6%), cocaine (1.8%), and amphetamines (1.7%) (Carlini et al., 2010). In relation to the general population, the II National Alcohol and Drug Survey (LENAD) showed a higher prevalence of licit drug use by adults. In 2012, 50% of those participants consumed alcohol and 16.9% tobacco. Considering personal drug use, the most cited drugs by adults were marijuana (6.8%), stimulants (2.7%), cocaine (3.8%), and solvents (2.2%) (Laranjeira et al., 2014). According to the II Home Survey on Psychotropic Drug Use in Brazil conducted in 2005 (Carlini et al., 2006), 12.3% of the Brazilian population was classified as alcohol dependent, a degree of alcohol dependence higher than the world's average, which ranges from 10% to 12% (Sordi et al., 2012).

Worldwide, the United Nations Office on Drugs and Crime (UNODC) estimates that approximately 35 million people suffer from substance use disorders (SUD), with only one to seven having access to treatment. International reports show an increase in the number of individuals with SUD and give special attention to the use of licit substances (such as alcohol and tobacco) and their adverse effects on the health of the population. They also discuss the opioid crisis in North America,[1] which is associated with an increase in the number of prescriptions and misuse of these substances, and with an increased number of related deaths (UNODC, 2019, 2020; WHO, 2009, 2018).

WHO epidemiological data showed that approximately 2.3 billion people worldwide consumed alcohol—recorded mainly in the form of distillates, beer, and wine—in 2016, with per capita consumption equivalent to about 6.4 l of pure alcohol. In the Americas, Europe, and the Western Pacific, alcohol was consumed by more than half the population. In this report, a decrease in the pattern of heavy episodic drinking (binge drinking)—consumption of 60 g or more of pure alcohol on one occasion at least once a month—was observed in the total population, given that in 2000 the prevalence was 22.6%, while in 2016 it was 18.2%. However, there were exceptions to some regions, such as Eastern Europe and Sub-Saharan Africa, where the prevalence was higher. This report also presented information on alcohol-related diseases and injuries, exposing that alcohol consumption was associated with 7.2% premature deaths, mainly of young people, between 20 and 39 years old. In addition, alcohol consumption was also associated to millions of deaths from

[1] The opioids were not addressed in the original text in Portuguese, because statistical-epidemiological data showed that its use is not so common in Brazil compared to other countries. These substances act mainly on the CNS by activating the mesolimbic reward system and sending signals to the ventral tegmental area (VTA), releasing dopamine (DA) in the nucleus accumbens (NAc). The main effects of this action are euphoria and analgesia. To better understand the neurobiological mechanisms of action of opioids and their possible health risks, we suggest reading Evans and Cahill (2016), Kakko et al. (2019), Koob (2020), Kosten and George (2002), and Napier and Persons (2019). To see more on the opioid crisis in North America, we suggest reading Bolliger and Stevens (2019), Boté (2019), and Stoicea et al. (2019).

digestive and cardiovascular diseases, cancer, traffic injuries, interpersonal violence, among others, in different ages (WHO, 2018).

Reports published in 2019, and 2020, by the United Nations Office on Drugs and Crime (UNODC) showed that there was an increase in drug use by the world population. In 2018, among the illicit substances, cannabis was the most used drug (192 million people), while opioids were related to greater health damage (UNODC, 2019, 2020). In 2017, the opioids were associated with 66% of the 167,000 deaths related to substance use disorders, in addition to millions of premature deaths and disability-adjusted life years (DALYs). As for cocaine use, it is estimated that 18.1 million people consumed it in 2017, and that the highest prevalence of its consumption was in North America (2.1%) and Oceania (1.6%) (UNODC, 2019, 2020). Regarding other drugs, many countries, especially in Western Europe, have shown concern with the use of over-the-counter tranquillizers. Its use has been more frequent among women and, in some countries, more prevalent than cannabis. In countries of Asia, especially Southeast Asia, there is a great concern with the use of methamphetamines, since according to those reports, the use of these substances varies between 0.5% and 1.1%, higher prevalence than global rates (UNODC, 2019).

Given the impacts of the COVID-19 pandemic (such as increased levels of unemployment and poverty and lack of opportunities), more attention is being paid to drug-related problems (such as harmful use patterns and dependence), due to its increased occurrence likelihood, around the world. That makes the formulation of prevention and treatment strategies accessible to the entire population even more important and urgent, taking into account the new context in which people are living and its several social and economic transformations (UNODC, 2020).

In adolescence, specifically, health organizations pay attention to the greater vulnerability to physical, psychological, and social harm resulting from early drug use, since adolescence is a phase of maturation of brain structures and functions and of cognitive, emotional, and social development. That stated, the importance of targeting attention to psychoactive substance use patterns and the need to develop and implement effective strategies to the prevention and treatment of drug abuse and, consequently, to mitigate its potential negative and harmful effects in all population is signaled. (Andrade et al., 2014; UNODC, 2019, 2020; WHO, 2009, 2018).

Consumption Patterns and Risk Factors

In relation to consumption patterns, it is necessary to reflect on the risk factors associated with the early and abusive use of licit and illicit drugs. In the family context, when there is a positive attitude of parents towards drug use, this influences the early use by their children. Therefore, it is important to identify how the relationships between users, types of drugs, and the permissive intrafamilial relationship system are established (Paiva & Ronzani, 2009; Schenker & Minayo, 2005). In addition to that, the role of group involvement, the search for risky situations, and the media's actions that encourage and praise the use of substances such as alcohol

(Cambron et al., 2018; Oliveira & Argimon, 2015; Schenker & Minayo, 2005) should also be taken into consideration when examining risk factors involved in drug use.

Factors such as incentive and permissiveness of family to drug use; stressful situations, such as family crisis; incentive and permissiveness of groups, in which the person interacts, to drug use; willingness to belong to certain groups that use drugs or have it as a symbol of status; and curiosity to experiment are also all well-known risk factors that collaborate for children and adolescents to start using drugs. The UNODC (2019) and several researches available in scientific databases also consider the following as potential vulnerabilities or risk factors to drug use: genetic predisposition, personality traits, presence of mental disorders, negligence or physical and emotional abuse, social norms and environmental stimuli, lack of knowledge about the substances and their effects and risks, among others.

Therefore, drug use behaviors involve multiple risk factors that deserve attention from health or related areas professionals. One of those risk factors is the probability of occasional use becoming a pattern of abuse and dependence, especially when experimentation occurs at an early stage of life, between childhood and adolescence, when neurobiological aspects are in process of development and more sensitive to the harmful effects of the psychoactive substances. Another factor refers to the probability of the use of licit drugs, such as alcohol, to predispose to the use of other substances, such as illicit ones—many of which have properties with high action potential to generate dependency. Also, the use of licit drugs can predispose to the use of more than one drug at once, which can potentialize the negative effects of the drugs and increase its risks. This information serves as an alarm for policies to prevent the use of alcohol and tobacco among the young population, since it is difficult for someone to begin consumption by trying cocaine or LSD, for example.

Another risk factor is the chemical property of the psychoactive substance and its specific mechanism of action in the CNS, especially when it occurs in the brain's reward system, situation in which the drug usually generates a sensation of pleasure and, consequently, a willingness to consume it again. This, together with personality factors, life history, environmental and cultural context, sets the user's "drug of choice."

According to the action in the brain, each substance will produce effects, desirable and undesirable, manifested under the form of signs and symptoms. The effects and risks of some of the main psychoactive drugs will be presented below.

Alcohol

Alcohol is a licit drug that has depressant action in the CNS. This means that the effect of its consumption is the reduction or inhibition of the activity of the CNS, especially, in the psychomotor activity. It is important to highlight that the level of alcohol consumption symptoms is directly related to the amount of alcohol ingested and present in the bloodstream (Abrahão et al., 2012; Nicastri, 2012). Initially, when there is low alcohol content in the blood, the first sensations are euphoria and disinhibition, as happens with CNS stimulant drugs, but these effects are due to the depressant action of alcohol in the prefrontal cortex, making inhibitory control, and some cognitive functions, slower.

Other common symptoms when there is little or moderate alcohol intake include impaired sensory functions, reduced motor coordination and speech and decreased attention. On the other hand, symptoms associated with high levels of the drug in the blood are usually associated with nausea and vomiting, double vision, coma, and, in extreme cases, hypothermia and death due to respiratory or cardiac arrest (Andrade et al., 2011; Diehl et al., 2019; Gilpin & Koob, 2008; Guimarães, 2013; Nicastri, 2012; Tabakoff & Hoffman, 2013). For this reason, from the point of view of its effects, alcohol is considered a biphasic substance since in low doses it produces euphoria and in high doses it produces CNS depression.

The continuous and abusive use of alcohol can increase the user's tolerance to the drug effects, impelling to the ingestion of larger quantities or to the increasing of use frequency of the drug in order to satisfy the needs or desires for it, and consequently, promoting its dependence. When it is intended to cease the drug use, the user can experience an abstinence syndrome, which can be characterized by the effects that occur with the user due to the lack of the drug in the body (Becker, 2008; Diehl et al., 2019; Simons et al., 2009).

Even when just the occasional use of alcohol occurs, there are still behaviors considered "at risk" linked to its consumption. For example, if a person drinks alcohol and drives, regardless of the amount, the effects produced can be fatal, since the reflexes become slower and the visual acuity decreases. Data suggest that in a range of 33 to 69% of fatal traffic accidents, drivers are under the influence of alcohol (Sordi et al., 2012). In addition, the chronic use alcohol can affect several organs and tissues, increasing the probability of development and aggravation of organic problems, such as gastritis, pancreatitis, cardiac arrhythmias, hepatitis, alcoholic cirrhosis, CNS lesions, changes in cognitive functions, among others (De Micheli et al., 2015; Diehl et al., 2019; Masur & Carlini, 2004; WHO, 2009, 2018).

Masur and Carlini (2004), from the question *"Cigarette, alcohol, marijuana, cocaine, heroin: which is the worst?* (p. 17), made a comparison of the short- and long-term damage caused by different psychoactive substances. The damages were evaluated in five dimensions: (1) organic consequences of chronic use; (2) abstinence syndrome; (3) social interaction deficits; (4) risk of overdose; and (5) consequences associated with the route of administration. In the items 1, 2, and 3 alcohol occupied a prominent position.

Furthermore, studies indicate positive correlations between chronic alcohol use and structural and functional changes in the brain. Neuroimaging tests suggest that abusive alcohol consumption, especially when started early, presents impacts on the development of certain brain regions, what can promote harmful cognitive changes and negative impacts on people's academic, professional, and social areas of life. With technological advances and the possibility of new researches, new studies have been exploring these indicators in order to better explain these correlations (Takagi et al., 2014) (Table 1.2).

Table 1.2 Combined use of alcohol and other substances

Alcohol + Combination	Effects and Risks
GHB, ketamine, and other depressants	It can generate major health risks such as cardiac arrest, reduced heartbeat, and coma.
Cocaine and other stimulants	It can cause a false sense of sobriety, and greater consumption of both can occur, causing risks of arrhythmia, coma, and cardiac arrest. the combined use of alcohol and cocaine causes the liver to produce an active metabolite called cocaethylene, a toxic substance to the cardiovascular system, associated with convulsions and damage to the liver.
Marijuana, LSD, MDMA, and other psychedelics	It can cause unusual reactions of perception, impacts in the analysis of the reality and in the judgment of situations and risk behaviors.

Source: É de Lei (Brazilian organization whose aim is to promote the reduction of health and social risks and harms through support in formulating drug-related policies. Site: https://edelei.org/)

Tobacco

There are several variations in tobacco consumption. The most common form is inhaled, which includes industrialized cigarettes, straw cigarettes, among others. However, there are also other consumable forms, such as vacuumed and chewed (Lopes et al., 2012; Pressman & Gigliotti, 2019). Regardless of its consumable forms, the substance present in its composition that is responsible for causing addiction is nicotine, a drug with a high potential for developing addiction. As the use of it becomes more frequent, the body's tolerance to nicotine increases and this makes the person need to ingest more and more to obtain the expected effect.

A person with nicotine addiction usually presents three types of symptoms: physical, behavioral, and psychological. The physical symptoms, such as insomnia, increased appetite, dizziness, and shortness of breath, usually occur when the person is a long period without smoking (abstinence syndrome). Behavioral dependence symptoms occur through associations between smoking and some daily behavior (e.g., coffee and cigarettes). Thus, if a person smokes a cigarette every time he/she wakes up in the morning, this behavior is likely to become a habit and the act of waking up in the morning, then, becomes a trigger for smoking behavior. Finally, psychological dependence symptoms refers to aspects about what role cigarettes play in a person's life (França et al., 2015). Thus, if someone smokes whenever they feel lonely, the cigarette occupies the function of company for these moments of loneliness. All these associations happen involuntarily and make the consumption cessation process difficult.

Due to the action of nicotine in the brain's reward system, occasional use can soon become abuse and evolve into addiction, called smoking addiction (APA, 2014), which is considered the world's largest avoidable cause of death (Pressman & Gigliotti, 2019). The Pan American Health Organization (PAHO) estimates that smoking is responsible for 12% of the world's adult mortality. It is also estimated that there are about 1 billion smokers worldwide and that most of them are concentrated in countries considered underdeveloped, which makes the low-income population the most affected by tobacco-related diseases (Santos et al., 2018).

The diseases associated with smoking are numerous and frequent, and generate high costs to the economy. Among them, cardiovascular diseases, respiratory diseases, effects related to reproductive functions (such as miscarriage), as well as several types of cancer (mouth, lung, pharynx, among others) (Lopes et al., 2012; Santos et al., 2018). In addition, research suggests that the effects of cigarette smoke for passive smokers are as harmful as they are for smokers, as they have a higher risk of developing the same tobacco-related diseases (Lopes et al., 2012; Pressman & Gigliotti, 2019).

Marijuana

Marijuana has been known and used by human beings for thousands of years for medicinal, religious, and recreational purposes, among others; it is also one of the illicit drugs most consumed by the Brazilian population and the world population to date (Sordi et al., 2012; UNODC, 2019, 2020). Like the other substances, its effects depend on factors such as quantity, preparation mode, and administration form (chewed leaf, inhaled or ingested via cake, among other forms), also of the sensitivity, expectations, and previous experiences of each person, besides the context in which the consumption occurs.

Its effects generate changes in cognitive, psychological, physical, and behavioral terms. They can include intensification of the perception of internal stimuli, such as light and fluctuating body sensations, and distortions in external stimuli, referring especially to time and space, with the possibility of causing hallucinations; as well as alterations in memory. The psychobehavioral effects usually include sensations of relaxation, euphoria and mood swings, disinhibition, and relaxation. The physical effects usually involve dry lips, tachycardia, conjunctival hyperemia (redness of the eyes), and bronchodilation, and also psychomotor and speech retardation (Barlow & Durand, 2015; De Luca et al., 2017; De Micheli et al., 2015; Guimarães, 2013; Masur & Carlini, 2004).

These changes occur as a consequence of the mechanism of action of tetrahydrocannabinol (THC, Δ^9-tetrahydrocannabinol), the main active component of marijuana, in cannabinoid receptors, substantially in regions such as the limbic and cortex system, associated with memory functions, perception, and sensation of relaxation and pleasure (Sordi et al., 2012). Interestingly, the body produces natural (endogenous) versions of cannabinoid substances, called endocannabinoids, such as anandamide, known in science as the neurotransmitter of happiness or bliss (Bedendo et al., 2017; Costa et al., 2011; Francischetti & Abreu, 2006).

According to some studies, the chronic or abusive use of marijuana can cause damage to short-term memory, concentration capacity, and reversible hormonal changes, as well as social, academic, and professional losses (Sordi et al., 2012).

There is also evidence that continued exposure to marijuana smoke can cause respiratory infections, as occur with people who smoke tobacco. However, further research is still needed to better investigate the relationship between marijuana use and these observed effects.

In addition, the long-term use of the substance may lead to the development of tolerance (more doses for the same effect) and abstinence, such as manifestation of anxiety, irritability, insomnia, and decreased appetite. However, these symptoms present low intensity and severity in comparison with other substances and also depend on the variables mentioned initially, such as the amount used before consumption cessation, period extension of use, and environmental factors (Barlow & Durand, 2015; Bonnet & Preuss, 2017; Guimarães, 2013; Masur & Carlini, 2004). In terms of psychological and behavioral dependence, marijuana seems to play important roles in social rituals and situations, presenting an especially strong influence among young people.

With regard to brain impacts resulting from the chronic use of marijuana, Crippa and collaborators (2005) indicated that the results of neuroimaging studies are inconclusive or divergent. Takagi et al. (2014) stated that the limitations of these studies refer to small, cross-sectional samples, which do not investigate drug abuse in a longitudinal manner. In addition, the authors note the association between drug abuse and psychiatric comorbidities, which may explain the morphological differences presented by the tests (the literature suggests that there are brain alterations in people with anxiety and depression, for example).

Based on this, it is possible that the observed alterations constitute a neurobiological risk factor for drug abuse and not the reverse. The same is true for psychosis, according to Ksir and Hart (2016a, 2016b). The authors state that although there are studies showing correlation, there is little evidence regarding the causal nature between psychosis and marijuana and that its use does not cause a psychotic disorder by itself. What seems to happen, based on reviews of studies, is that psychotic behaviors caused by marijuana use are more likely in subjects who have some prior history of mental disorder or predisposition to psychosis. However, further studies are needed to conduct an in-depth investigation of these issues (Table 1.3).

Besides the psychobiological aspects of marijuana use, social-political issues related to its use should be widely discussed, such as its classification as an illicit drug and, more recently, its resurgence as a substance with high medicinal potential. The social pressures responsible for this historical process need to be analyzed and discussed. Now, after years of research and evidence regarding its positive and

Table 1.3 Combined use of marijuana and other substances

Marijuana + Combination	Effects and Risks
Alcohol	It increases the probability of pressure drop, dizziness, and vomiting.
Psychedelics	It can intensify the effects of psychedelics, making them unpredictable and unpleasant.

Source: É de Lei (Brazilian organization whose aim is to promote the reduction of health and social risks and harms through support in formulating drug-related policies. Site: https://edelei.org/)

negative impacts on human health, decisions regarding regulatory policies, medicinal use, and interventions aimed at education, prevention, and treatment need to be scientifically grounded. This requires combining studies and experiments with critical discussions of the facts (Piomelli, 2016).

Solvents and Inhalants

This category includes drugs that are aspirated through the nose or mouth, such as shoemaker's glue, loló,[2] and perfume launcher, usually soaked in cloths or in the clothes. They can cause various effects, such as depression, stimulating, and hallucinogenic ones on the central nervous system. These effects can include: (a) initial excitement, due to the depression of functions in the prefrontal cortex (euphoria, exaltation, decreased critical judgment, impulsiveness, perceptual changes, etc.); (b) initial depression (confusion, obnubilation, headaches, etc.); (c) middle depression (reduced alertness, slow reflexes, lack of motor coordination, nystagmus, etc.); and (d) deep depression (intense alertness depression, state of unconsciousness with bizarre dreams and increased possibility of convulsions and alterations in the electroencephalogram) (Masur & Carlini, 2004).

The continuous abusive use of drugs of this category is associated with structural and functional alterations of brain regions and damages in cognitive functions, such as attention, memory, and learning, besides tiredness, headaches, motor damages, and mental confusion. In cases of overdose, it can lead to death by depression and cardiac or respiratory arrest. Despite this, the consumption of these substances is common in several places in the world, mainly by children and adolescents with fewer socioeconomic indexes. In Brazil, they are among the most popular drugs among public school students, according to studies (Carlini et al., 2010; Masur & Carlini, 2004; Takagi et al., 2014) (Table 1.4).

Table 1.4 Combined use of solvents or inhalants and other substances

Combination of Solvents or Inhalants +	Effects and Risks
Alcohol	Intensification of the depressant effect on the central nervous system, with the possibility of cardiorespiratory arrest and coma.

Source: É de Lei (Brazilian organization whose aim is to promote the reduction of health and social risks and harms through support in formulating drug-related policies. Site: https://edelei.org/)

[2] Loló, also known as Cheirinho-da-Loló (Loló's smell) is a street drug, common in Brazil region, which comprises an aerosol of chloroform in ether solution, which can cause cardiac arrest.

Amphetamines

Amphetamines are part of the group of CNS stimulant drugs and can produce feelings of euphoria and reduce fatigue, sleep, and appetite (APA, 2014). Their mechanism of action involves the release of dopamine, noradrenaline, and serotonin through the inhibition of the recaptation of neurotransmitters or through the inhibition of the enzyme monoaminoxidase (MAO), which causes feelings of pleasure, well-being, and euphoria (Calipari & Ferris, 2013; Faraone, 2018; Marcon et al., 2012). However, after the expected effects, people usually feel the opposite, i.e. a lot of tiredness, drowsiness, increased appetite, and more depressed mood (APA, 2014).

Disorders related to the use of these substances include physiological and behavioral symptoms, such as changes in heartbeat or blood pressure, sweating or chills, weight loss, muscle atony, euphoria or emotional blunting, changes in sociability, anxiety, tension, anger, and stereotyped behavior (Barlow & Durand, 2015; Muakad, 2013). It is important to note that tolerance to the use of amphetamines develops rapidly. Due to that, in Brazil, the National Health Surveillance Agency (Agência Nacional de Vigilância Sanitária – ANVISA) determined, on October 6, 2011, the prohibition of production, dispensation, import, export, prescription, and use of this drug because of the associated risks.

Cocaine and Crack

Cocaine is extracted from the plant *Erythroxylon coca* and can be consumed from different routes of administration: chewed, in the form of coca leaf; aspirated, in the form of powder (cocaine hydrochloride); injectable, cocaine hydrochloride dissolved in water; and smoked, in the form of crack or merla (coca paste) (Castro et al., 2015; Nicastri, 2012). Crack is the crystallized form of cocaine and can be quickly smoked and absorbed by the body as it reaches the bloodstream from the moment it reaches the lungs.

These CNS stimulant drugs interfere with the action of neurotransmitters. Their action mechanism involves the drug active property that blocks the receiving pump, enabling neurotransmitters, such as dopamine, noradrenaline, and serotonin, to remain in greater quantity and for longer periods in the synaptic clefts. The stimulant effects caused by cocaine/crack consumption involve brain regions such as the ventral tegmental area (VTA), accumbens nucleus, amygdala, hippocampus, and frontal cortex. Together (with the exception of the cortex), these regions make up what is called the "reward circuit" or "pleasure circuit," which plays a primary role in the repetitive characteristic of drug seeking and consumption behavior, given that the high levels of dopamine available in these regions, stand out greatly at levels related to stimuli/activities involving natural pleasures such as food and sex (Bedendo et al., 2017; Castro et al., 2015; Nestler, 2005).

From the stimulating action of cocaine/crack in the CNS, physical, cognitive, psychological, and behavioral effects are observed. The first two include

Table 1.5 Combined use of cocaine and other substances

Combination Cocaine +	Effects and Risks
Stimulant + depressant substances (alcohol, tranquilizers, or perfume launcher)	False sense of sobriety, increasing the sense of power and increasing the risks of accidents and involvement in other risk situations (violence, for example). In addition, it increases the risk of cardiac arrest.
Alcohol	The liver produces cocaethylene, a toxic substance to the liver, the cardiovascular system and that can cause convulsions.

Source: É de Lei (Brazilian organization whose aim is to promote the reduction of health and social risks and harms through support in formulating drug-related policies. Site: https://edelei.org/)

acceleration of heartbeats, pupils dilation, sweating, tremor, dry mouth, decreased appetite, insomnia, reduction of the critical sense and inhibitory control, alteration of time reaction, as well as of attention and sense of perception, which can generate hallucinations and cause panic attacks. The latter two involve feelings of euphoria, grandiosity and disinhibition, exaggerated alertness, aggressiveness, accelerated speech and gait, a state of arousal and reduction of tiredness (Castro et al., 2015; Nicastri, 2012). On the other hand, as the effects cease, unpleasant sensations may arise, such as intensification of anxiety and depression symptoms (Bedendo et al., 2017; De Micheli et al., 2015; Masur & Carlini, 2004; Rosário et al., 2019) (Table 1.5).

Ecstasy

3, 4 - methylenedioxymethamphetamine (MDMA), better known as ecstasy or "bullet," is a drug that generates both stimulant and hallucinogenic effects. This substance was initially called *empathy*, due to the increased sociability caused by its use. The most common form of administration of ecstasy is by oral route, from the ingestion of tablets of different colors and sizes. However, it can also be inhaled (by dismantling the pill and aspirating it through the nose). It is a fully synthetic drug, i.e. produced in the laboratory, so the tablets contain about 50 to 150 mg of the active substance. The mechanism of action is not yet well established, although it is known to have important action on serotonergic pathways (Meyer, 2013; Vegting et al., 2016; Xavier et al., 2008).

Its effects on the brain begin about 30 min after taking the pill and can be classified into three phases: (a) an initial feeling of disorientation, including changes in sense of perception, particularly in the sight and touch; (b) intense pleasure, such as increased positive emotions, extreme well-being, physical disposition, and reduced fear; and (c) a significant increase in socialization, including improved communication skills and decreased aggressiveness. Negative physical signs and symptoms include increased heartbeat, blood pressure, and body temperature, which can lead to an exacerbated intake of water, resulting in intoxication from excessive consumption and thus considerable changes in the body.

Table 1.6 Combined use of ecstasy and other substances

Ecstasy + Combination	Effects and Risks
Alcohol	Alcohol exacerbates dehydration caused by MDMA. Also, both substances overload the liver, kidneys, and raise body temperature.
Stimulants	Increased blood pressure, cardiac risk, and stroke.

Source: É de Lei (Brazilian organization whose aim is to promote the reduction of health and social risks and harms through support in formulating drug-related policies. Site: https://edelei.org/)

In extreme situations, the use of this drug can lead to malignant hyperthermia (excessive increase in body temperature), organ failure, induction of coma and death, risks intensified by the fact that it is an illicit drug manufactured in clandestine laboratories without regulation and quality control (De Micheli et al., 2015). After the effects, enormous fatigue, muscle pain, nausea, and depressive symptoms may appear. According to Garcia et al. (2014), the chronic use of this substance is correlated with changes in the functioning of neurotransmitters such as serotonin and in cognitive functions such as processing, memory, attention, and learning (Table 1.6).

LSD

Like ecstasy, LSD (*Lysergsäurediethylamid*: Lysergic Acid Diethylamide) is a synthetic drug, of the class of those that generate problems to the CNS. The form of presentation of LSD is also in tablets or small papers (stamps) that contain the synthesized acid. Doses between 75 and 200 mg of this drug are already capable of causing changes in the state of consciousness and hallucinogenic effects. The duration of the effects is quite prolonged when compared to cocaine/crack, for example, and can vary between 4 and 12 h, being more intense after 2 h of ingestion (Passie et al., 2008). The user's goal is usually to obtain hallucinations, changes in the state of consciousness and perception.

The mechanism of action is not well known, what is known is that it acts in the CNS disturbing qualitatively and quantitatively the functioning of the brain and provoking physical, cognitive, psychological, and behavioral alterations. The main physical signs and symptoms include pupil dilation, increased blood pressure and heartbeats, dry mouth, loss of appetite, and sleepiness. The others involve changes in consciousness, perception (of time and space, alteration of senses, colors, shapes, and contours), and thinking, including persecutory delusions and hallucinations, as well as mood swings and states of exaltation, which can be positive or negative ("good or bad travel").

Toxic or negative effects commonly reported are intense crises of anxiety, distress, panic, depression, and psychotic conditions, including "flashbacks," which are presentations of sudden signs and symptoms of the psychic effects of the drug experience without having consumed the substance again. On the other hand, there

Table 1.7 Combined use of LSD and other substances

LSD/NBOM Combination +	Effects and Risks
Alcohol	The effects can be diverse and make the experience unpredictable.
Stimulants	It can amplify the stimulating effects of LSD and related drugs and generate risks such as increased blood pressure and cardiorespiratory arrest.
Psychedelics	Intensification of the effects, which can generate, in some cases, states of mental confusion, delirium, and psychotic crisis.

Source: É de Lei (Brazilian organization whose aim is to promote the reduction of health and social risks and harms through support in formulating drug-related policies. Site: https://edelei.org/)

is no consistency in the literature on substance dependence on LSD, and the greatest risk related to its consumption is associated with the triggering of psychosis and mood swings in individuals predisposed to these disorders (Nicastri, 2012; Passie et al., 2008) (Table 1.7).

Final Considerations

In order to avoid reductionism on a multifactorial issue such as the use of psychoactive substances, it is important to emphasize that their effects and risks are influenced by the interaction of a series of biological, psychological, and sociocultural factors. It is, thus, a biopsychosocial issue. Therefore, in order to assess the damage resulting from the drug use, the context, the quantity used, the frequency, the age of initiation, the level of damage in work, in academic and in social activities, and other several variables must be taken into consideration.

In the political-criminal context of drugs, which starts from the prohibitionist perspective and the incessant and inefficient fight against consumption, it becomes more difficult to measure the effects and risks resulting from the use of psychoactive substances and their original active principles, since there is no formal regulation and control of the production process of these drugs. In other words, there is a lack of knowledge about the composition of most substances that are widely used in various contexts of socialization. This, in addition to hindering research and, consequently, the formulation of effective intervention strategies, can generate a series of damages to human health (as observed throughout this chapter), which could/can be avoided or reduced with policies of control, prevention, and reduction of risks and harm.

In any case, when talking about potential risks associated with drug use, one can compare the behavior to common everyday habits, as the American neuroscientist Carl Hart (2019) does.[3] According to the researcher, for everything in life there is a

[3] Lecture given at the VII International Congress of the Associação Brasileira Multidisciplinar de Estudos sobre Drogas / Brazilian Multidisciplinary Association of Drug Studies (ABRAMD), in Curitiba (Paraná, Brazil) in June 2019.

risk; and what maintains a behavior is its function. Driving cars and traveling by plane, for example, are habits that, in some way, may represent certain risks, but they are maintained because they are functional for human life; the same occurs in relation to the use of substances. In this sense, as well as education and awareness about other habits that can mean some risk to physical or psychological integrity, the conscious use of psychoactive substances should be discussed in order to prevent adverse consequences to the users and others. To this end, prevention and health care programs should be implemented in various areas of society, especially in educational settings. It is essential that these programs are evidence-based and periodically evaluated to measure their results.

References

Abrahao, K. P., Quadros, I. M. H., Andrade, A. L. M., & Souza-Formigoni, M. L. O. (2012). Accumbal dopamine D2 receptor function is associated with individual variability in ethanol behavioral sensitization. *Neuropharmacology, 62*(2), 882–889. https://doi.org/10.1016/j.neuropharm.2011.09.017

American Psychiatric Association (APA). (2014). *Manual diagnóstico e estatístico de transtornos mentais* (5th ed.). Artmed Editora.

Andrade, A. L. M., Abrahao, K. P., Goeldner, F. O., & Souza-Formigoni, M. L. O. (2011). Administration of the 5-HT2C receptor antagonist SB-242084 into the nucleus accumbens blocks the expression of ethanol-induced behavioral sensitization in Albino Swiss mice. *Neuroscience, 189*, 178–186. https://doi.org/10.1016/j.neuroscience.2011.05.028

Andrade, A. L. M., De Micheli, D., Silva, E. A., Souza-Formigoni, M. L. O., & Goeldner, F. O. (2014). Desenvolvimento neural na adolescência. In D. De Micheli, A. L. M. Andrade, E. A. Silva, & M. L. O. Souza-Formigoni (Eds.), Neurociências do abuso de drogas na adolescência: o que sabemos? (pp. 21–30). São Paulo, Brazil: Atheneu.

Barlow, D. H., & Durand, V. M. (2015). *Psicopatologia: uma abordagem integrada* (2nd ed.). Cengage Learning.

Becker, H. C. (2008). Alcohol dependence, withdrawal, and relapse. *Alcohol Research & Health: The Journal of the National Institute on Alcohol Abuse and Alcoholism, 31*(4), 348–361.

Bedendo, A., Andrade, A. L. M., & Noto, A. R. (2017). Neurobiologia da ação das drogas de abuso. In A. L. M. Andrade & D. De Micheli (Eds.), *Inovações no tratamento de dependência de drogas* (pp. 19–39). Atheneu.

Bolliger, L., & Stevens, H. (2019). From opioid pain management to opioid crisis in the USA: How can public-private partnerships help? *Frontiers in Medicine, 6*, 106. https://doi.org/10.3389/fmed.2019.00106

Bonnet, U., & Preuss, U. W. (2017). The cannabis withdrawal syndrome: Current insights. *Substance Abuse and Rehabilitation, 8*, 9–37. https://doi.org/10.2147/SAR.S109576

Boté, S. H. (2019). U.S. opioid epidemic: Impact on public health and review of prescription drug monitoring programs (PDMPs). *Online Journal of Public Health Informatics, 11*(2), e18. https://doi.org/10.5210/ojphi.v11i2.10113

Calipari, E. S., & Ferris, M. J. (2013). Amphetamine mechanisms and actions at the dopamine terminal revisited. *The Journal of Neuroscience: The Official Journal of the Society for Neuroscience, 33*(21), 8923–8925. https://doi.org/10.1523/JNEUROSCI.1033-13.2013

Cambron, C., Kosterman, R., Catalano, R. F., Guttmannova, K., & Hawkins, J. D. (2018). Neighborhood, family, and peer factors associated with early adolescent smoking and alcohol use. *Journal of Youth and Adolescence, 47*(2), 369–382.

Carlini, E. A., Galduróz, J. C., Noto, A. R., Carlini, C. M., Oliveira, L. G., & Nappo, S. A. (2006). *II Levantamento domiciliar sobre o uso de drogas psicotrópicas no Brasil: estudo envolvendo as 108 maiores cidades do país*. SENAD.

Carlini, B. (2010). *Drogas: cartilha sobre maconha, cocaína e inalantes*. Secretaria Nacional de Políticas sobre Drogas.

Carlini, E. A., Noto, A. R., Sanchez, Z. M., Carlini, C. M. A., Locatelli, D. P., Abeid, L. R., … Moura, Y. G. (2010). *VI Levantamento Nacional sobre o Consumo de Drogas Psicotrópicas entre Estudantes do Ensino Fundamental e Médio das Redes Pública e Privada de Ensino nas 27 Capitais Brasileiras*. SENAD.

Castro, R., Ruas, R., Abreu, R., Rocha, R., Ferreira, R., Lasmar, R., et al. (2015). Crack: Pharmacokinetics, pharmacodynamics, and clinical and toxic effects. *Revista Médica De Minas Gerais, 25*(2). https://doi.org/10.5935/2238-3182. 20150045.

Cho, S. B., Su, J., Kuo, S. I., Bucholz, K. K., Chan, G., Edenberg, H. J., McCutcheon, V. V., Schuckit, M. A., Kramer, J. R., & Dick, D. M. (2019). Positive and negative reinforcement are differentially associated with alcohol consumption as a function of alcohol dependence. *Psychology of Addictive Behaviors: Journal of the Society of Psychologists in Addictive Behaviors, 33*(1), 58–68. https://doi.org/10.1037/adb0000436

Costa, J., Maia, L., Orlandi-Mattos, P., Villares, J., & Esteves, M. (2011). Neurobiologia da Cannabis: do sistema endocanabinoide aos transtornos por uso de Cannabis. *Jornal Brasileiro de Psiquiatria, 60*(2), 111–122. https://doi.org/10.1590/S0047-20852011000200006

Crippa, J., Lacerda, A., Amaro, E., Busatto Filho, G., Zuardi, A., & Bressan, R. (2005). Efeitos cerebrais da maconha: resultados dos estudos de neuroimagem. *Revista Brasileira de Psiquiatria, 27*(1), 70–78. https://doi.org/10.1590/S1516-44462005000100016

De Luca, M. A., Di Chiara, G., Cadoni, C., Lecca, D., Orsolini, L., Papanti, D., Corkery, J., & Schifano, F. (2017). Cannabis; epidemiological, neurobiological and psychopathological issues: An update. *CNS & Neurological Disorders Drug Targets, 16*(5), 598–609. https://doi.org/10.2174/1871527316666170413113246

De Micheli, D., Silva, E. A., Noto, A. R., Camargo, B. M. V., & Renner, C. O. (2015). *Diálogos com os adolescentes sobre uso, abuso e dependência de drogas*. Casa do Psicólogo.

Diehl, A., Cordeiro, D., & Laranjeira, R. (2019). Álcool. In A. Diehl, D. Cordeiro, & R. Laranjeira (Eds.), *Dependência Química: prevenção, tratamento e políticas públicas* (2nd ed., pp. 92–108). Artmed.

Evans, C. J., & Cahill, C. M. (2016). Neurobiology of opioid dependence in creating addiction vulnerability. *F1000Research, 5*, F1000 Faculty Rev-1748. https://doi.org/10.12688/f1000research.8369.1

Faraone, S. V. (2018). The pharmacology of amphetamine and methylphenidate: Relevance to the neurobiology of attention-deficit/hyperactivity disorder and other psychiatric comorbidities. *Neuroscience and Biobehavioral Reviews, 87*, 255–270. https://doi.org/10.1016/j.neubiorev.2018.02.001

França, S., Neves, A., Souza, T., Martins, N., Carneiro, S., Sarges, E., & Souza, M. (2015). Factors associated with smoking cessation. *Revista de Saúde Pública, 49*(0). https://doi.org/10.1590/S0034-8910.2015049004946

Francischetti, E., & Abreu, V. (2006). O sistema endocanabinóide: nova perspectiva no controle de fatores de risco cardiometabólico. *Arquivos Brasileiros de Cardiologia, 87*(4), 548–558. https://doi.org/10.1590/S0066-782X2006001700023

Garcia, F., Moreira, L., & Assumpção, A. (2014). Neuropsicologia das dependências químicas. In D. Fuentes, L. F. Malloy-Diniz, C. H. P. Camargo, & R. M. Cosenza (Eds.), *Neuropsicologia: teoria e prática* (pp. 241–248). Artmed.

Gilpin, N. W., & Koob, G. F. (2008). Neurobiology of alcohol dependence: Focus on motivational mechanisms. *Alcohol Research & Health: The Journal of the National Institute on Alcohol Abuse and Alcoholism, 31*(3), 185–195.

Guimarães, F. S. (2013). Substâncias psicoativas. In R. Lent (Ed.), *Neurociência da mente e do comportamento* (pp. 324–348). Guanabara Koogan.

Kakko, J., Alho, H., Baldacchino, A., Molina, R., Nava, F. A., & Shaya, G. (2019). Craving in opioid use disorder: From neurobiology to clinical practice. *Frontiers in Psychiatry, 10*, 592. https://doi.org/10.3389/fpsyt.2019.00592

Koob, G. F. (2020). Neurobiology of opioid addiction: Opponent process, Hyperkatifeia, and negative reinforcement. *Biological Psychiatry, 87*(1), 44–53. https://doi.org/10.1016/j.biopsych.2019.05.023

Kosten, T. R., & George, T. P. (2002). The neurobiology of opioid dependence: Implications for treatment. *Science & Practice Perspectives, 1*(1), 13–20. https://doi.org/10.1151/spp021113

Ksir, C., & Hart, C. (2016a). Correlation still does not imply causation. *The Lancet Psychiatry, 3*(5), 401. https://doi.org/10.1016/S2215-0366(16)30005-0

Ksir, C., & Hart, C. L. (2016b). Cannabis and psychosis: A critical overview of the relationship. *Current Psychiatry Reports, 18*(2), 12. https://doi.org/10.1007/s11920-015-0657-y

Laranjeira, R., Pinsky, I., Caetano, R., & Mitsuhiro, S. (2014). *II Levantamento Nacional de Álcool e Drogas (LENAD) – 2012*. Instituto Nacional de Ciência e Tecnologia para Políticas Públicas de Álcool e Outras Drogas (INPAD) /Universidade Federal de São Paulo (UNIFESP).

Lopes, F., Kreische, F., Sordi, A., & Von Diemen, L. (2012). Tabaco. In *Brasil, Tratamento da Dependência de crack, álcool e outras drogas: aperfeiçoamento para profissionais de saúde e assistência social* (pp. 85–98). Secretaria Nacional de Políticas sobre Drogas.

Marcon, C., Silva, L. A., Moraes, C., Martins, J., & Carpes, A. (2012). Uso de anfetaminas e substâncias relacionadas na sociedade contemporânea. *Disciplinarum Scientia, Ciências da Saúde, 12*(2), 247–263.

Masur, J., & Carlini, E. A. (2004). *Drogas: subsídios para uma discussão*. Brasiliense.

Meyer, J. S. (2013). 3,4-methylenedioxymethamphetamine (MDMA): Current perspectives. *Substance Abuse and Rehabilitation, 4*, 83–99. https://doi.org/10.2147/SAR.S37258

Muakad, I. B. (2013). Anfetaminas e drogas derivadas. *Revista da Faculdade de Direito, Universidade de São Paulo, 108*, 545–572.

Napier, T. C., & Persons, A. L. (2019). Using modern neuroscience to inform opioid use and abuse liability in adolescents. *Orthopedic Nursing, 38*(2), 166–171. https://doi.org/10.1097/NOR.0000000000000527

Nestler, E. J. (2005). The neurobiology of cocaine addiction. *Science & Practice Perspectives, 3*(1), 4–10. https://doi.org/10.1151/spp05314

Nicastri, S. (2012). Drogas: classificação e efeitos no organismo. In *Brasil, Tópicos especiais em policiamento e ações comunitárias, TEPAC: redes de atenção e cuidado* (pp. 43–67). Secretaria Nacional de Segurança Pública.

Oliveira, M., & Argimon, I. (2015). Terapia cognitivo-comportamental em grupo: adolescentes e dependência química. In C. B. Neulfeld (Ed.), *Terapia cognitivo-comportamental em grupo para adolescentes* (pp. 189–201). Artmed.

Paiva, F., & Ronzani, T. (2009). Estilos parentais e consumo de drogas entre adolescentes: revisão sistemática. *Psicologia Em Estudo, 14*(1), 177–183. https://doi.org/10.1590/S1413-73722009000100021

Passie, T., Halpern, J. H., Stichtenoth, D. O., Emrich, H. M., & Hintzen, A. (2008). The pharmacology of lysergic acid diethylamide: A review. *CNS Neuroscience & Therapeutics, 14*(4), 295–314. https://doi.org/10.1111/j.1755-5949.2008.00059.x

Piomelli, D. (2016). Introduction to *Cannabis and Cannabinoid Research*. *Cannabis and Cannabinoid Research, 1*(1), 1–2. https://doi.org/10.1089/can.2015.29002.edi

Pressman, S., & Gigliotti, A. (2019). Nicotina. In A. Diehl, D. Cordeiro, & R. Laranjeira (Eds.), *Chemical dependence: prevention, treatment, and public policy* (2nd ed., pp. 109–124). Artmed.

Rangé, B. P., & Marlatt, G. A. (2008). Terapia cognitivo-comportamental de transtornos de abuso de álcool e drogas. *Revista Brasileira de Psiquiatria, 30*(2), 88–95.

Rosário, B., de Nazaré, M., Estadella, D., Ribeiro, D. A., & Viana, M. B. (2019). Behavioral and neurobiological alterations induced by chronic use of crack cocaine. *Reviews in the Neurosciences, 31*(1), 59–75. https://doi.org/10.1515/revneuro-2018-0118

Santos, S., Bittencourt, A., Silva, M., Stacciarini, T., Engel, R., & Cordeiro, A. (2018). Perfil e fatores associados ao sucesso terapêutico de tabagistas atendidos em um serviço público especializado. *Revista Enfermagem UERJ, 26*, e17381. https://doi.org/10.12957/reuerj.2018.17381

Schenker, M., & Minayo, M. (2005). Fatores de risco e de proteção para o uso de drogas na adolescência. *Ciência & Saúde Coletiva, 10*(3), 707–717. https://doi.org/10.1590/S1413-81232005000300027

Simons, J. S., Carey, K. B., & Wills, T. A. (2009). Alcohol abuse and dependence symptoms: A multidimensional model of common and specific etiology. *Psychology of Addictive Behaviors: Journal of the Society of Psychologists in Addictive Behaviors, 23*(3), 415–427. https://doi.org/10.1037/a0016003

Sordi, A., Kreische, F., Lopes, F., & Von Diemen, L. (2012). Maconha. In *Brasil, Tratamento da Dependência de crack, álcool e outras drogas: aperfeiçoamento para profissionais de saúde e assistência social* (pp. 49–54). Secretaria Nacional de Políticas sobre Drogas.

Stoicea, N., Costa, A., Periel, L., Uribe, A., Weaver, T., & Bergese, S. D. (2019). Current perspectives on the opioid crisis in the US healthcare system: A comprehensive literature review. *Medicine, 98*(20), e15425. https://doi.org/10.1097/MD.0000000000015425

Tabakoff, B., & Hoffman, P. L. (2013). The neurobiology of alcohol consumption and alcoholism: An integrative history. *Pharmacology, Biochemistry, and Behavior, 113*, 20–37. https://doi.org/10.1016/j.pbb.2013.10.009

Takagi, M., Youssef, G., & Lorenzetti, V. (2014). Principais achados em adolescentes dependentes de substâncias a partir de exames de neuroimagem: implicações no diagnóstico, tratamento e prevenção. In D. De Micheli, E. A. Silva, A. L. M. Andrade, & M. L. O. S. Formigoni (Eds.), *Neurociências do abuso de drogas na adolescência: o que sabemos?* (pp. 64–85). Atheneu.

Uhl, G. R., Koob, G. F., & Cable, J. (2019). The neurobiology of addiction. *Annals of the New York Academy of Sciences, 1451*(1), 5–28. https://doi.org/10.1111/nyas.13989

UNODC. (2019). *World drug report 2019*. United Nations Office on Drugs and Crime.

UNODC. (2020). *World drug report 2020*. United Nations Office on Drugs and Crime.

Vegting, Y., Reneman, L., & Booij, J. (2016). The effects of ecstasy on neurotransmitter systems: A review on the findings of molecular imaging studies. *Psychopharmacology, 233*(19–20), 3473–3501. https://doi.org/10.1007/s00213-016-4396-5

Whitesell, M., Bachand, A., Peel, J., & Brown, M. (2013). Familial, social, and individual factors contributing to risk for adolescent substance use. *Journal of Addiction, 2013*, 579310. https://doi.org/10.1155/2013/579310

WHO. (2009). *Alcohol and injuries: Emergency department studies in an international perspective*. World Health Organization.

WHO. (2018). *Global status report on alcohol and health 2018*. World Health Organization.

Xavier, C., Lobo, P., Fonteles, M., Vasconcelos, S., Viana, G., & Sousa, F. (2008). Êxtase (MDMA): efeitos farmacológicos e tóxicos, mecanismo de ação e abordagem clínica. *Archives of Clinical Psychiatry (São Paulo), 35*(3), 96–103. https://doi.org/10.1590/S0101-60832008000300002

Chapter 2
Behavioral Analysis of Substance Use and Dependence: Theoretical-Conceptual Aspects and Possibilities for Intervention

Richard Alecsander Reichert, Simone Martin Oliani, and Roberto Alves Banaco

Introduction

The use of substances to alter behavior, whether in terms of perception, degree of consciousness, or emotional state, is an ancient social practice in the history of mankind. Substance consumption took on a greater proportion in Western society at the end of the nineteenth century, spreading from the 1960s and on (Bergeron, 2012). Currently, harmful use and dependence are a major public health concern, insofar as they can have effects at the individual and social level (UNODC, 2019; WHO, 2018). Problems regarding the use of these substances are related to daily behaviors, such as drinking alcohol, smoking cigarettes, and consuming other drugs. Although common, these behaviors can progress from substance use to substance dependence and generate or intensify adverse consequences, represented by personal, family, academic, professional, financial, emotional, and social losses (Barlow & Durand, 2015).

Drug addiction was once considered a moral problem or character deficit. According to the popular notion, predominant mainly in the mid-nineteenth century, substance-dependent individuals consumed substances by free will, being

R. A. Reichert (✉)
Department of Psychobiology, Universidade Federal de São Paulo (UNIFESP), São Paulo, SP, Brazil
e-mail: reichert@unifesp.br

S. M. Oliani
Centro Integrado de Neuropsiquiatria e Psicologia Comportamental (CINP), Londrina, PR, Brazil
e-mail: simoneoliani@portalcinp.com.br

R. A. Banaco
Paradigma – Centro de Ciências e Tecnologia do Comportamento, São Paulo, SP, Brazil
e-mail: roberto@paradigmaac.com.br

S. M. Oliani et al. (eds.), *Behavior Analysis and Substance Dependence*,
https://doi.org/10.1007/978-3-030-75961-2_2

stigmatized as indecent or sinful. In this perspective, it was believed that people could decide whether or not to ingest drugs and, due to the immoral character, consumed them (Garcia-Mijares & Silva, 2006). Bergeron (2012) indicates, in this explanatory conception for the problem with drugs, a dualistic notion, which values notions of integrity, conscience, autonomy, and the sovereign nature of the human being. This view of dependency as a deviation or immoral standard of conduct may be based on the notion of free will, which Baum (2018) describes as simply being a name for the lack of knowledge regarding the determinants of behavior.

Several theoretical models have been developed with the goal of explaining the use and dependence on substances that alter behavior in terms of consciousness, perception, and emotions. However, many of these theoretical models approached the subject in a quite reductionist and simplistic manner, disregarding the variability of personal and contextual factors and the different dimensions involved. Different perspectives on substance use and dependence have emerged over time, some of which are shown in Table 2.1.

As Table 2.1 shows, there are many conceptions about substance abuse that have been associated for a long time. Several studies have been carried out in order to better understand the issues related to substance use. In addition to confirming its complexity and its multifactorial nature, these researches demonstrated the role of

Table 2.1 Theoretical models of substance use and dependence

Moral model	In the moral model, both substance use and dependence are considered personal choices. This behavior is believed to be a disregard for social norms. for this reason, users are the target of criticism, inattention, and punishment.
Temperance or sobriety model	The temperance model emerged at the end of the nineteenth century, being the first structured attempt to understand the etiology of alcohol dependence. According to this model, addiction is not a moral failure or a sin, but a habit to be unlearned through a balance in consumption.
Neurological degeneration model	According to this model, based on a study published in 1849, in Sweden, alcohol dependence should be understood as a pathology, and the treatment should be similar to other diseases of the time (steam baths, using leeches, etc.).
Spiritual model	In this model, alcohol dependence is seen as a condition in which the individual becomes unable to overcome by oneself, being necessary to surrender one's life to a higher power to then proceed with the recovery.
Psychological model	The psychological model encompasses several schools of thought that seek to explain the development of substance dependence, such as the cognitive-behavioral model, the psychoanalytic school, the social learning model, the systemic model, among others.
Biological model	The biological model suggests physiology and genetics as factors responsible for the etiology of substance dependence.
Biopsychosocial model	The biopsychosocial model states that substance dependence is multifactorial and therefore, a multilevel analysis (integrating different theories) would be necessary to understand the etiology of substance dependence.

Sources: Cordeiro (2018) and Perrenoud and Ribeiro (2019)

the social context in the installation and maintenance of these behavior patterns. An important study, known as "Rat Park," was carried out by Alexander, Coambs, and Hadaway in the 1970s. Upon realizing that experimental subjects used in laboratories were kept in environments quite different from their natural habitat, the researchers investigated whether environmental conditions as social isolation and the absence of alternative reinforcers would be predictors of substance use and dependence and if the presence of these stimuli could interfere with the choice of using drugs.

The goal of the study was to compare the rates of self-administration of morphine between two groups: (A) isolated and stimulus-deprived rats in laboratory cages and (B) rats living socially in an environment with the availability of alternative reinforcers. The results showed that rats that were isolated and without access to other reinforcers ingested significantly higher rates of the morphine solution available in both cages, which can be explained by the potentiation of the reinforcing effects of morphine in relieving aversive sensations resulting from adverse environmental conditions (Alexander et al., 1978; Gage & Sumnall, 2018). In line with these data, studies by other theorists from different fields of knowledge, such as Howard Becker (*Outsiders: Sociology of Deviation Studies*, 1963) and Norman Zinberg (*Drug Set and Setting: The Basis for Controlled Intoxicant Use*, 1984), reiterate the need to consider contextual aspects, in addition to the pharmacological characteristics of substances, when analyzing behaviors and social practices such as the drug use.

Further research and discussions highlight some methodological weaknesses of some similar experiments, in addition to the fact that other studies present divergent results. Regardless, there is a consensus in the scientific literature the idea that the behavior must be analyzed, in this case different patterns of substance use, considering the environmental influence, thus adopting a biopsychosocial perspective, that is, considering the interrelation between biogenetic and psychosocial variables. This new perspective enables the development of more integrative and effective protection, prevention, and treatment strategies at the individual and collective level.

The Approach Proposed by Behavior Analysis

A theoretical approach that recognizes the multidetermination and complexity of the behavior, covering psychosocial variables, in addition to biological ones, is the explanatory model of behavior analysis. This approach is a behavioral science based on the philosophical assumptions of radical behaviorism, of which Burrhus Frederic Skinner (1904–1990) was the driving force.

One of his influences was I. M. Sechenov (1829–1905), a Russian physiologist who developed one of the first explanatory models of behavior through the concept of reflex. His doctoral thesis, published in 1860, was entitled *"Data for the future physiology of alcohol intoxication."* The researcher sought to explain the behavior through organism–environment interaction, considering historical-environmental factors, because, in his perception, an organism cannot live without the external environment. Therefore, a scientific explanation of the organism must consider the context in which it is inserted. Sechenov was an influence for Ivan Pavlov (known for his studies on classical/respondent conditioning) who, in turn, was an influence for Skinner (Pessotti, 2016).

Skinner (2006) defines behaviorism as the philosophy of behavioral science. This means that when talking about behaviorism, philosophical issues are on the agenda, that is, questions that guide and clarify the way we understand the world. The conception of human beings in radical behaviorism starts from the principle declared by Bertrand Russell, in his 1927 book *"Outlines of Philosophy."* In the chapter entitled *"The role of the environment,"* Russell questions Watsonian behaviorism, which followed the same principles already described earlier by Sechenov and Pavlov: the relationship in which the environment determines the activity of organisms was only a part of the complex existing relationships. There were also the relationships in which organisms change the environment through their actions, and this altered environment, in turn, would also affect human activities… (Botomé et al., 2018).

These assumptions, supposed and developed by Skinner, refer to an approach to the functioning of the organism from a broader perspective, taking in consideration the organism and also the environment in which it is inserted, and which operates on it, as previously described (Moreira & Hanna, 2015; Pessotti, 2016; Skinner, 1957, 2003, 2006).

The behavior analysis, a science of behavior based on the philosophical principles of radical behaviorism, was inspired by the Darwinian concept of evolution of the species, which proposes the occurrence of morphological, physical, and intra- and intergenerational variations of individuals, and it is up to the environment to select individuals with characteristics better suited for survival. For this approach, science, more specifically the science of behavior, must look for the relationships between the natural events that influence human action, and are influenced by it, and that is why it is mandatory to recognize the role of the environment.

At the behavioral level, all individuals have variations in the way they behave, and the environment selects and maintains the most appropriate responses to that environment. Finally, given that the environment outside the organism is essentially composed of other humans, the social level must also be considered in the analysis to be elaborated (Banaco & Montan, 2018; Baum, 2018; Moreira & Medeiros, 2018; Skinner, 2003, 2006). Behavior is determined by multiple factors and, for this reason, a multilevel analysis is essential.

This theoretical model considers, therefore, the interaction between phylogenetic, ontogenetic, and sociocultural variables as determinants for the behavior. According to Skinner (1974/2006, p. 163), "*a scientific analysis of behavior must […] assume that a person's behavior is controlled more by his genetic and environmental history.*" For Skinner (1951/2003), what the human being does is the result of conditions that can be specified. The author points out that "*circumstances beyond the individual are important*" (p. 9) as opposed to the tendency to seek explanations for behavior exclusively within the organism.

Admitting that the role of science is to relate events, making arrangements of variables and verifying their changes, as well as establishing new relationships, it is a role of behavior analysis—the science of behavior—to identify the variables that control behavior, to then predict the likelihood of its occurrence. For that purpose, what people do, talk, think, or feel must be contextualized. That is why, behavior analysts define psychology as the science that studies the behavior of organisms in relation to the environment in which they are inserted, that is, the behavior–environment interactions are studied (Lombard-Platet et al., 2015; Moreira & Hanna, 2015).

In summary, the radical behaviorist and analytical-behavioral perspective (a) takes determinism in consideration when explaining facts of human nature, adopting a monist conception and favoring direct observation; (b) understands introspection as a way of recognizing private human events, and not as an investigative method or procedure; (c) proposes studying behavior in the context of the relationship between organism and environment; (d) highlights the importance of an accessible and functional form of research and, above all, that is applicable to any contexts where there are relationships between organism and environment that explain the installation and maintenance of behavior; (e) adds the functional possibility of the principles that guide behavior science, making it possible to solve both individual and collective/social issues; (f) reveals the existence of the operant behavior and takes it as the main focus of the investigations, recognizing and describing the several schedules and operations that can alter the probability of the behavior occurring and explaining its functionality; (g) starts from the assumption that, under certain contextual conditions, consequences follow responses; (h) sees the applicability of the three-term contingency paradigm to the analysis of social issues and cultural practices; and (i) has developed essential concepts such as modeling, social behavior, verbal behavior, and other essential terms for behavioral analysis (Carrara, 2016).

The analytical-behavioral theory studies the behaviors through the experimental method, and its interventions are based on the findings obtained through it. The behavior analysis, therefore, seeks to understand the relationships between the actions of the organism and the changes in the environment in which the latter is inserted, investigating the conditions responsible for the recurrence of certain responses. As for substance use and dependence, a broad and varied interpretation is sought, understanding that the behaviors are multifunctional. From the identification of environmental variables that influence behavior, it is possible to manipulate them and develop assertive behavioral strategies for the management of contingencies previous to problem behavior (Banaco & Montan, 2018) (see Fig. 2.1).

Behavior analysis has a wide range of research and evidence that define behavior as a product of mutual and complex interactions between phylogenetic, ontogenetic, and sociocultural variables. This theoretical model allows a broader understanding of behaviors such as drug use and dependence and emphasizes the context and environmental factors as the focus of more effective interventions, identifying and modifying the contingencies responsible for the installation and maintenance of behaviors, thus providing environments that facilitate learning new responses favorable to both individual and collective well-being.

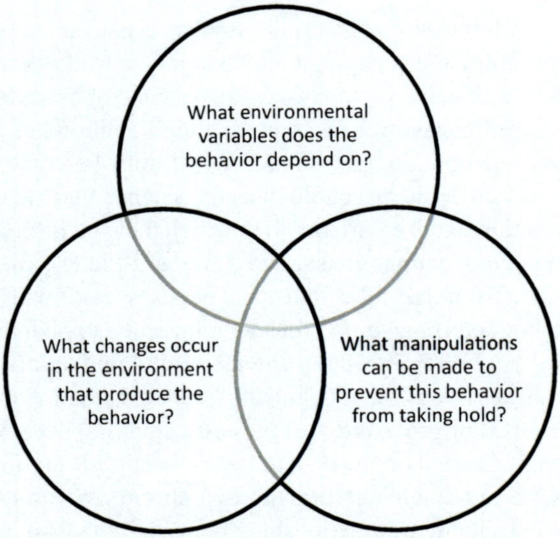

Fig. 2.1 Issues that guide the work of behavior analysts. (Source: Banaco and Montan 2018)

A topic which was previously understood in a restricted way has begun being analyzed scientifically in a broader way (biopsychosocial). Understanding the phenomenon from the analysis of the relationships established between the organism and environment and by identifying the variables that control the behavior, as well as recognizing the specific changes occurred in the central nervous system using psychoactive drugs, Skinner's maxim is recognized: the behavior is multidetermined. The integration of neuroscience with behavioral theories and approaches is a highly relevant interdisciplinary field and is part of the changes regarding the progressive understanding of substance use and dependence. The functional definition of addiction emerged as an alternative perspective based on scientific evidence, breaking with views that, being partial and limited, have not, so far, found good answers to this problem. The attempt to recognize the multifunctionality of human behavior tries to fill this knowledge gap regarding different sciences, since the subject is too broad to fit within one science only. Behavioral pharmacology, for example, is a field of study that starts from these premises and demonstrates the complementarity between behavior analysis and physiology, also showing how environmental variables can play a role in the effects created by psychoactive substances, as it is understood that setting some boundaries to the study on the functioning of drugs to merely neurobiological aspects produces incomplete knowledge on the subject. These advances make it possible to develop new behavioral and pharmacological technologies for the treatment of disorders related to substance use (Garcia-Mijares & Silva, 2006; Leonardi & Bravin, 2012; Maté, 2010).

This book aims to demonstrate several ways of approaching such a plural subject. Part I covers introductory aspects and main concepts, and approaches it in a more general and comprehensive perspective. Distinct ways of identifying substance abuse are presented, as well as the excessive aspect that classifies it as pathological (Chap. 1); behavioral use and dependence as well as possibilities for intervention are analyzed (Chap. 2); in addition to analyzing the diagnostic criteria for substance use disorders from an analytical-behavioral perspective (Chap. 3). Also in this Part, the basic concepts of behavioral pharmacotherapy can be found (Chap. 4); as well as the functional analysis of substance use and dependence (Chap. 5); and a discussion regarding the establishment and abolition of contingencies for the use of crack (Chap. 6). fvNext, in Part, the reader will find chapters that focus on contributions from clinical and social interventions, where they deal with the case analysis and demonstrate how to identify, develop a case formulation and proposals for treatment, as well as to evaluate the results of the interventions. The proposals listed are Contingency Management (Chap. 7), Exposure Therapy with Response Prevention (Chap. 8), Functional Analytic Psychotherapy - FAP (Chap. fv9), Dialectical Behavior Therapy – DBT (Chap. 10), Acceptance and Commitment Therapy – ACT (Chap. 11), Reinforcement Contingency Therapy (Chap. 12), and Motivational Interviewing (Chap. 13). Finally, in Part, special topics are presented: the interfaces between neurosciences and behavior analysis on drug use and dependence (Chap. 14); behavioral proposals to provide guidance and solution to issues related to the analysis of other behavioral excesses in humans (Chap. 15); marital narratives in detecting and developing substance abuse (Chap. 16); effects of substance use in romantic relationships and their relationship to violence against women (Chap. 17); and the availability and difficulty of detecting alcohol and tobacco abuse at the clinical level (Chap. 18).

References

Alexander, B. K., Coambs, R. B., & Hadaway, P. F. (1978). The effect of housing and gender on morphine self-administration in rats. *Psychopharmacology, 58*(2), 175–179.

Banaco, R., & Montan, R. (2018). Teoria analítico-comportamental. In N. Zanelatto & R. Laranjeira (Eds.), *O tratamento da dependência química e as terapias cognitivo-comportamentais: um guia para terapeutas* (2nd ed., pp. 115–132). Artmed.

Barlow, D., & Durand, V. (2015). *Psicopatologia: uma abordagem integrada* (7th ed.). Cengage Learning.

Baum, W. (2018). *Compreender o behaviorismo: comportamento, cultura e evolução* (3rd ed.). Artmed.

Becker, H. (2008). *Outsiders: Estudos de sociologia do desvio*. Zahar. (Originally published in 1963).

Bergeron, H. (2012). *Sociologia da droga*. Ideias & Letras.

Botomé, S. P., Kubo, O. M., Otero, V. R. L., & Banaco, R. A. (2018). *A Construção da Análise do Comportamento como orientação fundamental para intervir: técnicas e receitas ou procedimentos referenciais basilares para atuar*. Curso dirigido para a Acreditação como Analista do Comportamento, oferecido pelo ABPMC, São Luís, Maranhão, Brasil.

Carrara, K. (2016). O essencial em B. F. Skinner (1904–1990). In D. Zilio & K. Carrara (Eds.), *Behaviorismos: reflexões históricas e conceituais* (pp. 19–32). Centro Paradigma de Ciências do Comportamento.

Cordeiro, D. (2018). Transtornos por uso de substâncias: conceituação e modelos teóricos. In N. Zanelatto & R. Laranjeira (Eds.), *O tratamento da dependência química e as terapias cognitivo-comportamentais: um guia para terapeutas* (2nd ed., pp. 3–13). Artmed.

Gage, S. H., & Sumnall, H. R. (2018). Rat Park: How a rat paradise changed the narrative of addiction. *Addiction, 114*(5), 917–922.

Garcia-Mijares, M., & Silva, M. (2006). Dependência de drogas. *Psicologia USP, 17*(4), 213–240. https://doi.org/10.1590/s0103-65642006000400012

Lombard-Platet, V., Watanabe, O., & Cassetari, L. (2015). *Psicologia experimental: manual teórico e prático de análise do comportamento*. Edicon.

Leonardi, J., & Bravin, A. (2012). Uma introdução à farmacologia comportamental. *Interação em Psicologia, 15*(2). https://doi.org/10.5380/psi.v15i2.20514

Maté, G. (2010). *In the realm of hungry ghosts: Close encounters with addiction*. North Atlantic.

Moreira, M., & Hanna, E. (2015). Bases filosóficas e noção de ciência em análise do comportamento. In M. Hübner (Ed.), *Temas clássicos da psicologia sob a ótica da análise do comportamento* (pp. 2–19). Guanabara Koogan.

Moreira, M., & Medeiros, C. (2018). *Princípios Básicos de Análise do Comportamento* (2nd ed.). Artmed.

Perrenoud, L., & Ribeiro, M. (2019). Etiologia dos transtornos relacionados ao uso de substâncias. In A. Diehl, D. Cordeiro, & R. Laranjeira (Eds.), *Dependência química: prevenção, tratamento e políticas públicas* (2nd ed., pp. 9–14). Artmed.

Pessotti, I. (2016). I. M. Sechenov (1829-1905) e os “reflexos do cérebro”. In D. Zilio & K. Carrara (Eds.), *Behaviorismos: reflexões históricas e conceituais* (pp. 33–51). Centro Paradigma de Ciências do Comportamento.

Skinner, B. F. (1957). *Verbal behavior*. Appleton-Century-Crofts.

Skinner, B. F. (2003). *Ciência e comportamento humano*. Martins Fontes.

Skinner, B. F. (2006). *Sobre o behaviorismo*. São Paulo, SP: Cultrix. (Originally published in 1974).

UNODC. (2019). *World drug report 2019*. United Nations Office on Drugs and Crime.

WHO. (2018). *Global status report on alcohol and health 2018*. World Health Organization.

Zinberg, N. (1984). *Drug, set, and setting: The basis for controlled intoxicant use*. Yale University.

Chapter 3
Criteria for Substance Use Disorders Diagnosis (SUD): An Behavioral-Analytic Perspective

Fábio Henrique Baia, André Amaral Bravin, Wilson Benício Martins, and Rogério Guaita dos Santos Baia

Introduction

The Diagnostic and Statistical Manual of Mental Disorders - DSM-V (APA, 2014) and the ICD-10 Classification of Mental and Behavioral Disorders (WHO, 1993) present diagnostic criteria for "substance-related disorders" or "mental and behavioral disorders due to the use of psychoactive substance," respectively. The criteria used in these manuals conflict with the perspective of radical behaviorism (RB) [1]. However, Souza (2003) points out that, despite these problems, the manuals facilitate communication among professionals in different areas. The objective of this work is to present to analytical-behavioral therapists possible functional understandings of diagnostic criteria for substance use disorders. The understanding of the variables involved in determining these behaviors can facilitate the practice of therapists and allow improved communication with other health professionals.

[1] See Banaco et al. (2010) and Cavalcante and Tourinho (1998).

F. H. Baia (✉)
Universidade do Rio Verde (UniRV), Rio Verde, GO, Brazil

Universidade de São Paulo (USP), São Paulo, SP, Brazil
e-mail: fabio@unirv.edu.br

A. A. Bravin
Universidade Federal de Jataí, Jataí, GO, Brazil

W. B. Martins · R. G. dos Santos Baia
Universidade do Rio Verde (UniRV), Rio Verde, GO, Brazil

S. M. Oliani et al. (eds.), *Behavior Analysis and Substance Dependence*,
https://doi.org/10.1007/978-3-030-75961-2_3

Disorders Related to Substance Use

There are two reasons for choosing DSM-V (APA, 2014) as the main thread of this analysis, namely its recenticity and its harmonization with the International Classification of Diseases (ICD). It is known that in addition to the task of classifying diseases, both manuals present statistical, epidemiological, developmental aspects. Considering that the most current version of the DSM (APA, 2014) was published 20 years after the most current version of the ICD (WHO, 1993), this is the most recent of the two manuals, and this is the first reason that justifies the present choice. The second reason is the recognition that one of the objectives of the DSM-V was its harmonization with the ICD (APA, 2014). Thus, the professional who eventually needs the ICD-10 codes for his or her trade will be able to do so by consulting the new version of the DSM (APA, 2014), the opposite being impossible. This harmonization makes it possible to extend the behavioral interpretations carried out here to include the descriptors of ICD-10 (WHO, 1993).

The diagnostic criteria for substance dependence of DSM-V follow a descriptive logic, and were organized among those behaviors that indicate (a) "low control over substance use" (criteria 1 to 4), (b) "social harm" (criteria 5 to 7), (c) "risky substance use" (criteria 8 and 9), and (d) "pharmacological criteria" (criteria 10 and 11) (APA, 2014). However, this organization appears to rely more on topographic than functional aspects of behavior[2]. The following are the diagnostic criteria agglutinated by possible functional interpretations of the behavioral processes involved.

Criterion (1): The substance is often consumed in larger quantities or over a longer period than intended.

The use of the substance in quantities or periods longer than intended may lead to interpretations of forces explaining behavior as "intention." Intention as a causal force is incompatible with the behaviorist radical notion of the determinant variables of behavior. Radical behaviorism advocates explanations based on functional relationships between behavior and the environment, so it rejects any explanation that establishes mental causes as determinants of behavior (Moore, 2008). According to Hineline (2003), it is possible to understand intentional verbalizations as long as no causal forces are attributed to these statements. According to the author, "*statements of intent are in themselves behavioural events, and should be considered as such*" (p. 210). To understand intentional statements the author uses verbal relations. Declaring intention is a verbal behavior controlled by environmental events. When someone says they will consume only two shots of whiskey, this verbal behavior is controlled by past environmental events. To give an example,

[2] The current version of DSM-V presents diagnostic criteria that "cover 10 distinct classes of drugs: alcohol; caffeine; cannabis; hallucinogens [...]; inhalants; opioids; sedatives, hypnotics, and anxiolytics; stimulants (amphetamine-type substances, cocaine, and other stimulants); tobacco; and other substances". For the preparation of this chapter, the criteria that are repeated in most of the diagnoses for substances were chosen. Thus, specific criteria such as gastrointestinal discomfort of caffeine were discarded from the synthesis presented here.

saying "I will only drink two shots" to a given individual can be functionally equivalent to saying "in the past, when I was at a party and whiskey was present, I drank two shots and had my behavior reinforced by social acceptance from my wife, so when I am in similar situations such as party, whiskey and wife, I am likely to reemerge the two shots behavior." Note that the intent is neither causal force nor verbal descriptions controlled by future events.

Still according to Hineline (2003) when someone declares an intention to do something, it is possible that such a declaration alters the probability of the declared behavior occurring. Thus, when a person arrives at the party who has previously declared that he would only consume two shots of whiskey, he may have his behavior controlled by such a declaration. The previous declaration can act as a function altering stimulus, since consuming more than the declared one can lead to positive punishments such as fights by the wife for the lack of correspondence between what was said and what was done.

Thus, verbal correspondence studies can help to understand the determinant variables of verbal statements (saying behavior) and their correspondence/non correspondence with doing behavior (Beckert, 2005). The understanding of events that determine the verbal correspondence of the type say-do helps in the functional interpretation of the symptom of consuming substance above the intended. Non-correspondence may occur due to contingent reinforcements to this situation. For example, the verbal response of declaring a given consumption may be under control of events as social reinforcement. However, the behavior of consuming substance is controlled by reinforcements produced by the substance itself (e.g., the relief of withdrawal symptoms). In this case, verbal responses (intention to consume) and nonverbal responses (consumption) have different controls, which may lead to a mismatch between saying and doing. It is up to the behavioral therapist to understand how reinforcements produced by ingestion of substance outweigh reinforcements of the tell-to-do correspondence. A possible strategy for treatment could involve scheduling boosters for verbal tell-to-do correspondence so that such boosters compete with the consequences of consuming the drug at higher doses than declared.

Criteria 2 and 4: (2) There is a persistent desire or unsuccessful effort to reduce or control the use of the substance; and (4) There is a crack or a strong desire or need to use the substance

Both criteria, 2 and 4, point to the role of "desire" in the diagnosis of substance dependence. While criterion 2 argues for a desire to reduce or control substance use, criterion 4 argues for a strong desire to use it. This strong desire (designated as a craving) is defined as an uncontrollable need for drug use and has been held responsible for relapses, i.e. unsuccessful efforts to reduce or control use. Thus, a relationship is observed between both diagnostic criteria, and for this reason it seems more appropriate to present them on the same topic.

Skinner (1974/2006) states that the term desire should be understood as the probability of the behavior occurring. Thus, when referring to the existence of a persistent desire, the individual reports the control that an environmental event exerts over its response. Saying that he wishes to consume substance describes that there is a high probability of the consumption behavior occurring. Therefore, the behavior analyst should investigate the factors that are determining the probability of the behavior occurring.

The lower interruption or consumption behavior depends on environmental events. The interruption may occur by positive social reinforcement such as compliments released by other people (e.g., the companion, children or friends may say how they observed improvement in user behavior due to interruption or reduced use), or nonsocial reinforcement (e.g., improved attendance and frequency at work or improved ability to operate machines), both reinforcements incompatible with the use of the substance.

Another possibility is that the reduction or interruption occurs due to aversive events produced by substance consumption. Again, social and nonsocial environmental events may act as determinants of this behavior. Fights, reduction of invitations to social occasions, and problems with control agents such as police can become motivational operations for the reduction of drug use behavior. Once one understands what types of events can determine "desire," it is necessary to understand what events are the determinants of the failure of attempts to interrupt or reduce substance use.

Unsuccessful efforts to control substance use can be classified as relapse. According to Álvarez (2007), relapse is defined as a return to substance use. The understanding of the behavior of returning to substance ingestion involves reflex and operative processes. Usually, the reflexes have been attributed to the explanation of the fissure (aversive conditioned respondents, known as conditioned abstinence), and to the operant, the relapse (self-administration behavior of drugs). In this sense a respondent–operant interaction helps to understand the role of the *crack* in the unsuccessful effort to control use.

Among the reflex phenomena that help in the understanding of relapse are spontaneous recovery, resurgence, reinstatement, and renewal (Bouton, 2002). In the case of reflexes, the recovery of the value of CS after reflex extinction is investigated. In the case of the operant, there are the phenomena of (1) induction, in which after extinction, free reinforcements are released, promoting the return of the operant response; (2) reestablishment, recurrence of extinct operant responses if previous stimuli or stressing events are reappeared after extinction; and (3) resurgence, characterized by the reappearance of previously extinct operant responses when another operant response is put into extinction (Epstein et al., 2006). The interaction between reflexes and operants helps to understand how the resumption of a CS can lead to the recovery of operant responses.

For example, in a therapeutic group one client was asked to speak or imagine drugs without the effects of consumption being present, reflex extinction was in effect. After therapeutic follow-up the client stopped consuming alcohol and engaged in a stable love relationship. However, after several fights, the client and his girlfriend broke up the relationship. The weekend after the end the client went with friends to a nightclub. After frustrated attempts to start conversations with girls, the client reported a need to consume alcohol. After consumption, the client felt relaxed and was able to interact with other people. To the client's misfortune, consumption was not restricted to the nightclub and, 15 days later, he returned to consume alcohol daily, about eight cans a day. This example illustrates a case of resurgence. Besides the recovery of functioning responses, the use of alcohol can reestablish the value of other environmental events (smell of alcohol, friends, or nightclub) such as CS.

Other operative processes are also responsible for the "persistence" of drug use. In this scenario, the concept of stimulus equivalence can also help to understand the persistence/recurring use of the substance (Albuquerque & Melo, 2005). Equivalence of stimuli is characterized by situations in which one class of stimuli causes responses evoked by another class of stimuli (Pierce & Cheney, 2008). DeGrandpre et al. (1992) demonstrate how events not directly related to substance use can acquire, through stimulus equivalence, the ability to evoke drug consumption behavior. For example, the use of drugs correlated to a specific friend is sufficient for the mere presence of the friend to elicit the compensatory responses typical of the substance. If this same friend is also correlated to a location, such as a bar, it is possible that exposure to the bar elicits compensatory responses even if the bar–drug correlation has never occurred. Thus, even after the interruption of consumption, if the user returns to the bar correlated to the friend, when arriving at the place he may experience sensations typical of the abstinence syndrome, which can lead to lapse and relapse.

The interaction between reflexes and operants can be interpreted in two ways: (a) as a behavioral chain, where reflex responses (the crack) function as S^d's that evoke operant responses (relapse) that remove it from the environment (negative reinforcement), or (b) as a motivational operation, where the crack functions as a transitive conditioned motivating operation. The above-mentioned behavioral and operative response processes, as well as their interaction, contribute to the elucidation of both the "persistent desire," the "need to use the drug" (i.e., crack), and the "unsuccessful efforts to control substance use" (i.e., relapse). At the same time, self-control studies can also help to understand the return to consumption. For this reason, the behavior of choices and self-control will be presented together in the next diagnostic criterion.

Criteria 3, 5, and 7: (3) Much time is spent in activities necessary to obtain the substance, use it, or recover from its effects; (5) Recurrent use of the substance resulting in failure to meet important obligations at work, school, or home; and (7) Important social, occupational, or recreational activities are abandoned or reduced because of substance use.

DeGrandpre and Bickel (1993) point out that substance dependence refers to a process in which there is a proportional increase in the individual's demand behavior and self-administration of drugs, to the detriment of other behaviors that are not related to the consumption of the substance. Thus, it is possible to state that the above criteria involve situations characterized by choices.

It is in this sense that the criteria complement each other, since the functional class outlined above is that the organism stops doing something due to substance use (criterion 7), spends a lot of time with repertories related to drug use (search, acquisition, consumption, and recovery of drug use) (criterion 3), and in fact, this recurrent use results in failures in daily relationships (criterion 5).

In terms of search, acquisition, consumption, and recovery of use, operating controls and unconditioned respondents are present. The time required for recovery from the effects of drug use (half-life period) depends on the type of substance, its dosage, and route of administration. Therefore, in order to understand the recovery of the effects of the drug, it is necessary to understand physiological aspects and the mechanisms of action of each substance (pharmacokinetics and pharmacodynamics). It is not the purpose of this work to discuss the physiological processes of each drug, therefore we suggest reading Meyer and Quenzer (2005). On the other hand, operative processes are those that can help in the understanding of the so-called search, acquisition, and consumption of the substance. And according to the diagnostic criteria, these behaviors are analyzed in light of the time spent for their search, acquisition, and use.

As Todorov and Hanna (2005, pp. 159) state, "to choose is the response to one of two or more accessible stimuli and to prefer to spend more time answering [...], or to respond more to one of them. In this way, the time spent on obtaining and using drugs is likely to be proportional to their relative reinforcing value. Therefore, the above-mentioned processes that determine choices allow the interpretation of the time spent in obtaining and using drugs. Traditionally, the behavioral theory for choice is the "Law of Equalisation" (Herrnstein, 1970). The general statement of the law of equalization proclaims that when an organism can repeatedly choose between at least two different sources of reinforcement (e.g., drugs vs. labor), the proportion of responses from a given source tends to equal the proportion of reinforcements obtained from that source. Thus, the proportion of responses in each alternative (e.g., drugs, work, family, friends) tends to match the frequency, probability, proportion, magnitude, and immediacy of the reinforcements obtained, and is further affected by the "quality" of the reinforcement and topography of the required response (Herrnstein, 1970; Todorov & Hanna, 2005).

For reasons explained by natural selection, organisms have a better chance of survival when they behave in a way that maximizes the achievement of reinforcements possible in a situation over time. Authors such as Heyman (1996), characterize substance dependence as a process in which repeated drug use reduces the reinforcing value of other activities such as family, work, and friends, in relation to the activities involving substance use. Czoty et al. (2005) conducted an experiment in which cocaine user monkeys decreased their drug use due to food. This study used a choice procedure in which responses to produce cocaine and food competed. Thus, the study illustrates how therapists can interpret drug use as a choice and schedule interventions that make other reinforcements capable of controlling the substance use response. However, the delay of reinforcements can affect these choices. This will be examined below.

Criteria 6, 9, and 8: (6) Continued use of the substance despite persistent or recurrent social or interpersonal problems caused or exacerbated by the effects of its use; (9) Use of the substance is maintained despite awareness of

a persistent or recurrent physical or psychological problem that tends to be caused or exacerbated by it; and (8) Recurrent use of the substance in situations where it presents a danger to physical integrity

A particular situation of choice occurs when competing response alternatives produce different reinforcements—quantitatively or qualitatively. Thus, an "A" alternative could bring reinforcement of lesser and immediate magnitude, while a "B" alternative could bring reinforcement of greater magnitude, but delayed. This competing contingency of choice establishes a particular type of "conflict," and the choice of immediate alternatives of lesser magnitude has been called "impulsive choice," as opposed to its counterpart, which is called "self-contained choice."

To some degree drug use fits this description, where the immediate pleasure (or relief from abstinence) caused by substance use is preferred to maintaining health and good family and social relationships in the long term. Preferring immediate drug use over other backward reinforcements would be a way to characterize the impulsive behavior of drug users (Madden et al., 1997), and their perseverance would bring about the "social, interpersonal, physical, or psychological problems" described by the diagnostic criterion.

The relationship between the delay and the control produced by the reinforcement of the response is investigated in an area called "delay discount." Madden et al. (1997) demonstrated that nonusers of drugs had less subjective devaluation of the reinforcement value, due to their delay, when compared to opioid users, for the hypothetical reinforcement "money." Taking the results of this study as an example of the criteria, it is possible to understand that despite the long-term gains that could eventually occur (e.g., physical, psychological, social, or interpersonal health), the addict's behavior of choice is more under control of immediate gains (i.e., the effect provided by the drug) than the laggards. More than that, when the choice is for the drug itself, this choice becomes even more impulsive (predilection for the immediate drug). This model would explain, at least in part, both the continued use of the substance in spite of problems derived from the use, and the exacerbation of impulsiveness that starts to be caused by the use.

Still taking as an example the impulsivity/self-control paradigm, the counterpart of this logic is taken when analyzing the moment of choice for reinforcement of greater or lesser magnitude. Imagine the individual who has just recovered from a hangover by proposing abstinence from the drug (i.e., has just quenched it). The reinforcement of greater and later magnitude (e.g., family, health, and work) presents a greater subjective value when compared to that of lesser and immediate magnitude (e.g., alcohol; after all, he has just quenched himself of alcohol). As time passes and moments approach when the drug is available (e.g., beginning of next month and receipt of salary), its subjective value increases to the point of exceeding the subjective value of the once preferred delayed consequences (Madden et al., 1997; Tucker, 2004). In summary, even if the individual considers his family, health, and employment more important, when drug availability is signaled (e.g., receipt of wage, *happy hour* from work), its value suddenly becomes higher because it is immediately available (Tucker, 2004). According to Tucker (2004), the consequences of remaining abstemious only occur after a very extended period of time (delay of reinforcement), so that the value of choosing the immediate alternative is higher.

Given this reversal of preference, the predilection for the substance continues despite the problems caused by its use. Despite the individual having serious health problems, and/or social problems with his family and at work, and despite the subject's awareness of his problems or the risks he faces in obtaining the drug, the use of the substance persists. This can cause a further aggravation in social or health problems, which would virtually amount to further delaying the recovery from these aggravations. Once this delay becomes even greater, the greater will be the tendency for the individual to make impulsive choices when these immediate reinforcements are available, as in a kind of vicious circle.

Criterion 10: Tolerance

Tolerance is characterized in two ways: (a) it involves the necessity of larger doses to obtain the effect previously produced by uses of smaller doses of substances, and (b) the marked reduction of the effect with the continued use of the same amount of substance. Both can be understood as fruits of the same behavioral process.

Benvenuti (2004) highlights that through studies on reflex conditioning it has become more feasible to understand the mechanisms underlying the phenomena of development of behavioral tolerance. Rescorla (1988) describes that the determining factor for changing the function of a neutral stimulus (NS) in a CS is the contingent relationship between US and NS, that is, how much the CS predicts the occurrence of US. Siegel (1976) conducted an experiment that suggests that the use of a substance elicits compensatory (metabolic) responses that are opposed to the effect of the drug. When environmental events are contingent on the drug, such responses are controlled by the environment, even before the use of the substance. Thus, the compensatory responses (S^Rs) decrease the effects of the substance, generating the aforementioned behavioral tolerance. This is only reversed with the increase in the dosage of the drug. The understanding of the mechanisms that generate tolerance syndrome helps to understand abstinence syndrome.

Criterion 11: Abstinence

Abstinence syndrome is characterized by symptoms produced by the decrease of the substance in the body, either by its suspension or its metabolism. The symptoms produced are specific to each substance. As described above the reflex conditioning explains the tolerance. Thus environmental events elicit compensatory responses even before the ingestion of the drug. In fact the individual experiences symptoms caused by the suspension of drug use. Thus, the understanding of reflex conditioning helps to determine how environmental events can act as CS that elicit CR (such as tearing, hand shaking, headaches) that are characterized as withdrawal symptoms.

O'Brien (1976) conducted an experiment that suggests that the conditioning reflex of abstinence also helps to understand situations in which the individual consumes the substance in order to eliminate or relieve symptoms of abstinence. The environmental CS elicited by CS characteristic of abstinence symptoms, as a rule, it has aversive components. In this case, operant responses that result in the suspension of these symptoms may occur. Using substances that produce attenuation or suspension of symptoms (aversive stimulation) are classified as operating behaviors maintained by negative reinforcement. If such interoceptive stimulation (abstinence) is aversive, the behavior of using drugs will be maintained by reducing/eliminating the symptoms.

Final Considerations

This work presented possible functional interpretations of diagnostic criteria for substance dependence (i.e. substance use disorders), with the clarity that these are some possible alternatives, and that the interpretations provided here do not exhaust the subject. The elucidation of these elementary processes can be a first step towards the understanding of other more complex processes that involve interaction between some of the above-mentioned processes. We reiterate that these analyses do not exhaust the subject, but can contribute to other functional analyses of drug–behavior interactions.

It is also worth mentioning that the agglutination of criteria and the behavioral phenomena and processes suggested for their understanding has a didactic character. Therefore, the reader should not take a given situation as watertight. For example, variables that affect choices may be influenced by other phenomena such as reinstatement. In this case, the renewal of a stimulus such as CS can alter the subjective value of the drug. In any case, it is expected that the text has made clear the importance in recognizing analyses that involve respondent-operating interactions and/or that encompass biological factors.

Acknowledgments The authors thank Fundação de Amparo à Pesquisa do Estado de Goiás (FAPEG) for funding the research from which this product came (edital 06/2012, process n° 201210267001219).

References

Albuquerque, A. R., & Melo, R. M. (2005). Equivalência de estímulos: Conceito, implicações e possibilidades de aplicação. In J. Abreu-Rodrigues & M. R. Ribeiro (Eds.), *Análise do Comportamento: Pesquisa, teoria e aplicação* (pp. 245–264). Artmed.

Álvarez, A. M. A. (2007). Fatores de risco que favorecem a recaída do alcoolismo. *Jornal Brasileiro de Psiquiatria, 56*, 188–193.

American Psychiatric Association (APA). (2014). *Manual diagnóstico e estatístico de transtornos mentais* (5th ed.). Artmed.

Banaco, R. A., Zamignani, D. R., & Meyer, S. B. (2010). Função do comportamento e do DSM: Terapeutas analítico-comportamentais discutem a psicopatologia. In E. Z. Tourinho & S. V. Luna (Eds.), *Análise do Comportamento: Implicações históricas, conceituais e aplicadas* (pp. 175–191). Roca.

Beckert, M. E. (2005). Correspondência verbal/não verbal: Pesquisa básica e aplicações na clínica. In J. Abreu-Rodrigues & M. R. Ribeiro (Eds.), *Análise do Comportamento: Pesquisa, teoria e aplicação* (pp. 229–244). Artmed.

Benvenuti, M. F. (2004). Condicionamento respondente: Algumas implicações para o desenvolvimento de tolerância, síndrome de abstinência e overdose. In C. N. Abreu & H. J. Guilhardi (Eds.), *Terapia Comportamental e Cognitivo-comportamental: Práticas clínicas* (pp. 186–193). Roca.

Bouton, M. E. (2002). Context, ambiguity and unlearning: Sources of relapse after behavioral extinction. *Bilogical Psychiatry, 52*, 976–986. https://doi.org/10.1016/s0006-3223(02)01546-9

Cavalcante, S. N., & Tourinho, E. Z. (1998). Classificação e diagnóstico na clínica: Possibilidade de um modelo analítico-comportamental. *Psicologia: Teoria e Pesquisa, 14*, 139–147. Retrieved from http://periodicos.unb.br/index.php/revistaptp/article/view/17319

Czoty, P. W., McCabe, C., & Nader, M. A. (2005). Assessment of the relative reinforcing strength of cocaine in socially housed monkeys using a choice procedure. *The Journal of Phamracology and Experimental Therapeutics, 312*(1), 96–102. https://doi.org/10.1124/jpet.104.073411

DeGrandpre, R. J., & Bickel, W. (1993). Stimulus control and drug dependence. *The Psychological Record, 43*, 650–666. https://doi.org/10.1007/BF03395905

DeGrandpre, R. J., Bickel, W. K., & Higgins, S. T. (1992). Emergent equivalence relations between interoceptive (drug) and exteroceptive (visual) stimuli. *Journal of the Experimental Analysis of Behavior, 58*, 9–18. https://doi.org/10.1901/jeab.1992.58-9

Epstein, D. H., Preston, K. L., Stewart, J., & Saham, Y. (2006). Toward a model of drug relapse: An assessement of the validity of the reinstatement procedure. *Psychopharmacology, 189*, 1–16. https://doi.org/10.1007/s00213-006-0529-6

Herrnstein, R. J. (1970). On the law of effect. *Journal of the Experimental Analysis of Behavior, 13*, 243–266. https://doi.org/10.1901/jeab.1970.13-243

Heyman, G. M. (1996). Resolving the contradictions of addiction. *Behavioral and Brain Sciences, 19*(4), 561–610. https://doi.org/10.1017/S0140525X00042990

Hineline, P. N. (2003). When we speak of intentions. In: Em K. A. Lattal & P. N. Chase (Orgs.), *Behavior theory and philosophy* (pp. 203–222). Kluwer Acadmic/Plenum Publishers.

Madden, G. J., Petry, N. M., Badger, G. J., & Bickel, W. K. (1997). Impulsive and self-control choices in opioid-dependent patients and non-drug-using control participants: Drug and monetary rewards. *Experimental and Clinical Psychoparmacology, 5*(3), 256–262. https://doi.org/10.1037/1064-1297.5.3.256

Meyer, J. S., & Quenzer, L. F. (2005). *Psychopharmacology: Drugs, the brain, and behavior*. Sinauer Associates, Inc..

Moore, J. (2008). *Conceptual foundations of radical behaviorism*. Sloan Publishing.

O'Brien, C. P. (1976). Experimental analysis of conditioning factors in human narcotic addiction. *Pharmacological Reviews, 27*, 533–543. Retrieved from http://pharmrev.aspetjournals.org/content/27/4/533.long

World Health Organization (WHO). (1993). *Classificação de Transtornos mentais e de comportamento da CID-10* (10th ed.). Artmed.

Pierce, W. D., & Cheney, C. D. (2008). *Behavior analysis and learning* (4th ed.). Psychology Press.

Rescorla, R. A. (1988). Pavlovian conditioning: It's not what you think it is. *American Psychologist, 43*, 151–160. https://doi.org/10.1037/0003-066X.43.3.151

Siegel, S. (1976). Morphine analgesic tolerance: Its situation specificity supports a pavlovian conditioning model. *Science, 193*, 323–325. https://doi.org/10.1126/science.935870

Skinner, B. F. (2006). *Sobre o behaviorismo*. Cultrix. (Original work published in 1974).

Souza, A. C. A. (2003). Transtorno de personalidade borderline sob uma perspectiva analítico-funcional. *Revista Brasileira de Terapia Comportamental e Cognitiva, 5*, 121–137. https://doi.org/10.31505/rbtcc.v5i2.76

Todorov, J. C. & Hanna, E. S. (2005). Quantificação de escolhas e preferências. In: Em J. Abreu-Rodrigues & M. R. Ribeiro (Orgs.), *Análise do Comportamento. Pesquisa, teoria e aplicação* (pp. 159–174). Artmed.

Tucker, J. A. (2004). Contributions of behavioral economics for understanding and resolving substance use disorders. *NAD Publications, 44*, 35–48.

Chapter 4
Basic Concepts of Behavioral Pharmacology

Fábio Leyser Gonçalves

Introduction

The relationship between human beings and various psychoactive substances has been the object of curiosity and study throughout much of history. Magic elixirs, substances used in rituals or recreational drugs such as alcohol have been used by several people throughout history (Escohotado, 1995). The phenomenon of substance dependence, although it began to be systematically described in the mid-nineteenth century (Hancock & McKim, 2012) had a great advance with the development of research methods developed by the Experimental Analysis of Behavior (EAB). It was during the 1950s that the use of these methods, together with the methods of pharmacology, gave rise to behavioral pharmacology (Barrett, 2002, 2006, 2008; Hancock & McKim, 2012). The birth of this new area of knowledge made it possible to study the interaction between the effect of substances, such as drugs of abuse and the effects of environmental contingencies. This chapter intends to present some of the concepts and methods, besides the contributions of behavioral pharmacology to the understanding of the dependence phenomenon.

Behavioral pharmacology arises mainly from the work of Peter Dews, Roger T. Kelleher, and William H. Morse in the Harvard Medical School Laboratory of Psychology throughout the 1950s (Barrett, 2002). At the same time, pharmacologists and neurophysiologists were beginning to change the conception that communication in the central nervous system was chemical, and not electrical, as was thought until then (Valenstein, 2002). Psychiatric drugs such as the antipsychotic chlorpromazine and the benzodiazepine anxiolytics came on the market and began

F. L. Gonçalves (✉)
Universidade Estadual Paulista (UNESP), Bauru, SP, Brazil

Programa de Pós-graduação em Neurociências e Comportamento, Instituto de Psicologia da Universidade de São Paulo (USP), São Paulo, SP, Brazil
e-mail: fabio.leyser@unesp.br

S. M. Oliani et al. (eds.), *Behavior Analysis and Substance Dependence*,
https://doi.org/10.1007/978-3-030-75961-2_4

to be used clinically (Barrett, 2002). The combination of all these factors made behavioral pharmacology an extremely fertile area, contributing both to the advancement of what is now called neuroscience and to the improvement and refinement of methods and concepts of Experimental Analysis of Behavior (Branch, 2006).

Basic Concepts of Pharmacology

In order for a substance to have an effect on an organism, the first step is to be absorbed by the organism through one of the routes of administration. Each route of administration corresponds to the place or tissue where the drug will be received. When one thinks of medicines, the most remembered are the oral route and the parenteral routes (injections). Some medications are well absorbed by the digestive system and therefore the oral route seems a good option. Others need quick action and then administration directly into the circulatory system (intravenous route) may be more indicated. Another route associated with rapid absorption, widely used by dependents, is the pulmonary route, in which the substance is transformed into its gaseous state and enters the bloodstream through the mechanism of gas exchange associated with breathing, as in the case of tobacco, in the form of cigarettes. The various routes of administration are related to different absorption processes, i.e., the process of passage of the substance from the tissue into the bloodstream. The absorption is affected both by the chemical properties of the substance and by the properties of the tissues in which it is administered.

Once the substance enters the bloodstream, it will be distributed throughout the body. Once again, its physical-chemical properties will determine in which organs this substance will act. While liposoluble substances (i.e., those that dissolve in fat) will tend to remain in organs and fat tissue, water-soluble substances will spread more easily into the bloodstream. Also, depending on the size of the molecule, it may be confined to blood vessels and not reach some organs. This is the case of our central nervous system (CNS) where the blood vessels are covered by other cells and only smaller molecules can penetrate this organ (this protection is called the blood-brain barrier). After distribution, it is necessary to understand that a good part of these substances will be metabolized and/or excreted. While metabolization concerns the chemical transformation of the substance into smaller or easier to eliminate molecules (the main organ involved in this process is the liver), excretion concerns the elimination of the substance or its metabolites (products of metabolization) through feces, urine, or even through the pores on the skin, as is the case with volatile substances such as alcohol.

Neurotransmission

In the case of substances that affect behavior, a limiting step is the arrival to the CNS, crossing the blood-brain barrier. Although many of the drugs that act in the CNS also have some peripheral activity, the main effect on behavior is through central action. To understand how they work, it is fundamental to understand the functioning of the neurotransmission process. The CNS is formed by billions of cells, the *neurons* being the best known. Neurons are cells that function as central communication centers, all the activity of the CNS could be summarized, in a very simplified way, to the mediation between the activities of neurons that are in contact with the environment and the neurons that guide activities of effector organs. This mediation is done through communication between neurons. This communication becomes quite complex, since one neuron can communicate with several others, just as it can receive communication from several others. Initially, the main hypothesis is that this communication was made through the electrical transmission of nervous impulses, but as seen above, today it is widely known that most communication takes place through chemical substances, called *neurotransmitters* (Valenstein, 2002). These substances, synthesized inside the neurons, are released, and will connect to specific receptors in other neurons (and, even, in the neuron that released it). The neuron that releases the neurotransmitter is called *pre-synaptic*, the one that receives is called *postsynaptic,* and the place where there is proximity between the neurons is called *synapse*. Most drugs that act on the CNS will somehow affect the neurotransmission process. There are substances that facilitate the process of release of the neurotransmitter, increasing its availability in the synaptic cleft and therefore its effect. There are substances that bind directly to the receptors. Those that produce a similar effect to the neurotransmitter are given the name *agonists*, those that bind but do not produce *an* effect, preventing the neurotransmitter from acting, are called *antagonists*. Other drugs can increase the availability of the neurotransmitter preventing them from being recaptured by the neuron through the inhibition of the process known as reuptake. Other processes may be affected, but are outside the scope of this chapter.

Some Methods of Behavioral Pharmacology

The first studies in the area of behavioral pharmacology sought to investigate the effect of drugs such as pentobarbital (commonly referred to as a sedative) or d-amphetamine (a psychomotor stimulant) on the performance of pigeons in different reinforcement schedules (Barrett, 2002, 2006; Dews, 1955, 1958). With these experiments, Dews demonstrated that the depressant or stimulant effect depends on the reinforcement schedule used. While pentobarbital reduced responses in a Fixed Interval schedule (FI, where the reinforcement becomes available after a time interval), it increased the response rate in a Fixed Ratio schedule (FR, where the reinforcement availability depends on the number of responses), d-amphetamine produced the opposite effect, decreasing the rate in FR and increasing in FI. This effect became known as rate dependence, since, depending on the initial response rate, the effect is different (Barrett, 2002; Dews, 1955, 1958; Quisenberry et al., 2016). This discovery has several implications for both pharmacology and EAB. If, on the one hand, pharmacologists are faced with the fact that in order to study an effect of a substance on behavior, it is necessary to know more about the relations of the organism with its environment, on the other hand, behavior analysts have to consider that drug interferences, or other interferences on the organism, can alter the relationship that the organism establishes with the environment (Branch, 2006).

Still in this early period of behavioral pharmacology, some studies began to demonstrate that laboratory animals issued operant responses whose consequence was the administration of a series of drugs related to abuse and addiction, such as morphine (Thompson & Schuster, 1964), for example. The discovery that drugs such as morphine, cocaine, and alcohol could act as reinforcers in animal experiments led to a great leap in the knowledge of the dependence phenomenon (Hancock & McKim, 2012). Initially seen as an exclusively human phenomenon, the development of self-administration procedures for drugs in nonhuman animals allowed the advancement of knowledge of brain regions, neurotransmitters and receptors involved in this process. Furthermore, this laboratory demonstration helps us reject the idea that substance dependence is an eminently moral problem. From a behavioral point of view, self-administration procedures have also allowed the evolution and refinement of concepts and methods for understanding the dependence phenomenon. A basic implication is that these substances can function as positive reinforcement stimuli and, therefore, behaviors related to self-administration can be understood from the operant paradigm (Gonçalves & Silva, 1999; Silva et al., 2001). The basic procedure corresponds to what is usually called a continuous reinforcement schedule (CRF), which simply indicates that each emitted response is followed by intravenous or oral administration of a dose of the drug under study. A peculiarity of this procedure is that, since the effect of the drugs studied has a varied duration, the simple comparison of the response rate does not inform about its reinforcement value, not least because some sedative substances, for example, may prevent the emission of the response (Panlilio & Goldberg, 2007). Other reinforcement schedules have also been used as fixed and variable ratio and fixed and variable interval schedules. A particularly common schedule is progressive ratio. In this schedule, the number of responses required to release the drug dose is gradually increased until the animal stops responding. This type of procedure allows us to evaluate the effectiveness of the drug as a reinforcer by comparing the maximum ratio of responses emitted (Panlilio & Goldberg, 2007).

Second-order schedules have also proved quite useful. In this type of schedule the response is reinforced by presenting a conditioned reinforcer stimulus according to a reinforcement schedule, and eventually, following a second schedule, this stimulus is followed by the presentation of the drug. This schedule has a great advantage by reducing the dose of the drug administered, and also by simulating search behaviors for the drug, which can be reinforced by other stimuli such as the behavior of asking for money. In addition, it demonstrates the possibility of forming conditioned reinforcers, having the administration/effect of the drug as a primary reinforcer (Hancock & McKim, 2012). This principle is also used in other procedures such as conditioned place preference (Gonçalves & Silva, 1999). The conditioned place preference procedure consists of placing the animal in a box divided into two sides, identified by different visual and tactile patterns, and assessing whether it is preferred (stays longer) on either side. Afterwards, the animal receives the drug administration and is confined to the less preferred side. The final evaluation is the same as the initial one and, if there is more preference on the side paired with the drug, it is understood that the drug has a potential for abuse, because it can act as a reinforcement stimulus (Gonçalves & Silva, 1999).

From the study of the reinforcement function, more complex experiments began to be performed, using concurrent schedules. The proposition of the Matching Law by Richard Hernstein (Garcia-Mijares & Silva, 1999; Herrnstein, 1961) allowed, from this type of arrangement, to analyze the distribution of behavior by several sources of reinforcement. Hernstein's proposal is that the distribution of an organism's activities is proportional to the distribution of reinforcement, that is, where there is more reinforcement, more behavior is emitted, where there is less reinforcement, less behavior is emitted, or, in other words, less is chosen. In behavioral pharmacology, this type of study allowed the analysis of competition between drugs and other reinforcers. This allows us to evaluate that, for example, the same drug can control different response rates depending on alternative reinforcers, indicating that the reinforcer value of drugs (as well as other stimuli) is always relative to other present reinforcers (Gonçalves & Silva, 1999; Silva et al., 2001). Thus, if a drug is available in an environment as one of several options, the reinforcer value will be lower than if there is only one other option. These research raise the question that, besides identifying the neurobiological, or even behavioral function of a drug, it is necessary to consider the context in which the relationship is established.

Some behavioral theories related to drug addiction are based on the relativity of the value of reinforcement and can be called choice-based theories (Garcia-Mijares & Silva, 2006; Heyman, 2018). It is important to note that the term "choice," as understood here, is not related to free will or a supposed decision-making process, but to the distribution of behaviors among various alternatives (Garcia-Mijares & Silva, 1999). An analysis of the distribution of drug-related behaviors has also benefited from a frontier field known as behavioral economics (Bickel et al., 1993). In particular, the use of demand curves, i.e., the variation of behavior as a function of response cost (or price, in economic language), helps to understand, for example, the effect of public policies such as surcharges on the consumption of alcohol, tobacco, or even soft drinks and food (Epstein et al., 2012).

Understanding the Relationship Between Drugs and Behavior

As already mentioned, the studies in behavioral pharmacology also require extended analyses, both from a pharmacological and behavioral point of view. While the chemical structure of drugs and their neurobiological effects are not sufficient to predict their behavioral effects, the contingencies alone do not allow the prediction of behavior, without considering the effects of the drug. Thus, behavioral

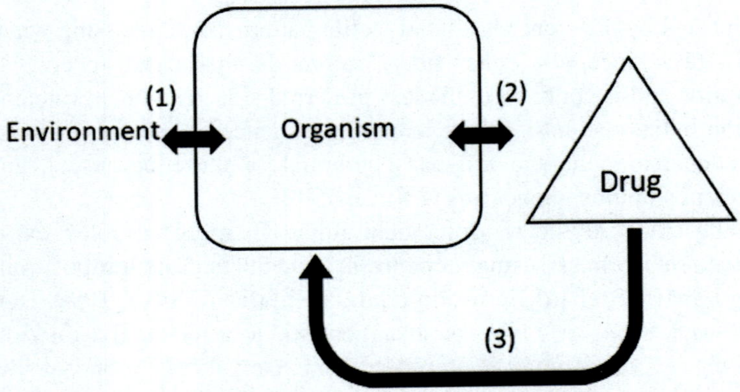

Fig. 4.1 Proposal of integration of the relations among drugs, organism, and environment

pharmacology brings an integrated point of view, in which it is necessary to take into account the environment in interaction with the alterations of the organism caused by the drug. Figure 4.1 presents a proposal of how it is possible to integrate this knowledge. One can understand behavior as the interaction between an organism and the environment, represented by the bidirectional arrow on the left (identified by 1). A first extension brought by behavioral pharmacology is that drugs, as part of this environment, can interact with the organism (2), exerting several stimulus functions such as reinforcement stimulus, conditioned stimulus, and discriminatory stimulus (Leonardi & Bravin, 2012). Finally, it is necessary to consider that the effect of the drug on the organism, represented by the lower arrow (3), modifies the functioning of that organism, also altering the way it interacts with the environment in general, or with the drug itself, in particular. This last point, although not obvious, was already present in the first studies of the effect of drugs on reinforcement schedules (Dews, 1955, 1958), since the same organism behaves differently under the same contingency when under different drugs. Thus, beyond an analysis of the stimulus functions, it is necessary to understand how the changes made by the drug in the organism alter its responses to the environment.

Behavioral Pharmacology of Some Addiction-Related Drugs

This section presents some information on the main substances related to dependence in Brazil. The information is based on the book *Drugs and Behavior: An Introduction to Behavioral Pharmacology* (Hancock & McKim, 2012), but it is considered useful to present this information in a summarized and prominent way, to facilitate the reader's access to the area. Information from other sources will be indicated throughout the text.

Ethanol

Ethanol, better known as alcohol, is one of the most widely used psychoactive substances in the world. It is normally administered orally and is absorbed by the digestive system and distributed equally throughout the body. Most alcohol is metabolized by the liver, but it is important to note that during the process an intermediate metabolite with toxic effects (called acetaldehyde) is produced, which helps to understand some effects of acute intoxication. Disulfiram is a substance that inhibits the enzyme responsible for metabolizing acetaldehyde, and has been widely used in the treatment of alcohol dependence, as it leads to a feeling of unease due to the accumulation of acetaldehyde. Alcohol acts on several neurotransmitter systems, but the main ones are the gabaergic systems (which involves gamma-aminobutyric acid, GABA) and glutamatergic (which involves the neurotransmitter glutamate). While GABA is the main inhibitory neurotransmitter, glutamate is the main excitatory neurotransmitter. The actions on these neurotransmitters are, in a way, complementary, since there is an increase in the gabaergic system and a decrease in the glutamate system's effect, causing, in general, a decrease in activity in the CNS, which can lead to coma or respiratory arrest, when ingested in excessive doses.

The general effects of alcohol are well known, but it is important to highlight some. The body develops tolerance to alcohol, i.e., decrease of its effect over the time of exposure. One of the mechanisms of tolerance is the increased production of enzymes responsible for metabolism, but there is evidence of behavioral mechanisms, also involved. Abstinence from alcohol is a condition that requires care and can be characterized by milder symptoms such as agitation and tremors, in an initial phase, and more severe symptoms such as hallucinations (usually with small animals or insects) and convulsions. The use of medication to control the symptoms may be necessary.

Ethanol can act as a discriminative stimulus and can therefore guide specific behaviors. Furthermore, it is self-administered by animals, acting as a positive reinforcer stimulus. With respect to interference in other behaviors, in low doses it increases the response rate in schedules such as FR and FI. In high doses, the response rate usually drops, evidencing its sedative effect. Another important effect is the increase in the frequency of punished behaviors and the decrease in the frequency of negatively reinforced behaviors (Galizio et al., 1984), changes that are usually called disinhibition and may be related to the increase in aggressive behavior, for example.

Tobacco

Tobacco originated in the American continent and its main component is nicotine. It is self-generated mainly by inhaling smoke from combustion as in cigarettes and cigars. This mode of administration is very efficient because the absorption occurs quickly through the lung, leading to a rapid increase in the amount of nicotine in the blood. Other modes of administration, such as transdermal adhesives, lead to slower and longer absorption, which has been used in the treatment of addiction. In addition, nicotine is also absorbed through the mucosa of the mouth, even in people who do not "bring in" smoke. Nicotine is metabolized by the liver and excreted by feces and by urine. The main neurotransmitter involved in the effect of nicotine is acetylcholine, a neurotransmitter involved in learning processes and the reinforcement process, for example. This is a neurotransmitter present in the CNS, and also in the peripheral nervous system, where, among other functions, it is present in the junction between nerves and skeletal muscles. When administered in low doses, nicotine works as an acetylcholine receptor agonist (called nicotinic receptors), exerting a stimulating effect. On the other hand, in high doses, these receptors become blocked, leading to an increase in the number of receptors in the long term.

In general, nicotine has vasoconstrictor effects, an appetite suppressing effect and an increased alert state. It also has some effect similar to antidepressants. Some effects develop rapid tolerance, such as the effects of nausea. Nicotine is self-administered by animals, presenting a reinforcer function. Moreover, nicotine seems to be quite efficient in the formation of conditioned reinforcers that play as important a role as nicotine in the process of maintaining self-administration. Nicotine can also act as a discriminative stimulus. In high doses, nicotine also acts as a punitive stimulus.

With respect to other behaviors, nicotine shows a rate-dependent effect on behaviors controlled by positive or negative reinforcement schedules, similar to what occurs with stimulants such as amphetamines. However, it hinders performance in DRL (*differential reinforcement of low* rates), a schedule where the response is reinforced after a period without response emission. This data appears after chronic administration and can be understood as a difficulty to stop emitting behaviors. Nicotine also facilitates the acquisition of delayed conditional discrimination in animals, in addition to other procedures that seek to evaluate cognitive functions such as memory[1].

Cocaine

Cocaine is extracted from the leaves of a bush called *coca* (*Erythroxylum coca*), native to the high regions of South America. The coca leaves were used by pre-Columbian people and are used in their chewed form until today. The active substance, cocaine, was only isolated in the middle of the nineteenth century and banned in the early twentieth century. Cocaine has a stimulating effect and is

[1] The term memory is used in its common sense, as the scope of the chapter does not allow a more detailed discussion of the term.

usually administered via the nose, where it is absorbed by the mucous membrane, intravenously or by inhalation of smoke, in the form of crack. Crack is nothing more than crystal cocaine, after association with sodium bicarbonate. The main difference between cocaine powder and crack is that the inhalation of smoke promotes a faster absorption, leading to a rapid increase of the drug in the bloodstream, making its effect more immediate, but more ephemeral. The excretion of cocaine occurs quickly, taking between 45 and 75 min to eliminate half of the dose (concept known as half-life). Cocaine acts mainly by inhibiting the reuptake of three neurotransmitters: dopamine; noradrenaline, and serotonin. Dopamine is the main neurotransmitter associated with the reinforcement process and motor control. Noradrenaline is the main neurotransmitter involved in the processes of attention, wakefulness and sleep, and eating behavior. Serotonin is a neurotransmitter that acts on aggressive behavior, mood, and appetite, for example.

The main peripheral effects of cocaine are an increase in heart rate and blood pressure, in addition to its local anesthetic effect. Cocaine also increases waking hours and promotes a sense of well-being, increased energy, clarity of thought, a sense of capacity, and power. It also has an anorexic effect, inhibiting the appetite and can lead to long-term malnutrition. In high doses it can lead to a transient psychotic state, with auditory and visual hallucinations and paranoid delusions.

Although drugs such as cocaine are classified as psychomotor stimulants, it is important to note that their effect is rate-dependent, as demonstrated by Dews' (1958) experiments mentioned above. The main functions altered by cocaine are related to the reinforcement process. Cocaine, like other stimulants, functions as a reinforcer, and its reinforcer value depends on the immediacy of the effect. This behavioral principle helps us to understand some of the differences between cocaine administered by different routes, such as crack and cocaine powder. Cocaine is self-administered in animals and its pattern of self-administration is similar to that of humans, intercalating more intense periods and periods of abstinence.

Final Considerations

In this chapter, the area of behavioral pharmacology was briefly presented. It arises from the interaction between pharmacology and Experimental Analysis of Behavior. When two areas meet, they both change and produce a new area. It is hoped that this chapter will serve as an invitation for some people to venture into this (not so) new field of study and, above all, will help to understand that the analysis of phenomena involving drugs and behavior requires a broad understanding and the contribution of multiple disciplines.

References

Barrett, J. E. (2002). The emergence of behavioral pharmacology. *Molecular Interventions, 2*(8), 470–475. https://doi.org/10.1124/mi.2.8.470

Barrett, J. E. (2006). Behavioral determinants of drug action: The contributions of Peter B. Dews. *Journal of the Experimental Analysis of Behavior, 86*(3), 359–370. https://doi.org/10.1901/jeab.2006.23-06

Barrett, J. E. (2008). Pioneer in Behavioral pharmacology: A tribute to Joseph V. Brady. *Journal of the Experimental Analysis of Behavior, 90*(3), 405–415. https://doi.org/10.1901/jeab.2008.90-405

Bickel, W. K., DeGrandpre, R. J., & Higgins, S. T. (1993). Behavioral economics: A novel experimental approach to the study of drug dependence. *Drug and Alcohol Dependence, 33*(2), 173–192. https://doi.org/10.1016/0376-8716(93)90059-Y

Branch, M. N. (2006). How research in behavioral pharmacology informs behavioral science. *Journal of the Experimental Analysis of Behavior, 85*(3), 407–423. https://doi.org/10.1901/jeab.2006.130-04

Dews, P. B. (1955). Studies on behavior. I. Differential sensitivity to pentobarbital of pecking performance in pigeons depending on the schedule of reward. *The Journal of Pharmacology and Experimental Therapeutics, 113*(4), 393–401.

Dews, P. B. (1958). Studies on behavior. IV. Stimulant actions of methamphetamine. *The Journal of Pharmacology and Experimental Therapeutics, 122*(1), 137–147.

Epstein, L. H., Jankowiak, N., Nederkoorn, C., Raynor, H. A., French, S. A., & Finkelstein, E. (2012). Experimental research on the relation between food price changes and food-purchasing patterns: A targeted review. *American Journal of Clinical Nutrition, 95*(4), 789–809. https://doi.org/10.3945/ajcn.111.024380

Escohotado, A. (1995). *Drogas, Las - de Los Origenes a la Prohibic*. Alianza Editorial.

Galizio, M., Smaltz, S. C., & Spencer, B. A. (1984). Effects of ethanol and naltrexone on free-operant avoidance behavior in rats. *Pharmacology Biochemistry and Behavior, 21*(3). https://doi.org/10.1016/S0091-3057(84)80105-7

Garcia-Mijares, M., & Silva, M. T. A. (1999). Introdução à teoria da igualação. In R. R. Kerbauy & R. C. Wielenska (Eds.), *Sobre comportamento e cognição vol. 4* (pp. 40–53). ARBytes.

Garcia-Mijares, M., & Silva, M. T. A. (2006). Dependência de drogas. *Psicologia USP, 17*(4), 213–240. https://doi.org/10.1590/S0103-65642006000400012

Gonçalves, F. L., & Silva, M. T. A. (1999). Mecanismos fisiológicos do reforço. In R. R. Kerbauy & R. C. Wielenska (Eds.), *Sobre comportamento e cognição vol. 4* (pp. 272–281). ARBytes.

Hancock, S., & McKim, W. A. (2012). *Drugs and behavior: An introduction to behavioral pharmacology*. Pearson Education.

Herrnstein, R. J. (1961). Relative and absolute strength of response as a function of frequency of reinforcement. *Journal of the Experimental Analysis of Behavior, 4*(3), 267–272. https://doi.org/10.1901/jeab.1961.4-267

Heyman, G. M. (2018). Deriving addiction: An analysis based on three elementary features of making choices. In H. Pickard & S. H. Ahmed (Eds.), *The Routledge handbook of philosophy and science of addiction* (pp. 23–33). Routledge. https://geneheyman.com/wordpress/wp-content/uploads/2013/06/DerivingAddiction2018gmh.pdf

Leonardi, J. L., & Bravin, A. A. (2012). Uma introdução à farmacologia comportamental. *Interação Em Psicologia, 15*(2), 193–201. https://doi.org/10.5380/psi.v15i2.20514

Panlilio, L. V., & Goldberg, S. R. (2007). Self-administration of drugs in animals and humans as a model and an investigative tool. *Addiction, 102*(12), 1863–1870. https://doi.org/10.1111/j.1360-0443.2007.02011.x

Quisenberry, A., Snider, S., & Bickel, W. (2016). The return of rate dependence. *Behavior Analysis: Research and Practice, 16*(4), 215–220. https://doi.org/10.1037/bar0000042

Silva, M. T. A., Guerra, L. G., Gonçalves, F. L., & Garcia-Mijares, M. (2001). Análise funcional da dependência de drogas. In H. J. Guilhardi, M. B. B. P. Madi, P. P. Queiroz, & M. C. Scoz (Eds.), *Sobre comportamento e cognição Vol. 7: expondo a variabilidade* (pp. 422–442). ESETec.

Thompson, T., & Schuster, C. R. (1964). Morphine self-administration, food-reinforced, and avoidance behaviors in rhesus monkeys. *Psychopharmacologia, 5*(2), 87–94. https://doi.org/10.1007/BF00413045

Valenstein, E. S. (2002). The discovery of chemical neurotransmitters. *Brain and Cognition, 49*(1), 73–95. https://doi.org/10.1006/brcg.2001.1487

Chapter 5
Functional Analysis of Substance Use and Dependence

Richard Alecsander Reichert, Eduardo José Legal, Simone Martin Oliani, and Denis Roberto Zamignani

Introduction

When using scientific methods for the analysis of human subjects, one must start from the assumption that behavior is ordered and determined (Skinner, 1953/2003). This perspective assumes that the actions of individuals result from processes of interaction that, once described, make it possible the prediction and, to a certain extent, the influence over behavior. Circumstances beyond the individual are, therefore, relevant—they can and must be identified, described, and managed in order to promote changes in actions. In other words, behaviors are understood as relationships between the subject (organism) and the environment in which it is inserted, and not just as actions devoid of history (Abib, 2004)..

Behavior analysis considers that behavior is multidetermined, the result of multiple functional relationships, in a process of reciprocal determination between environmental events and the actions of individuals. Behavioral processes can be

R. A. Reichert (✉)
Department of Psychobiology, Universidade Federal de São Paulo (UNIFESP), São Paulo, SP, Brazil
e-mail: reichert@unifesp.br

E. J. Legal
Universidade do Vale do Itajaí (UNIVALI), Itajaí, SC, Brazil
e-mail: edujlegal@univali.br

S. M. Oliani
Centro Integrado de Neuropsiquiatria e Psicologia Comportamental (CINP), Londrina, PR, Brazil
e-mail: simoneoliani@portalcinp.com.br

D. R. Zamignani
Paradigma – Centro de Ciências e Tecnologia do Comportamento, São Paulo, SP, Brazil
e-mail: denis@paradigmaac.com.br

S. M. Oliani et al. (eds.), *Behavior Analysis and Substance Dependence*,
https://doi.org/10.1007/978-3-030-75961-2_5

classified into two categories: (a) respondents or reflexes—involving an organism–environment relationship in which a response is elicited by a change in part of the environment (stimulus); and (b) operants—relationships in which one's actions operate on the environment, producing changes in that environment (called consequences) that, in turn, modify the likelihood that actions of the same class will occur on similar occasions, in a bidirectional process (Borloti et al., 2015; Costa & Marinho, 2002; Moreira & Medeiros, 2018; Nery & Fonseca, 2018)..

Behavior analysis therefore studies the relationships that select and maintain behaviors that contribute to one's adaptation and survival in the context. The concept of three-term contingency seeks to explain these relationships, conceptually representing the factors responsible for the occurrence of certain response classes or not. Therefore, the relationship between (a) antecedent context, situations which are present at the time of emitting the response, which, depending on the produced consequence, set the occasion for the emission of a behavior, is analyzed; (b) response (action) performed by the organism; and (c) consequent stimuli, which occur after the response is issued and alter the future likelihood of its occurrence in similar contexts (Lombard-Platet et al., 2015) (Table 5.1).

Behaviors are multidetermined, that is, there are a lot of relationships and factors involved that influence them. The causal model of behavior analysis is called the Consequence Selection Model, according to which any behavior is the result of the history of interaction between phylogenetic, ontogenetic, and cultural variables (Skinner, 1987). Substance use, for example, is determined by a complex interplay of biogenetic and psychosocial factors. To understand these patterns of behavior, it is necessary to analyze their pragmatic relevance, that is, the role they play in the lives of individuals. Discovering the functionality of the behavior enables its prediction and control, given that the variables that influence it can be managed (Borloti et al., 2015; Garcia-Mijares & Silva, 2006; Silva, 2007; Silva et al., 2001; Skinner, 2003; Vandenberghe, 2002).

When talking about problems related to substance use, the identification and management of the variables involved become essential for formulating the prevention and treatment interventions. To obtain this information, Silvares and Gongora (1998) suggest a functional analysis of behavior. And the objective of this chapter is to describe functional analysis as a central tool in the assessment and formulation of clinical cases related to substance use and dependence.

Table 5.1 Concepts of the three-term contingency

Sd (Discriminative stimulus)	R (Response)	Sc (Consequent stimuli)
Stimuli present at the time of emitting the response; situations in which an action occurs (context). They are also called "antecedent stimuli."	Action taken by the organism.	Stimuli produced by the response, which alter the probability of their emission in similar contexts (Sds).

Source: Lombard-Platet et al. (2015)

Functional Analysis of Behavior and Formulation of Clinical Cases

Functional analysis plays a key role in the formulation of clinical cases and behavioral therapy (Haynes & O'Brien, 1990; Nery & Fonseca, 2018). This process assesses the environmental aspects and the role that the behavior plays in certain contexts, or rather, the relationship of interdependency maintained between the behavior and the environmental variables. More directly, functional analysis is a way of identifying antecedents and consequences of behavior (Matos, 1999).

To perform a functional analysis is then to identify the function, that is, the survival value of a given behavior. For that, an analysis must always be contextualized—it is about answering what the function of a given response is for an individual, or what is the functional relationship between behavior and its immediate and long-term effects (Cruz, 2006; Neno, 2003). Regarding the drug use, this process makes it possible to identify the circumstances (antecedent stimuli) associated with substance use (response class) and the consequences (consequent stimuli) produced by these responses (Borloti et al., 2015; Spadin et al., 2018), as shown in Table 5.2.

Psychoactive substances can produce positive and/or negative reinforcers, increasing the probability of use due to the consequences produced by their consumption, or later leading to the search for treatment due to the long-term aversive effects, as exemplified in Table 5.2. Therefore, it is important to identify the reinforcing (and punishing) elements in the evaluation process. Thus, it is possible to understand what the relationship with the substance is, what the predisposing and maintaining factors of use are (peer pressure, interpersonal

Table 5.2 Model of Applied Functional Analysis

Sd (Discriminative stimulus)	R (Response)	Sc (Consequent stimuli)
Frequently visiting friends who have the habit of using cocaine.	Giving in to peer pressure and accepting using cocaine with friends.	Getting rid of peer pressure and/or creating sensations of Well-being, grandiosity, etc.
Going through a series of recurring personal issues that produce feelings of discomfort, stress, or anxiety.	Using alcohol and/or smoking cigarettes (tobacco).	Sensation of relaxation, getting away from problems, reducing anxiety, etc.
Being in a music festival.	Using ecstasy.	Disinhibition, euphoria, feeling closer to people.

Legend: Notice that the identification of the consequent stimulus (Sc) allows inferring the function of the response. In the first example, drug use has a dual function: (1) it is an escape-avoidance response (getting rid of or avoiding pressure from friends) and (2) it provides access to endogenous reinforcers (feelings associated with well-being, greatness). In the second example, on the other hand, the behavior of using the drug has also an escape-avoidance role, but of the deprived feelings of discomfort. Finally, the third example illustrates a relationship in which drug use produces negative (disinhibition) and positive (euphoria, sense of closeness) reinforcers, both of which are private. Eventually, an analysis of long-term consequences could indicate punishment, due to abuse and possible social, occupational, and economic losses conflicts) and what the consequences of this behavior are (social approval, reduction of symptoms of stress, or anxiety). The 5W's (Fig. 5.1), being when, where, why, with, and what happened, are questions to be answered in this process. Thus, it becomes possible to develop a plan to modify the contingencies responsible for the installation and the maintenance of drug use and dependence and to then teach new behaviors to replace the ones that result in personal and social losses (Spadin et al., 2018).

For the formulation of the case and in order to understand the relationship one establishes with the substance, or the function that it plays in one's life, some questions are essential, such as: When and how was the last time you used substances? Where were you? What were you doing? What happened before (in which situation and what did you feel)? What were the positive and negative consequences of the use? Do you use it alone or with other people? Who do you use it with? Where is the substance acquired? In addition, it is important to know one's family dynamics and professional and financial situation and ascertain the existence of health problems and psychiatric comorbidities. These questions are important to identify the variables associated with the installation and maintenance of use (such as social circumstances, for example) and, therefore, plan more effective interventions, such as the development of assertive coping skills (Spadin et al., 2018).

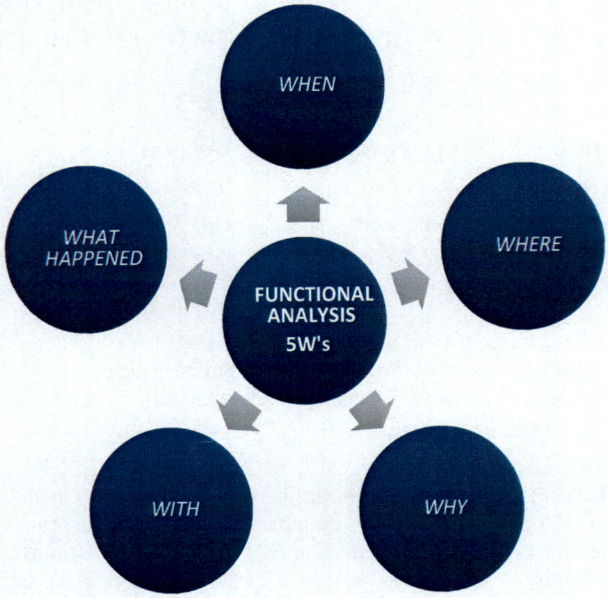

Fig. 5.1 5 W's. (Source: Based on Spadin et al., 2018)

Example of Cases[1]

V started using drugs as a teenager, at approximately 15 years old. The first use occurred at the birthday party of one of his schoolmates, where several people who were part of his daily life were present. At first, *V* declined the invitation. However, after several requests and under peer pressure, he could not resist and consumed a type of alcoholic beverage. Weeks after that, *V* went to someone's house to do school work. In that situation, they again asked him to drink alcohol. To avoid the same pressure and the embarrassing situation in which he found himself during the previous social event, he soon accepted the proposal and consumed the substance. Such behavior became frequent for *V* in several similar contexts, which illustrates the concept of social reinforcers (in this case, contingencies of negative social reinforcement—the behavior was issued with the function of eliminating aversive social consequences, such as embarrassment by colleagues). In contingencies involving social reinforcers, the behavior is maintained by social contingencies—more specifically, its effect on the behavior of other individuals—such as acceptance, affection, appreciation, rejection, intimidation, or approval from other people or groups. In addition to social reinforcement, the behavior of drinking alcohol has acquired other functions such as relaxing him, favoring social interactions, and creating an initial excitement (euphoria) (Table 5.3).

W is weekly invited to attend electronic music parties, contexts where the use of stimulating substances is tolerated, and often reinforced. To stay awake throughout the party and to facilitate interpersonal interaction, *W* makes use of ecstasy, a drug that provides disinhibition, euphoria, and a feeling of being close to other people (Table 5.4).

So far, the variables present in the current context have been mentioned, from immediate variables that serve as a "trigger" for using the drug to current variables that maintain the user's behavior based on contingencies of positive or negative reinforcement. However, when analyzing the clinical case, it is also important to identify what are called distal variables. Those variables that, throughout the individual's life history, contributed to the development of patterns of problematic behaviors and also of "healthy" behaviors that will favor the process of change.

Table 5.3 Functional analysis of V's alcohol-consuming behavior

Antecedents	Responses	Consequences	Processes	Effects
Birthday party	Consuming alcohol	Peer approval and acceptance	Positive reinforcement	Initial euphoria
Presence of friends				Relaxation
Peer pressure				

[1]The cases have been analyzed from the formulation model of Nery and Fonseca (2018)

Table 5.4 Functional analysis of the ecstasy use behavior in the context of electronic music parties by W

Antecedents	Responses	Consequences	Processes	Effects
Electronic music environment	Using ecstasy	Disinhibition	Negative reinforcement	Relaxation
Presence of friends who make use of the substances		Proximity to other people	Positive reinforcement	Excitement
Presence of unknown people		Interpersonal relationship		Euphoria

History and Development Data

When paying attention to one's life and development history, we look at variables such as the parenting practices prevalent in their life history, the history of exposure to intermittent reinforcement schedules, affective experiences of acceptance or rejection, history of overprotection or setting boundaries, among others (Banaco et al., 2012). Such variables play an important role in determining one's current patterns of interaction with the world.

Parental educational practices are behaviors from caregivers that seek to educate, socialize, and control their children's behavior. According to Gomide (2006), positive educational practices are characterized by positive monitoring, genuine parental interest in the child with displays of affection and praise; the teaching of moral behavior, empathy, and self-criticism, through examples from parents and discussions about books, TV programs, among others. Punitive/aversive educational practices, on the other hand, include neglect—inattention, absence, neglect, omission, and lack of parental love towards the child—; inconsistent punishment that depends on the parents' mood and not on the child's bad behavior; negative monitoring, with exaggerated inspection and surveillance by parents in relation to their children; high frequency of repetitive instructions; relaxed discipline—difficulties in establishing and enforcing rules; in addition to physical abuse—excessive physical punishment, usually accompanied by anger on the part of the parents (Rodrigues et al., 2011). Parental practices influence the child's development in many ways. Some of these aspects that may have implications in cases of alcohol abuse or dependence are highlighted in the text that follows.

In a very summarized way, parenting practices are studied in terms of two basic dimensions: responsiveness and demand (Ribas et al., 2003). The first dimension is about the parents' sensitivity to the child's demands and their immediacy in meeting their needs, both biological (food, cleanliness, temperature) and affective and cognitive (interacting verbally with the child, communicating that they believe in the child's ability to solve situations of challenge or conflict, to encourage the child to explore the environment in search of developing autonomy, etc.). Affective and responsive parents contribute to the child acquiring the experience of security when it comes to affection and trust in interpersonal relationships and in oneself as capable of producing satisfying social relationships. The second dimension, requirement, on the other hand, concerns the actions of parents who set boundaries and which control their children's behavior, so that they can be inserted into society, responding to the rules of social interaction. Demanding parents contribute to the development of self-control, tolerance to frustration, developing respect for boundaries, to the tolerance of waiting in situations where reinforcement is not immediate. A balanced combination of both factors (authoritative parenting style) results in the development of the basic repertoires necessary for a healthy interaction with the world. When either or both of these factors are lacking in parenting practices, there may be behavioral problems.

Regarding substance abuse, what is called permissive parenting is noteworthy—permissive parents are very responsive, but not demanding. They are warm and affectionate, are receptive to children's wishes, and available to satisfy their needs, while exercising little authority and limit, not favoring the learning of self-control, nor the opportunity for the child to exhibit self-management and behaviors of responsibility, in addition to a low ability of conflict resolution—important requirements for the development of autonomy. Permissiveness, when accompanied by overprotection, also tends to produce low tolerance to discomfort (Maccoby & Martin, 1983).

Positive parenting practices, in addition to involving the establishment of consistent boundaries, involve, to a greater or lesser extent, a history of exposure to intermittent reinforcement schedules. Contingencies of intermittent reinforcement teach that in order to achieve some goals, people have to persist and vary when things go wrong (especially in ratio schedules) or wait for the right time to act (interval schedules). Children who were exposed to moderate and controllable stressors in a gradual and monitored manner, tend to develop the necessary perseverance and variability to solve problems with autonomy, as well as the necessary tolerance to deal with situations whose solution is slow, difficult, or even impossible (Banaco et al., 2012).

In adulthood, the combination of a low tolerance for discomfort and low repertoire of self-management, self-control and conflict resolution results in a high risk for the use of tobacco and alcohol (Maccoby & Martin, 1983). When the individual is faced with difficult or conflicting situations and does not have sufficient skills to solve them, a condition of discomfort or suffering sets in. As its history also did not allow the development of tolerance to discomfort, it is necessary to seek something that relieves suffering - which is experienced as intense and uncontrollable. Therefore, alcohol plays a role in avoiding discomfort, while postponing the resolution of the situation.

The Developmental Variables Composing a Case Study[2]

X is 32 years old. His father passed away at 48 due to complications associated with harmful alcohol use. During childhood and part of teenagehood, *X* constantly witnessed scenes of domestic violence; his father beat his mother almost daily after returning from a bar near his home. In addition, *X* was harassed during the school years, being the victim of daily bullying among his peers. At the age of 27, he was diagnosed with depression, due to a history of neglect and physical and emotional abuse. Concomitantly, he was diagnosed with an alcohol use disorder, claiming that drinking alcohol would be a strategy to deal with life's adversities and relieve the symptoms of anxiety and depression. Currently, *X* does not undergo medical and psychological monitoring and continues to make harmful use of alcohol, which causes him a series of losses in various areas of his life. Among them, the end of his marriage about a year ago and the loss of his job 5 months ago. These losses intensify the symptoms of anxiety and depression and *X* uses alcohol to relieve them (Table 5.5).

Z is 53 years old. In his childhood, he suffered from physical and emotional violence, which created traumas and led to the decision of leaving home at the age of 14. He is currently on the street, exposed to a series of risks on a daily basis. He is a crack user, and says that the substance provides an intense state of momentary pleasure. In addition, to sleep, Z makes heavy use of alcohol, claiming that without it, he cannot fall asleep due to fear of being raped on the streets (Table 5.6).

Table 5.5 Functional analysis of X's behavior of using alcohol

History and development	Antecedents	Responses	Consequences	Processes	Effects
Alcohol use in the family (model)	End of marriage	Consuming alcoholic beverages	Easing/avoidance of feelings of discomfort and sadness	Negative reinforcement – Escape and avoidance	Relief
Intrafamily violence	Losing the job		Reducing symptoms of anxiety and depression		
	Symptoms of anxiety and depression (private events)		Avoidance of beginning tasks with a high response cost (e.g. looking for a job in the face of a history of alcohol abuse)		

[2] The cases were analyzed from the formulation model of Nery and Fonseca (2018).

Table 5.6 Functional behavior analysis

History and Development	Antecedents	Responses	Consequences	Processes	Effects
Intrafamily violence	Homelessness	Using crack	Contact with other people	Positive reinforcement	Euphoria
Childhood trauma	Risk of violence	Consuming alcoholic beverages	Reducing the state of fear and anxiety	Negative reinforcement	Momentaneous self-esteem increase
	Other several risks		Falling asleep		Relief
					Relaxation

Final Considerations

As it can be seen in the examples shown above, functional analysis allows us to understand the relationships that initiate and maintain behaviors, in this particular case, the use of psychotropic substances. Its clinical relevance is evident in that it shows how each story implies different variables and how they are of utter importance in understanding these behaviors, since they signal under which circumstances the use of a psychotropic substance is more likely. In this way, it shows which variables control the consumption of these substances.

In addition to being an important instrument for clinical evaluation, functional behavior analysis allows us to understand the diverse factors that influence drug use and dependence, breaking from moral models and simplistic views that attribute the etiology of disorders related to the use of substances only and exclusively to individuals and their biogenetic characteristics or the pharmacological effects of substances. Human behavior is multidetermined and, therefore, needs to be analyzed taking into account its complexity and dynamics. Based on the identification of variables that precipitate and maintain the behavior, such as substance use, it is possible to formulate not only individual clinical objectives but also more effective public policies and prevention and treatment interventions, based on scientific evidence.

References

Abib, J. (2004). O que é comportamentalismo. In M. Brandão (Ed.), *Sobre Comportamento e Cognição* (pp. 52–61). ESETec.

Banaco, R. A., Kovac, R., Martone, R. C., Vermes, J. S., & Zamignani, D. R. (2012). Psicopatologia. In M. M. C. Hübner & M. B. Moreira (Eds.), *Fundamentos de Psicologia: Temas clássicos de psicologia sob a ótica da Análise do Comportamento*. Guanabara Koogan.

Borloti, E. B., Haydu, V. B., & Machado, A. R. (2015). Crack: análise comportamental e exemplos das funções da dependência. *Acta Comportamentalia, 23*(3), 323–338.

Costa, S., & Marinho, M. (2002). Um modelo de apresentação de análises funcionais do comportamento. *Estudos De Psicologia (Campinas), 19*(3), 43–54. https://doi.org/10.1590/S0103-166X2002000300005

Cruz, R. (2006). Uma introdução ao conceito de autocontrole proposto pela análise do comportamento. *Revista Brasileira De Terapia Comportamental E Cognitiva, 8*(1), 85–94.

Garcia-Mijares, M., & Silva, M. (2006). Dependência de drogas. *Psicologia USP, 17*(4), 213–240. https://doi.org/10.1590/S0103-65642006000400012

Gomide, C. I. P. (2006). *Inventário de Estilos Parentais – IEP*. Vozes.

Haynes, S., & O'Brien, W. (1990). Functional analysis in behavior therapy. *Clinical Psychology Review, 10*(6), 649–668. https://doi.org/10.1016/0272-7358(90)90074-K

Lombard-Platet, V., Watanabe, O., & Cassetari, L. (2015). *Psicologia experimental: manual teórico e prático de análise do comportamento* (5th ed.). Edicon.

Maccoby, E., & Martin, J. (1983). Socialization in the context of the family: Parent-child interaction. In P. H. Mussen & E. M. Hetherington (Eds.), *Handbook of child psychology: Socialization personality and social development* (Vol. 4, pp. 1–101). Wiley.

Matos, M. (1999). Análise funcional do comportamento. *Estudos De Psicologia (Campinas), 16*(3), 8–18. https://doi.org/10.1590/S0103-166X1999000300002

Moreira, M., & Medeiros, C. (2018). *Princípios básicos de análise do comportamento* (2nd ed.). Artmed.

Neno, S. (2003). Análise funcional: definição e aplicação na terapia analítico-comportamental. *Revista Brasileira De Terapia Comportamental E Cognitiva, 5*(2), 151–165.

Nery, L. B., & Fonseca, F. N. (2018). Análises funcionais molares e moleculares: um passo a passo. In A. K. C. R. de-Farias, F. N. Fonseca, & L. B. Nery (Eds.), *Teoria e formulação de casos em análise comportamental clínica* (pp. 22–54). Artmed.

Ribas, A. F. P., Seidl de Moura, M. L., & Ribas, R. C., Jr. (2003). Responsividade materna: Levantamento bibliográfico e discussão conceitual. *Psicologia: Reflexão & Crítica, 16*, 137–145. https://doi.org/10.1590/S0102-79722003000100014

Rodrigues, O. M. P. R., Altafim, E. R. P., & Schiavo, R. A. (2011). Práticas parentais de mães adultas e adolescentes com bebês de um a doze meses. *Aletheia, 34*, 96–108.

Silva, J. (2007). *Autoconhecimento como técnica psicoterapêutica para a mudança comportamental* (Undergraduate thesis, Centro Universitário de Brasília). Retrieved from https://repositorio.uniceub.br/jspui/handle/123456789/2972

Silva, M. T. A., Guerra, L. G. G. C., Gonçalves, F. L., & Garcia-Mijares, M. (2001). Análise funcional da dependência de drogas. In H. J. Ghilardi, M. B. B. P. Madi, P. P. Queiroz, & M. C. Scoz (Eds.), *Sobre comportamento e cognição* (pp. 422–442). ESEtec.

Silvares, E., & Gongora, M. (1998). *Psicologia clínica comportamental: a inserção da entrevista com adultos e crianças*. EDICON.

Skinner, B. (2003). *Ciência e comportamento humano* (11th ed.). Martins Fontes. (Originally published in 1953)

Skinner, B. F. (1987). The selection by consequences. In B. F. Skinner (Ed.), *Upon further reflection*. Prentice-Hall. (Original work published in 1981).

Spadin, F. B., Chohfi, A. F., & Zanelatto, N. A. (2018). Análise funcional, formulação de caso e conceituação cognitiva. In N. A. Zanelatto & R. Laranjeira (Eds.), *O tratamento da dependência química e as terapias cognitivo-comportamentais: um guia para terapeutas* (2nd ed., pp. 383–401). Artmed.

Vandenberghe, L. (2002). A prática e as implicações da análise funcional. *Revista Brasileira De Terapia Comportamental E Cognitiva, 4*(1), 35–45.

Chapter 6
Establishing and Abolishing Contingencies of *Crack* Use: User Descriptions of a CAPSad

Eduardo Coelho Abreu and Elizeu Borloti

Introduction

The prevention of the (re)occurrence of risky use of psychoactive substances (SPAs) during the treatment of this use is of fundamental importance to the objective of the treatment. This importance is due to the fact that, to paraphrase White (2012), the (re)occurrence is more than a rule in the process called abuse/dependence of SPAs. Therefore, understanding the variables that favor or disfavor the maintenance of treatment gains is a central political, clinical, and scientific issue (p. 5). Thus, this chapter aims to describe what are the establishing/abandoning contingencies of the (re)occurrence of *crack* use in patients at a Center for Psycho-social Alcohol and Drugs Attention (CAPSad).

Contingencies are relationships of interdependence between drug use behavior and the environmental context of its (re)occurrence. Recurrence is the repetition of occurrences of use in a given period of time (Alemi et al., 2004). This indicates how much people who use drugs "want" the drug and how much they "work" to get it, that is, how much the use is "motivated" to occur and occur again (Michael, 2000). The technical term for this process is *motivational operation*, and can establish or abolish drug use behavior: *establishing operations* and behavioral demolishing *operations.*

OEs and OAs are events or conditions of stimuli prior to behavior that momentarily change: (a) the value of the consequences that act as specific types of boosters or punishers; and (b) the probability of evocation of behaviors that were previously associated with those consequences. As motivational operations (WMs), in the field of substance dependence, but not only, such events or antecedent conditions exert a

This chapter is part of the first author's master's dissertation: Abreu (2015).

E. C. Abreu (✉) · E. Borloti
Universidade Federal do Espírito Santo (UFES), Vitória, ES, Brazil

S. M. Oliani et al. (eds.), *Behavior Analysis and Substance Dependence*,
https://doi.org/10.1007/978-3-030-75961-2_6

powerful influence on the use of drugs and other related operating behaviors (e.g., calling friends, traveling, etc.) and therefore should be considered in the intervention on use (Langthorn & McGill, 2009). OMs should be envisioned in the analysis of historical factors that contribute to the understanding of the acquisition and maintenance of repertories related to the use of SPAs, indispensable to be functionally considered, in order to set unique goals in treatment (Dawson et al., 2009; D'Amico et al., 2009; Dios et al., 2009).

It is clear to see the relevance of WMs in drug dependence intervention from their two effects (Laraway et al., 2003). In the *altering effect of* the consequence *value*, a StateE establishes the efficacy of a specific type of reinforcement or punishment and a StateE abolishes the efficacy of a specific form of reinforcement or punishment. In the *behavioral altering effect*, a StateE evokes behaviors previously associated with the events it establishes as boosters, and a StateE decreases the frequency or suppresses behaviors associated with events that it abolishes itself as boosters. An example of these harm-reduction effects of drug use is when a person avoids using the drug on Sunday because it is important to feel well on Monday in order to go to work.

With these concepts understood, this chapter sheds light on two of the challenges related to research on recovery in substance dependence, described by White (2012): (a) the characteristics of the patient's life history, family, treatment path, and community that establish or end the recovery from drug dependence in the long term; and (b) the strategies used by him to promote the resolution of less-serious problems in his daily life, without the need for professional intervention. It also intends to collaborate in the development of better results from drug use treatments, since it addresses the function of variables prior to use and discusses the difficult task of maintaining long-term results by preventing recurrence of use (McLellan et al., 1994; Dennis et al., 2005). This prevention depends on the identification of both public and private drug use history events (Abreu, 2015).

There are differences of opinion about what the objectives of treatment should be and what can be evaluated as success or recovery. There is also no single explanation for the (re)occurrence of use during treatment. In the behavioral perspective characterized here—which defends the need for measurement and prediction (Alemi et al., 2004)—the description of aspects of the change in the use of SPAs allows us to anticipate possible (re)occurrences of use (Abreu, 2015). At this point is the merit of this field research.

Methodology

It is necessary to briefly summarize the methodology used in the study on which this chapter was based, in order to contextualize how its results were obtained. It was a descriptive study applied in a natural context, since, without deliberate interference, it sought to know variables of interest in the occurrences or recurrences of the use of SPA (its descriptive property) during the treatment of the dependency or abuse of

SPA (its applied property) in a CAPSad (the natural *setting of* the study). This knowledge and understanding of these variables are ultimately aimed, for practical reasons, at preventing such (re)occurrences. Abreu (2015) found little empirical explanatory knowledge accumulated on the recurrence of SPAs use in treatment contexts in CAPSad (it is important to mention that, in behavior analysis, the functional description of a behavioral phenomenon is already its explanation (Baum, 1999). To carry out the study that gave rise to this chapter, approval was required from the Committee on Ethics in Research with Human Beings (CEP/UFES) and by the municipal body to which CAPSad is linked.

The survey was conducted with five CAPSad users whose preferred drug is *crack*. The exclusion criteria were: (a) having severe psychiatric illness (i.e., schizophrenia or bipolar disorder) not stabilized by medication; (b) having physical disability not stabilized by medication; (c) being treated involuntarily or compulsorily; and (d) having another illicit substance used on the same preferential basis as *crack*.

The inclusion criterion was to be part of the daily care service, a fact that would ensure the maintenance of the participants in the treatment and, consequently, access to them for data collection. The inclusion of participants whose preferred drug is *crack is* justified in the same criteria of the Borloti, Haydu, and Machado (2015a) study: (a) the growing prevalence of its use as a preferential SPA among Brazilians (Carlini et al, (Carlini et al., 2006); (b) its considerable Brazilian consumer market, the largest in the world, which is reaching one million people (United Nations Office for Drug Control and Crime Prevention, 2010); and (c) the fact that, in general, these consumers do not believe that this use is a "problem," a belief that, also in general, is related to social exclusion, including the exclusion of the users themselves from public services for treatment (not to mention that the treatments in these services are usually not adjusted to their demands that, if not met, have as an outcome the severity and poor prognosis (Brazilian Psychiatry Association, 2012).

The instruments used for data collection were: (a) Multidimensional evaluation questionnaire, which aimed to evaluate the patient's reason for seeking treatment, the patient's situation in relation to the treatment, the characteristics of their behavior of *crack* use, their family relationships and other relationships, among other psychosocial aspects; (b) Inventory of drug use situations (ISCD), composed of 50 items, which provides a profile, on a 4-point Likert scale, of the estimates of the frequency of use in the last 3 months, questioned about being high-risk situations (Annis & Martin, 1985; Borloti & Cesar, 2015); and (c) Semi-structured interview, which complemented the data from other instruments, adding direct verbal reports of public and private environmental events related to the use during the data collection period, contemplating avoidance behaviors or strategies for maintaining the weekly gains of treatment.

After the survey was approved by CEP/UFES (Universidade Federal do Espírito Santo, Brazil) and the municipal health department, it was discussed with the coordination of CAPSad to define the other questions necessary for it to be carried out, such as the use of rooms for interviews, the presentation of the survey to the users of the service and the scheduling of visits by the researcher to the site. Later, interacting with the collective activities of CAPSad, the research was presented to all patients and for the five of them who showed interest in integrating the research as participants, meetings were scheduled in which the term of consent was presented in order to formalize the agreement with the participation, such as ensuring the confidentiality of personal data provided and the scheduling of interviews.

In the following weeks, six interviews were conducted with each of the five participants, which took place between 2 March 2015 and 25 May 2015. In the initial interview, the multidimensional evaluation and the first ISCD application were done. Later, every two weeks, the meeting was guided by the semi-structured interview to follow the progress of the patient's treatment at CAPSad. At the end of 3 months of collection, in the sixth interview, ISCD was applied again for future comparison with the results of the first application.

The multidimensional evaluation questionnaire has composed a simpler database. The content of its major topics allowed the grouping of participants' answers (P1, P2, P3, P4, and P5), indicating idiosyncratic situations of each one's treatment processes.

ISCD generated data that compared the usage pattern at the beginning and end of the collection period. The greater the outcome of a participant, the greater the number of situations of risk for the use of the drug experienced by him/her. Comparing the averages of these values in the first and second applications of the instrument, it was possible to estimate a percentage of recovery during the collection period and which situations were considered the most problematic (by the highest averages among all applications of the instrument, for all participants).

The interviews, conducted every two weeks, provided data that made up a database described according to their relevance to the objective of this study, since, as predicted by the recurrent and chronic characteristics of substance dependence (White, 2012), not all meetings would provide elaborate verbal reports of changes in drug-related behavior. The treatment of these reports involved grouping similar descriptions by the same participant in different weeks, or between different participants in the same week. In order not to repeat them on a case-by-case basis, they were grouped and discussed in general and functionally, indicating which participant explained which response and in which interview. Thus, the discussion was focused on the dynamics of the process of the most important events and exemplified with the most demonstrative answers of that dynamics.

In the interpretation of data, the theoretical reference was the analytic-behavioral. Therefore, this chapter brings a novelty to the field of "relapse prevention," in which the most common is to find studies with cognitive-behavioral interpretation (e.g., Alan Marlatt et al., 2002; Romanini et al., 2010; Tapert et al., 2004).

Results and Discussion

Table 6.1 summarizes the participants' profile.

It is important to emphasize that during the collection process, more than serving its original purpose, the Multidimensional Assessment Questionnaire has acquired

Table 6.1 Profile of participants

	Sex	Age	Personal goal in treatment	House	Health problem
P1	Male	57	Abstinence of use	In street situation	Hepatitis, Anemia, Insomnia.
P2	Male	35	Abstinence of use	Fixed residence	Dependency on alcohol
P3	Male	46	Reduction of damage from use	Shared residence ("republic")	Insomnia
P4	Male	49	Abstinence of use	Fixed residence	–
P5	Female	31	Abstinence of use	Shelter	–

Source: Reprinted from Abreu (2015, p. 49)

a function to the treatment. Its application cannot be, and should not have been, "nonclinical" (Madrid, 2009). The presentation of its items was done with sensitivity: (a) the ambivalence that usually accompanies the patient during treatment (Borloti et al., 2015b); and (b) the need to strengthen treatment adherence and participation in research. Therefore, it also served to establish a better relationship between researcher and participant, affecting the reinforcing value of the bond established between both, necessary for subsequent contacts, already with a therapist–patient relationship aspect. This clinical emphasis on research cautiously looks at verbal reports collected in questionnaires, inventories, or interviews. As the report is a perception of behaviors or facts, and not behaviors or facts that have occurred, its analysis, from the perspective of behavior analysis, always requires its understanding in its antecedent and consequent environmental variables (Ferreira de Mattos Silvares, 2006).

About the reason for the search and current treatment situation, although everyone described improvement plans, they did not describe problem situations when asked what motivated them to seek treatment. Rather, they described how they learned about CAPSad and how far they had come. The most common source of indication was the referral through the primary health care unit of their territories, followed by referrals by family members (P3), as well as referrals by the service at the reception center for drug users of the "Rede Abraço," Program of Integrated Actions on Drugs of the government of the State of Espírito Santo at the time (P5).

The majority of the participants considered the use itself as a determining factor in the state of their lives at the time of the research; and for this reason they intended, with the treatment, to be able to recover bonds with the family and/or children, and/or with the old activities of study and work, bonds that they considered "more worthy." P3, on the other hand, intended only to reduce the damage of use.

All reported motivation in, having progressed in treatment, achieving better living conditions and personal goals. The role that CAPSad has for these participants is from a place where they see themselves distant from the "reality of the streets," distant from use, closer to other patients in recovery. Being at CAPSad has been repeatedly described as being in a place "destined for learning" and which offers "security" from the different ways of accessing the drug outside.

The substance of preference, the focus of the treatment of all participants, is *crack*. The frequency and amount used varies widely among them and, in general, their reports on "how much" they use merge with others, such as those of the form of use (the "how"). The responses obtained were "I'm using very little" (P2, P4), "I'm not using as much as I used before" (P1), "I can't describe" (P3), and "I always use as much as I can" (P5). As for the form of use, P1, P2, and P4 said to make use alone from other people, while P3 only did so occasionally, sometimes making use with "some companion." P5, on the other hand, always used in the same place where he had access to the drug, which normally coincided with the place of prostitution, exchanging sex directly for *crack* or for money to buy *crack*.

As for the family relationship and other relationships, while P3 and P5 were completely estranged from their children and any other member of their family, P2 and P4 were living with family members and P1 had a good relationship with the former spouse. The proximity or distance from their families appeared as a variable that directly influenced the progress of the treatment, since the major supporters of the treatment were family members, nuclear (P1, P2 and P4) or former spouse (P1). In the case of P3 and P5, the distance from their families and their children generated sadness and discouragement, negatively interfering with the treatment. Despite this, the re-approximation of their loved ones was, according to the reports, an objective to be achieved as a consequence of the behaviors that define the control of the use of *crack* (P3) or the complete interruption of the use of any SPAs (P5).

For those who had family support, family members always ended up acting as providers of rules to be followed, explaining variables related to keeping away from the use and the problems it brought. However, the family also emerged as a problem, as in the case of P1 and P5, who saw the conflicts in it as intensifying the use. All the participants reported discomfort in the face of their relatives' distrust of them, both with the probability of "treatment leakage" and the lack of understanding of the difficulties in avoiding the use of *crack*.

Everyone could see when the *crack craving* started to bother, such as generating uncomfortable body sensations, headache, insomnia, nausea, and the urge to use. The most common strategies to avoid consumption varied topographies in attempts to get closer to the family and change the daily routine, seeking to get away from places and people related to use.

There was a constant complaint that the interests and objectives in the treatment differed greatly from person to person. Everyone was afraid that differences in goals and stages in treatment progress would become a problem for their treatment. This reinforced the elusiveness of the social approach in CAPSad, leading everyone to consider others (participants and nonparticipants) only as colleagues, not as friends.

As for the recurrence of use, P3 was the one that had more reports about this, being this recurrent use in motivational events present in daily life, allowing a greater understanding of the motivational operations of the use of *crack* and the motivational function that the instruments of data collection, already as an intervention, began to have on the use throughout the collection. For P3, the use of *crack* allowed him to feel relief from the tension of work as a tattooist and from the fatigue or boredom of everyday life. Several reinforcing consequences were attributed to his use behavior, making him assume that his goal in treatment was only to get back to control the amount used and the frequency of use. His treatment, however, did not become unfeasible for this reason. In the weeks that followed in data collection, P3 reported building new goals to be achieved, which gradually led him to develop a verbal repertoire skilled in describing amount and frequency of use. It seems that the research was interventionist in modifying behavior in relation to these properties of use, because goals could be set: initially to achieve the reduction to a certain daily amount and then to a weekly amount. Thus, P3 was able to bring its occurrences of use under control of quantitative properties that were not the focus of its attention before.

This change in behavior occurred as P3's behavior ceased to be under control reinforcing only the immediate effect of the drug. His behavior became more sensitive to the variables prior to *craving*. This sensitivity enabled him to anticipate and avoid situations in which *craving* would be so intense that use could not be avoided. The effects of SPA itself have never ceased to have reinforcing value, but P3 seems to have become more sensitive to the undesirable consequences of possible occurrences of use, and thus may choose to make the appropriate decision, either by the moments or by the places where such decision was discriminated as necessary (Martin & Pear, 2009).

This same behavioral process can be observed during the collection with P2 and especially P4. The latter justified that although the immediate effect of SPA use was desired, the negative effect used to last weeks: the disappointment of the family, the feeling of failure or the worsening that it felt when the use recurred.

It can also be observed that drug use by the participant with more–frequent-use reports (P3) and by the one with less-frequent-use reports (P4) occurred, but in a different behavior pattern. Both started to emit SPAs use behavior in a reduced frequency and intermittent reinforcement (Martin & Pear, 2009). This may have happened because, although this scheme is more commonly used to develop behavioral persistence, in some cases it can be used to reduce the frequency of an unwanted behavior, which, for some reason, has great reinforcing value and, thus, its recurrent evocation is quite likely. In both cases, the use of *crack* became something undesirable and therefore should be controlled or allowed only at regular intervals or, in the case of P4, very long, so as to no longer characterize a use with indiscriminate function, but with a negative reinforcing function (soften the negative bodily effects caused by long-term abstinence). For P3, this new function of use could be a beginning of the development of its improvement, while for P4 the strategy was progressively, or less and less, to use any substance, so as not to suffer from the uncomfortable effects of a total and abrupt interruption of use.

Total interruption of use is a strategy of behavior change that was often seen by patients themselves as the only way to recover a substance dependent, a report made by P1 during the first interview, by P2 during the second interview and by P5 during his fifth and last interview. However, this strategy implies some predictable problems to any extinction of behavior scheme, to be considered in drug addiction intervention. Initially it implies an abrupt increase in the frequency of behaviors aiming at reinforcement no longer presented to the disappearing behavior; later, a variety of behaviors were evoked in order to try to achieve the desired reinforcement (Martin & Pear, 2009).

For a substance dependent, this often implies what was reported by P1 during the fifth interview: his attempt to completely stop using any amount of *crack* ended up producing a crisis of abstinence so severe that he acted as an operation that established the reinforcing value of unwanted behavior never before issued, in this specific case, stealing money, punished with one week's detention. After his release from jail, the use of SPA occurred again, but in a more moderate way. The episode was related to the description of the objective of completely interrupting the use, only in a gradual manner.

The negative punishment scheme can be seen in P5's accounts, when he described that he stopped living with his family amidst the fights generated by his use of *crack*. Her mother expelled her from her home after recurrent disagreements, mainly for disagreement with the SPAs use behavior assumed by P5. In a way, this same kind of disagreement was the reason P2 separated from his wife and had to go back to live with his mother, and also P1 separated from his wife and went to live on the street.

On the other hand, positive reinforcement schemes of appropriate behaviors to increase their frequency were described initially by P2 and P4 (both during the second interview), and later by P1 (third interview) and P5 (fourth interview). Whether it was to improve the relationship with the family and get back in touch with the children, or to obtain better living conditions, get a good job (P5), or complete their studies, all, at some point, described reinforcements they intended to achieve. In this way, they focused on activities other than those of use. Gradually, they promoted the fading of the reinforcing quality of drugs in their lives as they sought to develop repertories of behaviors such as visiting family, walking, eating, and caring in order to produce positive reinforcements, such as the family members present, the good taste of food, a different place visited, sobriety, or improved physical conditions and appearance (clean body, without burns, with adequate weight and pleasant aspect).

All participants were able to hear reports on the development of behavioral persistence through an intermittent reinforcement scheme (Martin & Pear, 2009). In these cases, the persistence placed was to be able to withstand abstinence more and more as they gradually became aware of better life chances, the further away they got from risky use of *crack*. Some aimed at abstinence as the goal of treatment, others at harm-reduction, but all, at some point, stressed the importance of persevering in treatment, developing resistance to the frustration of the absence of the reinforcing effect caused by the drug, compensated by long-term gains.

It is essential to emphasize the demand for attention to variables that precede the behavior of use that can help both the patient in treatment and the service that serves them, in order to preserve the advances in patient recovery, avoiding recurrence of use. There were, in common, in the reports of the participants, descriptions of antecedent events that compose a specific type of variable for momentarily altering the reinforcing value of the consequence of a certain behavior and, consequently, evoking this behavior (Michael, 1993, 2000). This specific knowledge allows access to motivational variables of SPAs use behavior and, thus, describe the probability of use, providing an essential theoretical tool to prevent its (re)occurrence.

During data collection it was possible to notice frequent descriptions of these variables in the reports of the participants, as in the description made by P3, that the substances used by any chemical dependent have some positive effect, otherwise they would not be used. This fact is undeniable, since SPAs work as unconditioned boosters. Like food for a hungry person or water for a thirsty person, for a substance dependent abstinence implies an operation establishing the use of SPAs, increasing the probability that they will be used the more they are deprived (Martin & Pear, 2009).

A broad example of establishing operation is drug deprivation combined with discriminatory stimuli, such as people who are also users or places where the substance is commonly used. While for P1, P3, and P5 the occurrences of use are everyday events, either because, at the time of the study, they were living on the street or in shelters and had constant and inevitable contact with people who use the most varied drugs, for P2 and P4 the occurrences of use are sporadic events, because they tried to distance themselves from places and people whose presence, in the deprivation of the drug, made the emission of the use behavior more likely. For all participants, the environments of access to the drug, as discriminatory stimuli, become more powerful when combined with the deprivation of the drug in the organism as an establishing operation. This knowledge is part of self-control of use, and can act on the predisposition to frequent environments where they know they will be more prone to use, also by the presence of people who facilitate access to the drug. On the other hand, it has been reported that isolation can also serve as an establishing operation. P2 described a certain situation in which the occurrence of SPA use occurred because he distanced himself from home, after having spent a long time thinking about the effects and the substance itself, until he could no longer control himself in order to avoid use.

When they answered about the reasons why they made occasional use of *crack* between the periods of each interview, there were several reports of operations establishing the use: facing negative emotions (P1 and P5), sadness, or discouragement in everyday life, facing negative physiological states, such as *craving* provided by deprivation of the substance, or feelings of anxiety and "nervousness." P1 and P3 also considered that the use of *crack* was useful to "escape from reality," a means to achieve some momentary relief. On the other hand, P2 and P4's accounts of operations that were able to avoid use by staying at home or by surrounding themselves with people who supported them in their treatment serve as examples of use-abusing operations.

Other examples of SPAs can be seen in the P5 report, which describes that the better you feel, the less will you have to make use of any substance. When asked what this "feeling better" would be, or what would elicit it, P5 addresses the role that CAPSad plays for her in her treatment, functioning as a place where all activities are aimed at reducing as much as possible the likelihood that patients under treatment will feel the need to use some substance. In this case, the medication prescribed for the patients also performs the function of an establishing operation.

However, for the vast majority of participants, the operation that demolishes the most recurrent use is also the most controversial and can even be assessed as contradictory. For many, the only way to diminish the willingness to use some substance is by making use of some other substance that produces less damage. The harm-reduction policy contemplates this logic, in this case, replacing a drug such as *crack,* which causes extensive harm, with one with less-harmful effect.

The ISCD results shown in Table 6.2 were grouped into total values, adding the value of all inventory responses in each application, as well as average values (obtained by dividing the total value by the number of questions). In this way, the variation of results in percentage can also be calculated: how much each result varied in 3 months. The data in Table 6.2 do not correspond to the intensity or frequency of SPAs use itself, but to the self-assessment of the risk of use by each participant at the time of ISCD applications. The result of each participant was analyzed according to the stage of their treatment.

The analysis of the data in Table 6.2 allows one to follow the development of the treatment, for example, P2 obtained the greatest variation of results, going from a high total value to one of the lowest, coinciding with its solid change of routine, being less exposed to situations that would be at great risk of SPAs use. Throughout the data collection period, he received constant support and attention from his mother, and even at times when he felt he was closer to losing control, he managed to stay in the focus of his treatment.

It is noticeable that all the results correspond to values that, in the second application, are higher than 50. These values would be equivalent to average 1 in the answers to the inventory, corresponding to a behavior of complete abstinence from use, which despite being a goal for some participants, is not required in the work of CAPSad. They can be considered significant advances in the treatment of P1, P2, and P4, since the verbal report of their uses suffered a change in a period of 3 months of data collection, and even in the cases of P3 and P5, it is possible to notice that there were behavioral gains in the treatment. Despite these gains for some and not all, the probability of use was discriminated from the ISCD. Table 6.3 informs the previous context that may or could have acted as a motivational operation for (re)occurrences of *crack* use.

It is possible to verify in Table 6.3 that out of the 50 risk situations, 9 obtained mean responses equal to or greater than 3, indicating that these situations are the

Table 6.2 Total score, average, and change in responses at ISCD

Participant	1st application		2nd application		Variation
	Total	Average	Total	Average	
P1	134	2.68	107	2.14	−20.15%
P2	123	2.46	73	1.46	−40.65%
P3	131	2.62	132	2.64	0.76%
P4	65	1.3	58	1.16	−10.77%
P5	90	1.8	97	1.94	7.78%

Source: Reproduced from Abreu (2015, p. 64)

Table 6.3 Items, situations, and categories of situations with higher risk of (re)occurrences of drug use.

ISCD Item	High-risk situation for (re)use (ISCD issue)	Higher average response value	High-risk situation category
1	When I got depressed	3 (first application)	Facing negative emotions
4	When I felt I had nowhere to run	3 (first application)	
34	When I was overwhelmed and wanted to escape	3 (second application)	
24	When I felt anxious or tense	3 (both applications)	Facing negative physiological states
16	When I unexpectedly found one of these drugs or happened to see something that reminded me of these drugs	3.2 (first application)	Surrender to temptations and impulses in the absence of someone else
21	When I was alone	3 (first application)	
46	When I started thinking about the effect of the drug	3.4 (first application)	
37	When I had conflicts at home	3.2 (first application)	Confronting interpersonal conflict
48	When I was with a group of people and everyone was using these drugs	3 (first application)	Social pressure for the occurrence/recurrence of psychoactive substance use

Source: ISCD item extracted from Annis, H. M., & Martin, G. (1985). Inventory of Drug-Taking Situations. Toronto, Canada: Addiction Research Foundation. High-risk situation category extracted from Borloti & Cesar (in press). Drug relapse prevention strategies. In: Borloti, E., Balbi Neto, R. de Q. B., Machado, A. R., Andrade, A. da P. Crack, alcohol and other drugs: intervention strategies for ongoing formation

ones that offer the highest risk of use for the survey participants. These situations notoriously coincide with the different reports already described as operations establishing the use of *crack*: the aversiveness of negative emotions and deprivation of use, felt as *craving* in places where *crack* is used and in the presence of other people who use it, with a discriminatory function.

Final Considerations

Following CAPSad users in treatment for descriptions of common variables in the recovery process was a valuable experience. Through sequential interviews and other tools, new data can be achieved that describe the progress and difficulties faced during treatment. The results give several indicators of the importance of maintaining constant attention on the variables that control the behavior of participants to use drugs, emphasizing the need to access factors of the patient's history and motivational operations that influenced the emergence and maintenance of SPA use.

The constant attention to the control of stimuli and the motivational context of drug use allows us to predict the probability of both the emergence of (re)occurrences of use and the maintenance of the objective of treatment. By having such attention, behavioral changes may occur, such as those observed in this study. More than describing and discussing operations that establish and destroy the use of SPAs, this study described strategies for data collection that ended up contributing to the recovery process of participants, bringing greater self-knowledge about the variables that controlled their use behavior. It can be considered an empirical knowledge about the dynamics of treatment in substance dependence.

References

Abreu, E. C. (2015). *Contingências estabelecedoras e abolidoras do uso de crack: Descrições de usuários de um CAPSad*. Master's thesis, Universidade Federal do Espírito Santo, Brasil.

Alemi, F., Haackb, M., & Nemesc, S. (2004). Statistical definition of relapse: Case of family drug court. *Addictive Behaviors, 29*(4), 685–698. https://doi.org/10.1016/j.addbeh.2004.02.027

Annis, H. M., & Martin, G. (1985). *Inventory of drug-taking situations*. Addiction Research Foundation.

Associação Brasileira de Psiquiatria. (2012). Abuso e dependência: Crack. *Revista da Associação Médica Brasileira, 58*, 138–140.

Baum, W. (1999). *Compreender o Behaviorismo: Ciência, Comportamento e Cultura*. Artmed.

Borloti, E., & Cesar, B. (2015). Estratégias de prevenção de recaída no uso de drogas. In E. Borloti, R. R. Q. B. Balbi Neto, A. R. Machado, & A. P. Andrade (Eds.), *Crack, álcool e outras drogas: estratégias de intervenção para a formação permanente* (pp. 99–126). Editora GM.

Borloti, E. B., Haydu, V. B., & Machado, A. R. (2015a). Crack: análise comportamental e exemplos das funções da dependência. *Acta Comportamentalia, 23*(3), 323–338.

Borloti, E., Machado, A. R., & Balbi Neto, R. R. D. Q. (2015b). Intervenções motivacionais na dependência química. In E. Borloti, R. R. Q. B. Balbi Neto, A. R. Machado, & A. P. Andrade (Eds.), *Crack, álcool e outras drogas: estratégias de intervenção para a formação permanente* (pp. 107–128). Vitória.

Carlini, E. A., Galduroz, J. C., Silva, A. A. B. S., Noto, A. R., Fonseca, A. M., Carlini, C. M., … van der Sanchez, Z. M. (2006). *II Levantamento domiciliar sobre o uso de drogas psicotrópicas no Brasil: estudo envolvendo as 108 maiores cidades do pais* (p. 2005). SENAD/CEBRID. Retrieved from http://www.cebrid.epm.br

D'Amico, E. J., Ramchand, R., & Miles, J. N. (2009). Seven years later: Developmental transitions and delinquent behavior for male adolescents who received long-term substance treatment. *Journal of Studies on Alcohol and Drugs, 70*(5), 641–651. https://doi.org/10.15288/jsad.2009.70.641

Dawson, D. A., Li, T. K., Chou, S. P., & Grant, B. F. (2009). Transitions in and out of alcohol use disorders: Their associations with conditional changes in quality of life over a 3-year follow-up interval. *Alcohol, 44*(1), 84–92. https://doi.org/10.1093/alcalc/agn094

de Dios, M. A., Vaughan, E. L., Stanton, C. A., & Niaura, R. (2009). Adolescent tobacco use and substance abuse treatment outcomes. *Journal of Substance Abuse Treatment, 37*(1), 17–24. https://doi.org/10.1016/j.jsat.2008.09.006

Dennis, M. L., Scott, C. K., Funk, R., & Foss, M. A. (2005). The duration and correlates of addiction and treatment careers. *Journal of Substance Abuse Treatment, 28*(Suppl. 1), 51–62.

Laraway, S., Snycerski, S., Michael, J., & Poling, A. (2003). Motivating operations and terms to describe them: Some further refinements. *Journal of Applied Behavior Analysis, 36*(3), 407–414. https://doi.org/10.1901/jaba.2003.36-407

Madrid. (2009). *Protocolo de intervención psicológica*. Retrieved from http://www.madrid.es/UnidadesDescentralizadas/Salud/Publicaciones%20Propias%20Madrid%20salud/Publicaciones%20Propias%20ISP%20e%20IA/Folletos%20IA/Documentos%20tecnicos/protocolo_psicologico.pdf.

Marlatt, G. A., Parks, G. A., & Witkiewitz, K. (2002). *Clinical guidelines for implementing relapse prevention therapy*. University of Washington.

Martin, G., & Pear, J. (2009). *Modificação de comportamento: o que é e como fazer*. Editora Roca.

McLellan, A. T., Alterman, A. I., Metzger, D. S., Grissom, G. R., Woody, G. E., Luborsky, L., & O'Brien, C. P. (1994). Similarity of outcome predictors across opiate, cocaine, and alcohol treatments: Role of treatment services. *Journal of Consulting and Clinical Psychology, 62*, 1141–1158. https://doi.org/10.1037//0022-006x.62.6.1141

Michael, J. (1993). Establishing operations. *The Behavior Analyst, 16*, 191–206.

Michael, J. (2000). Implications and refinements of the establishing operation concept. *Journal of Applied Behavior Analysis, 33*, 401–410. https://doi.org/10.1901/jaba.2000.33-401

Romanini, M., Dias, A. C. G., & Pereira, A. S. (2010). Grupo de prevenção de recaídas como dispositivo para o tratamento da dependência química. *Disc. Scientia. Série: Ciências da Saúde, 11*(1), 115–132.

Ferreira de Mattos Silvares, M. (2006). *Psicologia clínica e comportamental: A inserção da entrevista com adultos e crianças*. Edicon.

Tapert, S. F., Ozyurt, S. S., Myers, M. G., & Brown, S. A. (2004). Neurocognitive ability in adults coping with alcohol and drug relapse temptations. *The American Journal of Drug and Alcohol Abuse, 30*(2), 445–460. https://doi.org/10.1081/ada-120037387

United Nations Office for Drug Control and Crime Prevention (UNODC). (2010). *Global illicit drug trends*. UNODCCP. Retrieved from: http://www.undcp.org/adhoc/report_2001-06-26_1/report_2001-06-26_1.pdf

White, W. L. (2012). *Recovery/Remission from Substance Use Disorders: An analysis of reported outcomes in 415 scientific reports, 1868–2011*. Retrieved from: http://www.williamwhitepapers.com/pr/2012%20Recovery-Remission%20from%20Substance%20Use%20DisordersFinal.pdf

Part II
Clinical and Social Interventions

Chapter 7
Contingency Management for the Treatment of Substance Use Disorders

Viviane Simões, Rodolfo Yamauchi, and André Q. C. Miguel

Introduction: Substance Use from an Operant Behavioral Perspective

Most academic areas that study substance use disorders (SUD) understand this phenomenon as a psychiatric disorder, where individuals develop a compulsive and uncontrolled use of substances, despite the various adverse effects that this consumption brings to themselves, their family and the community (APA, 1994). This understanding is supported by neurobiological findings that not only describe the mechanisms of drug action in the brain but also point to the structural and functional neurological changes caused by the chronic use of these substances (Kalivas et al., 2005; Volkow et al., 1997, 2000).

It is a consensus that SUD can cause diverse suffering and harm to individuals and, therefore, it is valid to characterize this behavioral repertoire as the product of a psychopathology. However, from a behavioral perspective, to understand substance consumption as pathological behavior is a misconception (Bigelow et al., 1998). It is understood that addictive behaviors may be considered inappropriate, undesirable promoters of the most diverse adverse consequences, potentially resulting in serious harm to the individual and to society (Higgins & Silverman, 1999). Nevertheless, such behaviors cannot be considered pathological from an operant behavior perspective since they follow the same principles and laws of any operant

V. Simões · R. Yamauchi
Department of Psychiatry, Federal University of Sao Paulo, Sao Paulo, SP, Brazil

A. Q. C. Miguel (✉)
Department of Psychiatry, Federal University of Sao Paulo, Sao Paulo, SP, Brazil

Analytics and PsychoPharmacology Laboratory (APPL) and the Program of Excellence in Addiction Research, Washington State University, Spokane, WA, USA
e-mail: andremiguel@wsu.edu

S. M. Oliani et al. (eds.), *Behavior Analysis and Substance Dependence*,
https://doi.org/10.1007/978-3-030-75961-2_7

behavior. That is, these behaviors are controlled by the functional relationships between the contingencies present in their environment (Bigelow et al., 1998). In the same direction, drug abuse can be considered compulsive, if by this we mean a high frequency of self-administered, but not uncontrolled behavior (Bigelow et al., 1998; Higgins & Silverman, 1999). On the contrary, it is strongly controlled by the immediate reinforcers produced by substance use (pharmacological effects), as well as by other delayed conditioned reinforcers, generally more difficult to observe (Higgins et al., 2004).

As will be seen below, substance self-administration responses can be considered as learned normal responses that lie some point along a *continuum* ranging from sporadic consumption, with little or no associated harm, to excessive consumption accompanied by numerous undesirable and adverse effects. A substantial body of studies provide the empirical basis for an operant understanding of SUD (Higgins & Silverman, 1999; Higgins et al., 2004). According to this perspective, the behavior of self-administering a substance should be considered the central problem in individuals with SUD, as this is the only response that is always present and is mandatory for anyone who closes a diagnosis of SUD (those who do not self-administer a substance cannot have the problems resulting from that use). Within this reasoning, if the environment can be changed in such a way as to reduce or extinguish substance use, it would most probably also reduce or eliminate the negative effects (aversive consequences) produced by this response.

Theoretical and Experimental Basis for the Self-Administration of Substances

Experiments on operant conditioning and behavioral pharmacology were first developed in the 1950s (Griffiths et al., 1980; Higgins et al., 2004). Initial studies demonstrated that the same substances abused by humans are spontaneously consumed by several other species (Aigner & Balster, 1978). In fact, without any previous exposure, will animals voluntarily consume a large amount of psychoactive substances (Griffiths et al., 1980). Animals also learn new and complex response that, as consequence, allow them access to the effects of a given substance (Griffiths et al., 1980). After some exposures, the reinforcing effects contingent to the consumption of these substances become so strong that these animals will give up other important reinforcers such as water and food in order to have access to these substances instead (Petry & Heyman, 1995). In summary, these experimental findings with animal models suggest that (1) for these species, substances of abuse act as unconditioned positive reinforcers; (2) these reinforcers are so strong that animals will emit high-cost responses in order to gain access to these substances; and (3) after some exposure these reinforcers will gain enough strength to compete with other important reinforcers (such as food and water).

Thus, substance use (self-administration) can be understood as learned operant behavior (behavior controlled by the consequences it produces) that is initially controlled by the unconditioned reinforcing effects (subjective and physiological effects) caused by the substance (Cahoon & Cynthia, 1972; Higgins & Petry, 1999). As with any reinforcer, the effects of the substance will reinforce any response that, as a consequence, allows access to the substance (in human natural contexts some examples would be going to the dealer, buying the drug, and using it).

These findings are important, but do not explain the interaction between self-administration and other contingencies present in the same environment where it occurs. It is known that all operating behaviors are sensitive to the presence of other contingencies in their environment (Skinner, 1969). Thus, the response of consuming substances should also be influenced by the presence of other contingencies.

In fact, experimental studies suggest that other environmental variables not related to reinforcers contingent to substance use may influence the reinforcing effects of substance use itself (Higgins & Petry, 1999). Aversive stimuli, such as shocks, social aggression, social exclusion, or reduced availability of food, liquids, or exercise, lead to an increase in the frequency of substance use among laboratory animals (Goeder & Guerin, 1991; Wolffgramm & Heyne, 1995). However, when animals are exposed to alternative sources of positive reinforcers, not related to substance use (e.g. access to female, nest building materials, appetizing foods), the frequency of substance use decreases significantly (Higgins, 1996, 1997).

Data obtained from animal models and clinical studies involving human volunteers suggest that humans behave similarly to other species with regard to the consumption of psychoactive substances. Humans learn and maintain new responses to access drugs, reach high levels of consumption (with risks of overdose), increase the frequency of use in the presence of aversive stimuli, and decrease this frequency if positive reinforcers are available in their environment (Higgins, 1997; Higgins & Petry, 1999). These findings suggest that: (1) the same operant conditioning processes present in substance use responses can be observed in several species, including humans; (2) as with all operant behaviors, substance use is also sensitive to the presence of other contingencies present in the environment where consumption occurs; (3) substance use can increase or decrease depending on possible changes in contingencies present in a specific environment; and (4) enriching the environment with other sources of positive reinforcement can promote a reduction in drug use.

As a rule, when an individual begins to use a substance, this consumption is controlled only by unconditioned positive reinforcers (e.g. effect of the substance) and conditioned positive reinforcers (e.g. friends of use). As substance use increases in frequency and becomes more generalized to other environmental contexts, new contingencies also come to control substance use. Unconditioned negative reinforcers (withdrawal symptoms) as well as conditioned negative reinforcers (aversive sensations produced by a fight with a friend or the end of a relationship) also come to control substance use (Higgins, 1997; Higgins & Petry, 1999). In other words, the reinforcers that control the substance use can be separated into four groups:

- *Unconditioned positive reinforcers* caused by the physiological effects induced by the substance (e.g. euphoria, relaxation, feeling of transcendence).
- *Conditioned positive reinforcers* linked to the social environment where consumption occurs (e.g. group of friends, bar table, football game).
- *Unconditioned negative reinforcers* (e.g. withdrawal, craving).
- *Conditioned negative reinforcers* linked to aversive aspects of the environment (e.g. fighting with a family member, loneliness).

Generally, one or more of these reinforcers are present during the initiation of substance use, and most likely all of these reinforcers are present when the individual presents an abusive and/or addictive pattern of substance use.

The more the reinforcing effects linked to substance use (either for pleasure or to alleviate cracking) are intensified, the greater the amount and frequency of substance use. During this process, the individual's repertoire is reduced as the individual is increasingly extinguishing responses that lead to other reinforcers (work, friends, family) in order to be able to emit only the responses that lead to the reinforcing effects of the drug.

It is usually at this time the individual starts to neglect the emission of other important response in order to use drugs that his friends, family members, and society start to consider him as having a substance use problem. In other words, the more a person stops to emit "appropriate and/or desirable" responses to the society and choose to emit "undesirable and/or inappropriate" behaviors related to substance use, the more they tend to consider their consumption problematic.

Contingency Management (CM)

The name contingency management (CM) describes the intervention proposal well. According to Skinner (1969), the term contingency can be understood as the relationship, or interrelationship, between antecedent stimuli (events that occur before a given response), the emission of a response or behavior, and the consequences produced by that response (consequent stimuli). These consequent stimuli can be either reinforcing, when they increase the frequency or probability of the response to be emitted in the future, or punitive when they reduce the frequency or probability of this response to be emitted in the future. Thus, as the name implies, CM treatment aims to manage contingencies (or even create new contingencies) in order to modify harmful behavior patterns present in the repertoire of the individual with SUD.

The maintenance of problematic drug use by an individual is a product of the presence of strong (unconditioned and conditioned) reinforcers contingent on drug use and the lack of other reinforcers contingent on alternative responses (Higgins et al., 2004). This unequal competition between reinforcers associated with drug use and reinforcers associated with alternative responses makes it difficult to modify the pattern of substance use.

As seen previously, experimental studies suggest that it is possible to reduce or eliminate certain problematic behaviors that in themselves generate reinforcing consequences (such as substance use) by reinforcing other behaviors that are incompatible with problem behavior (e.g., maintaining abstinence) (Higgins, 1996, 1997). Thus, CM aims to reduce or eliminate problematic behaviors (substance use) by reinforcing (offering prizes or tokens with a certain monetary value) behaviors that are incompatible with those considered a problem (abstinence) (Higgins & Petry, 1999).

The use of punishment (contingent on substance use) may be effective in some cases, but produces undesirable consequences (counter-control) such as treatment drop-out, aversive emotional states, and conflicts between patient and clinician(s) (Amass & Kamien, 2004). The use of positive reinforcement, in turn, does not produce this type of negative effects. Thus, in order to extinguish undesirable responses related to substance use, CM treatment aims to manipulate the contingencies present in the individual's environment by increasing the presence of positive reinforcers linked to alternative responses and, when possible, incompatible with substance use.

Creating new contingencies using natural reinforcers is always preferable as these contingencies tend to remain after the end of treatment. However, it is very common that the behavioral repertoire of substance users are quite impoverished (especially the most severe cases) and that most of the reinforcers linked to this repertoire are related to substance use. Thus, CM treatment develops new contingencies with arbitrary reinforcers (not naturally produced by the natural or social environment) that are contingent to responses alternative to substance use, and hence, promote abstinence and other desirable responses (Higgins & Petry, 1999; Petry, 2000).

For more than 30 years, CM has been applied in the treatment of cocaine and other drug addictions (Prendergast et al., 2006). Studies with this technique present high methodological rigor and systematically achieve the best results in terms of adherence to treatment, achievement, and maintenance of abstinence (Higgins et al., 1991, 1994; Stitzer & Bigelow, 1978).

One of the most studied methods of CM, with the greatest evidence of effectiveness, is termed vouchers CM (Higgins et al., 1993). In this method, vouchers with a certain monetary value (that can be exchanged for products present in the community) are given to a patient immediately after he/she emits a desired behavior (e.g., abstinence, adhering to pharmacological treatment). These vouchers act to reinforce a response that is incompatible with the emission of problematic response (e.g. maintaining abstinence is incompatible with consuming substances). An important point to consider regarding the use of tokens as reinforcers is that, because they represent the possibility of obtaining products and goods, these tokens act as generalized conditioned reinforcers (because they represent everything that can be obtained with that monetary value). Since they act as generalized reinforcers, they are not very sensitive to satiation (they do not reduce their reinforcing value) and are, therefore, ideal for this type of procedure.

In general, these reinforcers are given systematically (2–3 times a week) to increase the reinforcing magnitude of the consequences produced. As the patient performs these behaviors consecutively, the value received in tokens increases. This increase in reinforcing value aims to promote longer-lasting changes and the maintenance of abstinence on a continuous basis, as well as to highlight that longer periods of abstinence are more valued than shorter periods. When the patient cannot present these behaviors (e.g., cannot become abstinent/relapse) he/she is encouraged to try again, but does not receive vouchers in that given day.

Using this methodology, Higgins and colleagues developed in 1991 the first study that became a reference for all other CM studies that followed. To allow a better understanding of how the CM is applied, a description of the whole procedure, as well as the results obtained in this experiment, will be presented here. In this study, cocaine-dependent participants were randomized into two groups (one receiving standard treatment and the other receiving standard treatment plus CM). In both groups, participants were encouraged to leave 3 urine toxicological samples per week. While the control group did not receive any form of recompense for test results, the CM group could earn vouchers for submitting negative cocaine samples. For the CM group, the first test with a negative result (done immediately and in front of the patient) guaranteed the patient a $2.50 voucher gain. To encourage continued abstinence, each consecutive negative test increased in value by $1.25. However, if the patient failed to submit a test or the sample tested positive for cocaine, the patient did not receive a voucher that day and future voucher were reset to their original value. This reduction in voucher value was intended to punish cocaine use responses.

Since for individuals with a cocaine use disorder, money is directly associated with cocaine use, vouchers were not transformed into money, but rather into products and goods available in existing in the community (e.g., supermarket purchases, concert tickets). If the patient remained abstinent throughout the treatment (12 weeks) he would receive $997.00 in products and/or services.

Results obtained in this study showed that 85% of the patients receiving CM remained in treatment during the 12 weeks compared to only 33% of the control group patients ($p. < 0.05$). In addition, 46% of patients receiving CM remained abstinent for at least 8 weeks compared to zero in the control group ($p. < 0.05$). Subsequent randomized controlled trials replicated the same results (Higgins et al., 1993, 1994).

Effectiveness of Contingency Management in the Treatment of Substance Use Disorders

CM applied to SUD treatment is one of the most-studied psychosocial interventions. Randomized clinical trials in CM have been conducted in the United States (Higgins et al., 1991, 1993, 1994), Spain (Garcia-Fernandez et al., 2011;

Secades-Villa et al., 2015), United Kingdom (Weaver et al., 2014), Switzerland (Petitjean et al., 2014), China (Chen et al., 2013; Jiang et al., 2012), and Brazil (Miguel et al., 2016, 2019).

Meta-analysis studies suggest that CM applied alone, or in conjunction with other cognitive behavioral treatments, is effective in promoting continued abstinence and treatment adherence among individuals dependent on a wide variety of substances (Lussier et al., 2006, Prendergast et al., 2006). More specifically, meta-analysis studies have found that the CM has an effect size ranging from moderate to high (this being the largest effect size found for any psychosocial treatment for SUD) (Lussier et al., 2006).

The results obtained in CM studies were so positive that in 1998 the National Institute on Drug Abuse (NIDA) developed a practical manual on how to properly implement CM in open cocaine treatment programs (Budney, 1998). In 2007, the National Institute for Health and Clinical Excellence (NICE) recommended CM to the UK's National Substance Abuse Treatment Agency (Pilling et al., 2007).

Contingency Management for Crack Use Disorder in Brazil

Recently, the first study of CM in Brazil was performed (Miguel et al., 2016, 2019). In this study, which used the CM voucher's model, 65 crack-dependent individuals who sought treatment at the Vila Maria Medical Specialty Outpatient Clinic (AME-Vila Maria), in the North Zone of São Paulo, were randomized into two groups. In total, 32 subjects were allocated to the control group, and 33 were allocated to the experimental group. In this 12-week study, the control group received the standard intervention offered by AME-Vila Maria, while the experimental group received the same standard treatment offered by AME-Vila Maria in association with CM. The CM procedure consisted of reinforcing the abstinence from crack-cocaine. In this study, after the first crack-cocaine negative urine sample was submitted, the participant immediately received a voucher with a monetary value of R$ 5. This value increased by R$ 2 for each consecutive crack-cocaine negative sample, to a maximum value of R$ 15, thus increasing from R$ 5 to R$ 7, 9, 11, 13, and 15, respectively. If the participant left the three negative weekly samples for crack-cocaine, he also received a bonus of R$ 20.

The results of this study demonstrate that CM was more effective in reducing crack-cocaine use and promoting longer periods of crack-cocaine abstinence when compared to standard treatment. In CM treatment, 21.2% of subjects remained abstinent from crack-cocaine during all 12 weeks of the study, compared to none in the control group. CM was also more effective in promoting treatment retention. In total, 51.5% of subjects adhered to all 12 weeks of treatment compared to none of the control group (Miguel et al., 2016). Significant differences in favor of CM were also observed with respect to participation in treatment and in reducing marijuana, and alcohol use (Miguel et al., 2016). Furthermore, a greater reduction in depressive and anxious symptoms was observed among participants exposed to CM (Miguel et al., 2017). Finally, when asked about their experiences with CM treatment, the vast majority of participants highlighted that CM is easy to understand, that they liked to receive this type of treatment, that they thought CM was fundamental in their treatment response, and that they believed other crack- cocaine users would benefit from this intervention (Miguel et al., 2018).

Clinical Case

This will be a brief account of a family therapy where CM was effective in treating the cocaine use of one of the relatives.

In 2015, Marcos' parents sought psychological care as they had recently discovered that Marcos was using cocaine with a certain regularity. Marcos is 24 years old, single, and works promoting night-time events and parties in São Paulo, Brazil. As a child and adolescent he was always very sociable and cheerful, but had a lot of academic difficulties, which led him to repeat a school year twice and to change schools on three occasions. At the age of 17 he was diagnosed with Attention Deficit Hyperactivity Disorder (ADHD) and started to be medicated with Ritalin, using this medication until his college years. After graduating from high school, Marcos went to live in São Paulo city (his family lives in the countryside of the state of São Paulo) to go to business school. In a period of 2 years, Marcos studied and abandoned three different colleges, having always had a very weak academic performance.

During this period Marcos also began to work and stand out in the promotion of night-time events and parties (field where he works until today). Two years ago Marcos tried cocaine for the first time and started using it sporadically in the following months. In the last year, this use became more frequent (2–4 days per week) and Marcos began to have professional, financial, and family problems. In a few months, Marcos began to show a pattern of excessive spending (much higher than he earned), which culminated in a debt of R$ 100,000. It is worth mentioning that Marcos' family has a good economic condition and has always paid all of Marcos' living costs (house, car, house and car bills, cell phone, insurance, income tax, etc.), making this spending pattern even more problematic. During this period, his family found cocaine in his car and, while talking to one of his friends, discovered that Marcos was using cocaine regularly. After making this discovery they decided to seek treatment. Initially they encouraged Marcos to do individual therapy, but Marcos did not adhere and continued to use cocaine. Therefore, in order to ensure Marcos' participation, they sought family therapy.

In the first consultation with the family, Marcos denied that his use was frequent and reduced the negative impact that cocaine had in his life (quite common among substance users). At the same time he wanted his parents to pay his debts (a recurring pattern of response historically reinforced by his father). Understanding that Marcos' main complaint was the financial issue while his parents' complaint was cocaine use, the therapist proposed CM treatment using Marcos' need for financial help to reinforce his abstinence from cocaine. After a negotiation listening to all the points and considerations of the family members, a personalized CM strategy was developed based on a compromise after considering both Marcos and his family's needs/desire (it is very important that all those present in the therapy process participate and agree on the CM strategy to be employed).

The CM strategy developed consisted of the following actions: First, the debt was financed in 3 years with instalments of 4000 reais per month. From the renegotiation of the debt it was agreed that Marcos would do two urine tests per week until his debt was paid in full (a nurse was hired to do the urine tests since his family lives 3 h away from São Paulo). For each negative cocaine test Marcos would earn 150 reais. If the two tests of the same week were negative he would receive an additional 200 reais. Finally, if all the tests were negative during the month, Marcos would receive an additional 2000 reais. Thus, if all the tests of an entire month were negative for cocaine (total abstinence in this period), Marcos would earn exactly 4000 reais (value of the debt installment). On the other hand, a positive exam or not being submitted to an exam would result in a loss of 2350 reais in that month.

This reinforcement scheme was chosen to motivate total abstinence and not only the reduction of cocaine consumption. In addition, all of the amount earned by Marcos (paid by the parents in practice) would be destined directly to the payment of the debt. If Marcos could not remain 100% abstinent, it would be his responsibility to add the amount necessary for the payment of that month's installment. If this did not happen, Marcos' car would be taken by his parents and Marcos would only get it back after reaching one month of complete abstinence from cocaine. Finally, if he could not pay his debt (which in this case would also mean continuing to use cocaine), his car would be sold to pay his debt.

It is important to emphasize that Marcos, being of age, has the right to choose whether or not to use cocaine or to participate in the treatment. The main contingency that the treatment is proposing here is that Marcos' parents do not continue paying his expenses and debts if he continues using cocaine. In doing so, this contingency scheme uses positive (debt payment) and negative (withdrawal from the car) reinforcers to increase Marcos's abstinence response.

This treatment has been applied for exactly 15 months. In the first 3 months, Marcos showed an intermittent pattern and had 60% of his tests negative. During this period, he was able to use his own money to pay his total monthly debt in the first two months, but not in the third month (which led to losing his car in the fourth month). Since then, his performance has been excellent. In the 12 months that followed, Marcos was completely abstinent in 10 months, reached a 6-month sequence of continuous abstinence and at no time had more than two consecutive positive tests. Along with this, Marcos learned to control his spending and is paying his debt on time (either by demonstrating his abstinence or paying out of his own pocket). Finally, his professional career has improved, as has his relationship with his family members.

Final Considerations

CM is among the most effective treatments for SUD. CM is effective in promoting continued abstinence, decreasing substance use and increasing treatment adherence and participation.

Several studies in CM show that CM can be generalized to the treatment of several substances use disorders (e.g., cocaine, alcohol, heroin, tobacco) and different subpopulations (adolescents, pregnant women, individuals with severe mental health, homeless individuals). Efforts from the academic community, mental health providers, and society in general are needed to disseminate this form of treatment and encourage the implementation of CM as an integral part of the treatment offered in outpatient services for SUD in Brazil and abroad.

References

Aigner, T. G., & Balster, R. L. (1978). Choice behavior in rhesus monkeys: Cocaine vs. food. *Science, 201*, 534–535. https://doi.org/10.1126/science.96531

Amass, L., & Kamien, J. (2004). A tale of two cities: Financing two voucher programs for substance abusers through community donations. *Experimental and Clinical Psychopharmacoogy, 12*(2), 147–155. https://doi.org/10.1037/1064-1297.12.2.147

American Psychiatric Association (APA). (1994). *Diagnostic and statistical manual of mental disorders* (4th ed.). American Psychiatric Association.

Bigelow, G. E., Brooner, R. K., & Silverman, K. (1998). Competing motivations: Drug reinforcement vs non-drug reinforcement. *Journal of Psychopharmacology (Oxford, England), 12*(1), 8–14. https://doi.org/10.1177/026988119801200102

Budney, A. J. (1998). *National institute on drug abuse therapy manuals for drug addiction: Manual no. 2: A community reinforcement plus vouchers approach: Treating cocaine addiction*. National Institute on Drug Abuse.

Cahoon, D. D., & Cynthia, C. C. (1972). A learning approach to chronic drug use: Sources of reinforcement. *Behavior Therapy, 3*, 64–71. https://doi.org/10.1016/S0005-7894(72)80052-2

Chen, W., Hong, Y., Zou, X., McLaughlin, M. M., Xia, Y., & Ling, L. (2013). Effectiveness of prize-based contingency management in a methadone maintenance program in China. *Drug and Alcohol Dependence, 133*(1), 270–274. https://doi.org/10.1016/j.drugalcdep.2013.05.028

García-Fernández, G., Secades-Villa, R., García-Rodríguez, O., Alvarez-López, H., Sánchez-Hervás, E., Fernández-Hermida, J. R., & Fernández-Artamendi, S. (2011). Individual characteristics and response to Contingency Management treatment for cocaine addiction. *Psicothema, 23*(1), 114–118.

Goeder, N. E., & Guerin, G. F. (1991). Non-contingent electric footshock stress increases vulnerability to self-administer cocaine in rats. *Psychopharmacology, 114*, 63–70. https://doi.org/10.1007/BF02245445

Griffiths, R. R., Bigelow, G. E., & Henningfield, J. E. (1980). Similarities in animal and human drug-taking behavior. In N. K. Mello (Ed.), *Advances in substance abuse: Behavioral and biological research* (pp. 1–99). JAI Press, Inc..

Higgins, S. T. (1996). Some potential contributions of reinforcement and consumer-demand theory to reducing cocaine use. *Addictive Behaviors, 21*(6), 803–816. https://doi.org/10.1016/0306-4603(96)00037-8

Higgins, S. T. (1997). The influence of alternative reinforcers on cocaine use and abuse: A brief review. *Pharmacology, Biochemistry, and Behavior, 57*(3), 419–427. https://doi.org/10.1016/s0091-3057(96)00446-7

Higgins, S. T., & Petry, N. M. (1999). Contingency management. Incentives for sobriety. *Alcohol Research & Health: The Journal of the National Institute on Alcohol Abuse and Alcoholism, 23*(2), 122–127.

Higgins, S. T., & Silverman, K. E. (1999). *Motivating behavior change among illicit-drug abusers: Research on contingency management interventions*. American Psychological Association.

Higgins, S. T., Delaney, D. D., Budney, A. J., Bickel, W. K., Hughes, J. R., Foerg, F., & Fenwick, J. W. (1991). A behavioral approach to achieving initial cocaine abstinence. *The American Journal of Psychiatry, 148*(9), 1218–1224. https://doi.org/10.1176/ajp.148.9.1218

Higgins, S. T., Budney, A. J., Bickel, W. K., Hughes, J. R., Foerg, F., & Badger, G. (1993). Achieving cocaine abstinence with a behavioral approach. *The American Journal of Psychiatry, 150*(5), 763–769. https://doi.org/10.1176/ajp.150.5.763

Higgins, S. T., Budney, A. J., Bickel, W. K., Foerg, F. E., Donham, R., & Badger, G. J. (1994). Incentives improve outcome in outpatient behavioral treatment of cocaine dependence. *Archives of General Psychiatry, 51*(7), 568–576. https://doi.org/10.1001/archpsyc.1994.03950070060011

Higgins, S. T., Heil, S. H., & Lussier, J. P. (2004). Clinical implications of reinforcement as a determinant of substance use disorders. *Annual Review of Psychology, 55*, 431–461. https://doi.org/10.1146/annurev.psych.55.090902.142033

Jiang, H., Du, J., Wu, F., Wang, Z., Fan, S., Li, Z., Hser, Y. I., & Zhao, M. (2012). Efficacy of contingency management in improving retention and compliance to methadone maintenance treatment: A random controlled study. *Shanghai Archives of Psychiatry, 24*(1), 11–19. https://doi.org/10.3969/j.issn.1002-0829.2012.01.002

Kalivas, P. W., Volkow, N., & Seamans, J. (2005). Unmanageable motivation in addiction: A pathology in prefrontal-accumbens glutamate transmission. *Neuron, 45*(5), 647–650. https://doi.org/10.1016/j.neuron.2005.02.005

Lussier, J. P., Heil, S. H., Mongeon, J. A., Badger, G. J., & Higgins, S. T. (2006). A meta-analysis of voucher-based reinforcement therapy for substance use disorders. *Addiction (Abingdon, England), 101*(2), 192–203. https://doi.org/10.1111/j.1360-0443.2006.01311.x

Miguel, A. Q., Madruga, C. S., Cogo-Moreira, H., Yamauchi, R., Simões, V., da Silva, C. J., … Laranjeira, R. R. (2016). Contingency management is effective in promoting abstinence and retention in treatment among crack cocaine users in Brazil: A randomized controlled trial. *Psychology of Addictive Behaviors: Journal of the Society of Psychologists in Addictive Behaviors, 30*(5), 536–543. https://doi.org/10.1037/adb0000192

Miguel, A., Madruga, C. S., Cogo-Moreira, H., Yamauchi, R., Simões, V., Ribeiro, A., … Laranjeira, R. R. (2017). Contingency management targeting abstinence is effective in reducing depressive and anxiety symptoms among crack cocaine-dependent individuals. *Experimental and Clinical Psychopharmacology, 25*(6), 466–472. https://doi.org/10.1037/pha0000147

Miguel, A. Q. C., Madruga, C. S., Simões, V., Yamauchi, R., da Silva, C. J., Abdalla, R. R., … Laranjeira, R. (2018). Crack cocaine users views regarding treatment with contingency management in Brazil. *Substance Abuse Treatment, Prevention, and Policy, 13*(1), 7. https://doi.org/10.1186/s13011-018-0144-7

Miguel, A. Q. C., Madruga, C. S., Simões, V., Yamauchi, R., da Silva, C. J., McDonell, M., … Mari, J. J. (2019). Contingency management is effective in promoting abstinence and retention in treatment among crack cocaine users with a previous history of poor treatment response: A crossover trial. *Psicologia: Reflexão e Crítica, 32*(1), 14. https://doi.org/10.1186/s41155-019-0127-2

Petitjean, S. A., Dürsteler-MacFarland, K. M., Krokar, M. C., Strasser, J., Mueller, S. E., Degen, B., … Farronato, N. S. (2014). A randomized, controlled trial of combined cognitive-behavioral therapy plus prize-based contingency management for cocaine dependence. *Drug and Alcohol Dependence, 145*, 94–100. https://doi.org/10.1016/j.drugalcdep.2014.09.785

Petry, N. M. (2000). A comprehensive guide to the application of contingency management procedures in clinical settings. *Drug and Alcohol Dependence, 58*(1–2), 9–25. https://doi.org/10.1016/s0376-8716(99)00071-x

Petry, N. M., & Heyman, G. M. (1995). Behavioral economics of concurrent ethanol-sucrose and sucrose reinforcement in the rat: Effects of altering variable-ratio requirements. *Journal of the Experimental Analysis of Behavior, 64*(3), 331–359. https://doi.org/10.1901/jeab.1995.64-331

Pilling, S., Strang, J., Gerada, C., & NICE. (2007). Psychosocial interventions and opioid detoxification for drug misuse: Summary of NICE guidance. *BMJ (Clinical Research Ed.), 335*(7612), 203–205. https://doi.org/10.1136/bmj.39265.639641.AD

Prendergast, M., Podus, D., Finney, J., Greenwell, L., & Roll, J. (2006). Contingency management for treatment of substance use disorders: A meta-analysis. *Addiction (Abingdon, England), 101*(11), 1546–1560. https://doi.org/10.1111/j.1360-0443.2006.01581.x

Secades-Villa, R., García-Rodríguez, O., & Fernández-Hermida, J. R. (2015). Contingency management for substance use disorders in Spain: Implications for research and practice. *Preventive Medicine, 80*, 82–88. https://doi.org/10.1016/j.ypmed.2015.07.001

Skinner, B. F. (1969). *Contingencies of reinforcement: A theoretical analysis*. Meredith.

Stitzer, M., & Bigelow, G. (1978). Contingency management in a methadone maintenance program: Availability of reinforcers. *The International Journal of the Addictions, 13*(5), 737–746. https://doi.org/10.3109/10826087809039299

Volkow, N. D., Wang, G. J., & Fowler, J. S. (1997). Imaging studies of cocaine in the human brain and studies of the cocaine addict. *Annals of the New York Academy of Sciences, 820*, 41–55. https://doi.org/10.1111/j.1749-6632.1997.tb46188.x

Volkow, N. D., Wang, G. J., Fischman, M. W., Foltin, R., Fowler, J. S., Franceschi, D., … Pappas, N. (2000). Effects of route of administration on cocaine induced dopamine transporter blockade in the human brain. *Life sciences, 67*(12), 1507–1515. https://doi.org/10.1016/S0024-3205(00)00731-1

Weaver, T., Metrebian, N., Hellier, J., Pilling, S., Charles, V., Little, N., … Strang, J. (2014). Use of contingency management incentives to improve completion of hepatitis B vaccination in people undergoing treatment for heroin dependence: A cluster randomised trial. *Lancet (London, England), 384*(9938), 153–163. https://doi.org/10.1016/S0140-6736(14)60196-3

Wolffgramm, J., & Heyne, A. (1995). From controlled drug intake to loss of control: The irreversible development of drug addiction in the rat. *Behavioural Brain Research, 70*(1), 77–94. https://doi.org/10.1016/0166-4328(95)00131-c

Chapter 8
Cue Exposure Therapy for Substance Use: A Complement to Functional Analysis

Rodrigo Noia Mattos Montan and Roberto Alves Banaco

Introduction

Substance use disorder (SUD) manifests itself as a harmful condition in the lives of millions of Brazilians, and it has become an area of study of different approaches that investigate the acquisition and maintenance of drug use and drug dependence. In 2015, the Brazilian population showed a significant number of people who needed treatment: around 2.3 million people between the age of 12 and 65 showed dependence to alcohol and 1.2 million to other substances (marijuana, solvents, benzodiazepine tranquilizers, amphetamine-type stimulants, cocaine, crack, opiates, and ketamine—except alcohol and tobacco). These numbers represent a prevalence of 1.5% of the population for alcohol dependence and 0.8% for other substances dependence (Bastos et al., 2017). An estimate of 1.6 million individuals received treatment in their lifetime for substance use, which accounts for 1.1% of the Brazilian population (Bastos et al., 2017, p. 141).

Among the different approaches and theoretical models that study SUD, we can find cognitive behavioral therapy (CBT) (Zanelatto & Laranjeira, 2018), motivational interviewing (Miller & Rollnick, 2012), psychopharmacological intervention (McKim & Hancock, 2012), contingency management (Higgins et al., 2007), and behavior-analytic approach (Banaco & Montan, 2018). The last one focuses on the topic incorporating practices from different clinical models, namely functional analytical psychotherapy (FAP) (Souza & Oshiro, 2019), acceptance and commitment therapy (ACT) (DuFrene & Wilson, 2012), contingency management (Miguel et al., 2016), dialectical behavior therapy (DBT) (Melo et al., 2018), and cue exposure therapy (CET) (Conklin & Tiffany, 2002). CET is an intervention proposal that is

R. N. M. Montan (✉) · R. A. Banaco
Associação Paradigma – Centro de Ciências e Tecnologia do Comportamento (Paradigma Association – Center for Sciences and Technology of Behavior), São Paulo, Brazil
e-mail: roberto@paradigmaac.org

S. M. Oliani et al. (eds.), *Behavior Analysis and Substance Dependence*,
https://doi.org/10.1007/978-3-030-75961-2_8

still scarcely used in the clinic for substance abuse, and its effectiveness remains under investigation (Conklin & Tiffany, 2002; Martin et al., 2010).

Despite being a topic of debate, CET studies with SUD have contrasting results from those obtained by exposure and response prevention (ERP)[1] in psychological treatments applied to other psychiatric disorders. ERP has proven effective in the treatment of phobias, posttraumatic stress disorders, and obsessive-compulsive disorder (Botella et al., 2017; Maples-Keller et al., 2017; Opriş et al., 2012). Given this scenario, we must investigate the gaps present in studies on the topic and develop methodological designs to fill such gaps. This chapter aims to shed light on the theoretical model on which CET is based, its clinical implications in substance use, and methodological issues present in CET studies.

Theoretical Model of Cue Exposure Therapy

Classical Conditioning on the Substance Effect

In literature, CET is referred to as different terms, the most common being: *cue exposure* and *cue exposure therapy*. The term *cue exposure* refers to a method that assesses the degree of dependence (referred to as *cue reactivity)* and assists the patient to identify high-risk stimuli to relapse. In experimental models, the same terms are used to study responses of the organism in the presence of conditioned stimuli (Childress et al., 1988; Saladin et al., 2006). The term *cue exposure therapy* is commonly used in studies that aim to habituate or extinguish conditioned responses, both at operant and respondent levels (Mellentin et al., 2017).

The term cue exposure (CE) refers to a basic process contemplated by the classical conditioning theory (or Pavlovian conditioning). To elucidate this process, let us take cocaine –an unconditioned stimulus (US)— as an example. When administered by any access route (intranasal, intravenous, or pulmonary/smoked), it elicits unconditioned responses (UR) that require no previous learning history. Any organism that ingests cocaine will show URs such as altered heart rate and body temperature, and feelings of euphoria. A neutral stimulus that has been previously paired with cocaine use acquires properties of a conditioned stimulus (CS). For instance, if cocaine is always administered where there is a "bag of cocaine" –inside a restroom,

[1] Here, the results from the studies of both treatments are compared because in Brazil, ERP and CET are treated as the same therapy, being different from the international literature that understand them as different treatments. The international literature specifies ERP as a therapy offered for treating posttraumatic stress and anxiety disorders, such as phobias and obsessive-compulsive disorder, while CET is referred to as a treatment offered only for SUD. Despite having different names, ERP and CET base their practice on a process, contemplated by the classical conditioning theory, that includes extinction training through stimulus exposure and response prevention. Therefore, in Brazil, for having the same theoretical basis and methods, ERP and CET are seen as the same and both are referred to under the same term "*exposure and response prevention therapy.*"

in the presence of a user friend etc.—it will cause these environmental cues –if repeatedly associated to drug use—to acquire a CS function. When the organism is reexposed to these stimuli –even in the absence of the US (cocaine)—a conditioned response (CR) is elicited, which may consist of a change in heart rate and body temperature, and a feeling of euphoria. The more often the stimulus is paired with cocaine, the more likely the CR is to occur and greater is its intensity when the organism is reexposed to it. According to Drummond et al. (1995), when a CS is presented, its related CR depends on the organism's history with it. As they have eliciting and evoking properties, drug-related CSs increase the probability of active drug-seeking and self-administration. (Drummond et al., 1995). This happens because stimuli paired with substance use are followed by aversive bodily changes, which only cease after its ingestion. Thus, a history of operant conditioning begins, involving seeking and finding the substance, followed by its use, which removes aversive body states. For this reason, they acquire the function of motivating operations (MOs), given that, in the presence of CSs, substance-seeking and self-administration are more strongly evoked –that is, their occurrence becomes more likely when CSs are present rather than absent. To assess the strength of a response, elements such as latency, rate, and (when subjected to extinction) resistance can be measured (Michael, 1980). MOs acquire control over responses because the operant conditioning history of ingesting the drug produced both negative and sometimes positive reinforcing consequences. A probable positive reinforcing consequence – which further strengthens substance-seeking and self-administration—is the effect the substance has on the organism, producing states of pleasure. A probable negative reinforcing consequence, on the other hand, is the removal of CRs due to their aversive properties – and this is proof that they are aversive: they become the MO for their own removal, through the operant response of substance-seeking and use.

Pavlov (1927) was the first to demonstrate and suggest studies on classical conditioning and drug use in an experiment that administered morphine into dogs. Other researchers –contrary to mentalist approaches of the time—demonstrated that stimuli that signal the opportunity for substance use elicit CRs at a respondent level, as well as evoke operant drug-seeking responses (e.g., Siegel, 1979; Stewart et al., 1984; Wikler, 1948). Theorists present three basic ways in which CSs can control substance use by eliciting: (1) CRs similar to withdrawal symptoms (e.g., Wikler, 1948); (2) CRs that occur in the opposite direction of the effect caused by the substance (Siegel, 1975); and (3) CRs that occur in the same direction as the effect caused by the substance (Stewart et al., 1984).

The effect of substances on the responses of organisms help us to understand some aspects of SUD such as substance-seeking, withdrawal symptoms, substance craving,[2] and relapses. As shown previously, whereas one theoretical model infers that CRs are opposite to the effects caused by the drug, the other shows CRs to be drug-like and similar to those effects. Wikler (1948) described in his studies that

[2] According to Banaco and Montan (2017) drug-seeking itself (operant behavior) to eliminate withdrawal symptoms is referred to as *craving*.

stimuli preceding drug use can elicit reflex responses and evoke operant responses similar to the effects of the drug itself and noted that antecedent stimuli can cause opposite effects to those of the drug. When studying dogs self-administering morphine, he observed that substance use was maintained due to its pleasurable effects, thus having a positive reinforcing function on the response. He also noted that the use of morphine was maintained due to its ability to attenuate and remove aversive symptoms from the withdrawal effects, negatively reinforcing the response. In an attempt to explain relapse, the author proposed the *conditioned withdrawal model* contributing to the understanding of the role of respondent conditioning on substance use –a view that influences behavioral approaches until today. Wikler (1948) demonstrated that several morphine CSs elicited CRs that resemble morphine withdrawal symptoms, and relapse was interpreted as a response that produces relief from aversive withdrawal symptoms.

When proposing a similar model, Siegel (1975) stated that drug-related CRs occur in the opposite direction to their unconditional effects –model commonly known as the *conditioned preparatory* or *compensatory response*. Although Siegel (1975) conceptualizes and observes drug CRs in an alternative way, his view seems to have been influenced mainly by Winkler's model. On the other hand, Glautier and Remington (1995), when analyzing the two models, explain that Wikler's *conditioned withdrawal model* and Siegel's *conditioned compensatory response model* are similar. Firstly, both recognize that the substance has a biphasic action –that is, the initial effects of the substance on the organism are identical to the effect of the substance itself. Secondly, in both models, negative reinforcement is the primary mechanism by which CRs contribute to substance use. That is, compensatory response processes are given as aversive –just as the symptoms of conditioned withdrawal—in a way that the aversive state is reduced by ingesting the substance, thereby negatively reinforcing its use. However, Siegel (1989, p. 158) argues that the term *conditioned compensatory response* can in fact be called *withdrawal symptom*. Nevertheless, Cunningham (1998, p. 250) classifies both models as parts of the same whole. Although similar, Siegel's model presents an essential characteristic regarding the interaction of tolerance upon the effect of the substance and how it is modulated by the presence of CSs during substance use. It is argued that drug-opposite CRs added to the drug URs result in the *conditioned tolerance effect*. (Glautier & Remington, 1995).

Conversely, a second alternative model exposed by Cunningham (1998) regard CRs as similar to the effects of the substance. The model suggests that USs, when paired to substance use such as alcohol and morphine, elicit physiological responses equal or similar to the effects of the substance itself (Lynch et al., 1973). This was observed by Pavlov (1927) when studying the effect of respondent conditioning on substance use. He observed in his experiment that a hypodermic morphine injection resulted in nausea, salivary secretion, followed by vomiting and sleepiness. After 5–6 days of morphine administration, stimuli prior to morphine injections –such as the presence of the experimenter, the opening of the syringe box, fur-trimming over a small skin area, alcohol sterilization, and even the injection of other fluids—sufficed to produce CRs similar to URs.

Although Pavlov registered supposedly aversive symptoms, the second model also shows that exposure to drug CSs elicit drug-like CRs that increase the reinforcing value of the stimulus associated to it. Thus, CSs promote the evocation of drug-seeking or self-administration responses just as priming doses of the substance do, along with reinstating responses of self-administration after extinction (Cunningham, 1998; de Wit & Stewart, 1981). In a study by De Wit and Stewart (1981), mice were trained to self-administer cocaine (1 mg/kg/injection), and trained in daily test sessions of self-administration and extinction. This stage was followed by either the administration of priming doses of cocaine or exposure to drug CSs during extinction, and measurement of the first self-administration response latency. They observed that drug CSs restore self-administration responses just as priming doses of cocaine reinstate self-administration after extinction.

Stewart et al. (1984) argued that "compulsive drug use, even of opiates, is maintained by appetitive motivational processes, that is, by the generating of positively affective motivational states" (p. 252). This model assumes that appetitive and pleasurable effects of drug CRs establish the use of the substance as reinforcing, thus referring less to the effects of negative reinforcers produced from the relief of aversive withdrawal symptoms. However, despite being different models, one assuming CRs as drug-opposite and the other drug-like, both emphasize that reexposure to CSs associated to the context of drug use produces relapses during prolonged periods of abstinence. In other words, both models explain relapse (Cunningham, 1998). On the other hand, only the *compensatory response model* explains the tolerance process, which is described as the need for a gradually greater intake of substance, during the opportunities for its use, in order to obtain its same effects (see a more detailed description below).

Besides constituting theoretical models that entail behavioral processes involved in substance use, the literature still has been studying the direction of CRs starting from psychological or physiological states in the organism (e.g., Niaura et al., 1988; Schwarz & Cunningham, 1990; Siegel, 1979).

Glautier and Remington (1995) suggest that the variable of interest in CE studies should be the substance use itself, since it is in the interaction between respondent and operant behavior that the behavior of drug-seeking and self-administration of substance occurs. Therefore, when we consider the variables that influence not only substance use and the role of tolerance upon the increase of drug intake but also the patient's relapse during abstinence, it is known that respondent and operant conditioning play an important role in the acquisition and maintenance of abusive substance use.

Conditioned Compensatory Response and Its Role in Tolerance, Relapse, and Overdose

The same mechanisms that explain conditioned compensatory responses also explain tolerance. When performing manipulations to assess the effect of drugs, Siegel (1975, 1979, 1989) observed that drug CSs increase motivation for their use as they elicit CRs in the opposite direction of URs, and that the presence of CSs interferes in the effect of the drug –which helps to understand the development of drug tolerance by the organism. When a subject is said to have acquired tolerance to a substance, it means that he or she must use progressively larger doses to achieve the desired effects. The use of larger doses has an effect in determining abusive substance use (Glautier & Remington, 1995). We can assume that if substance use happens in the presence of CSs, its effect would be attenuated by compensatory CRs that precedes the systemic stimulation of the substance in the organism. When the pairing between the stimuli present in the context of substance use during its administration and the systemic stimulation of the drug in the organism is strengthened by frequent use, the substance is expected to have its effects increasingly cancelled, given the increased magnitude of compensatory CRs (Siegel, 1979). In this theoretic model, tolerance to drug effects is determined by situational factors (Glautier & Remington, 1995). This effect was demonstrated in a study by Siegel et al. (1978) in which mice showed larger tolerance to morphine's analgesic effects when the administration occurred in situations in which the administration had been paired with the contexts of use. They also found that tolerance to morphine effects was cancelled when the drug administration setting suffered changes.

To illustrate an interaction between the effects of the substance and compensatory CRs, Banaco and Montan (2018) adapted and transformed a figure from Siegel (1979) (see Fig. 8.1). Figure 8.1 shows the effects of substances (panel A); the CSs

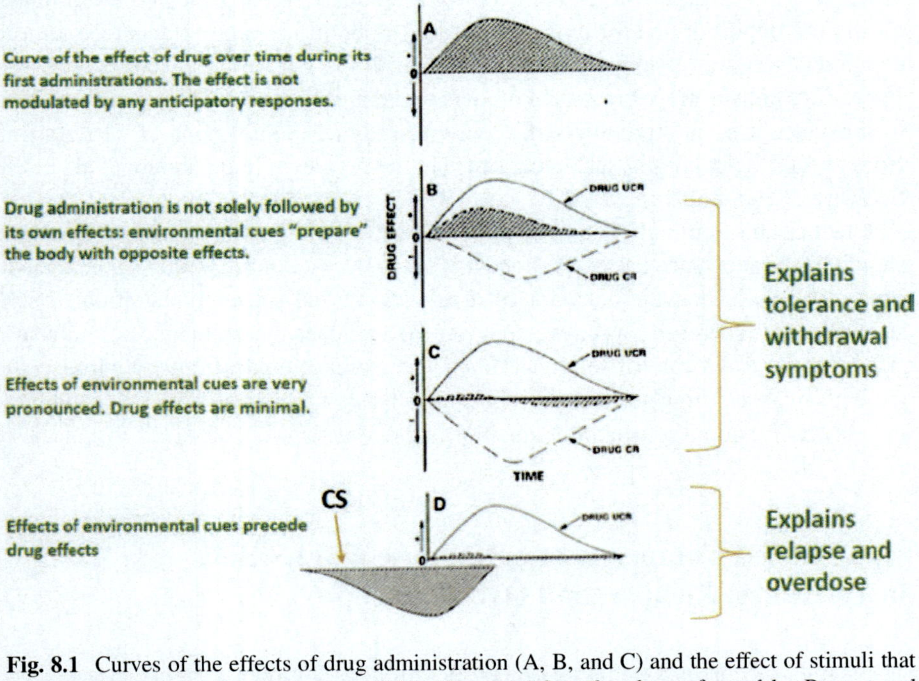

Fig. 8.1 Curves of the effects of drug administration (A, B, and C) and the effect of stimuli that consistently precede drug intake (graph D). (Source: Adapted and transformed by Banaco and Montan (2018) from Siegel (1979))

that precede drug intake and their effects on tolerance (panel B); and withdrawal symptoms, relapse, and overdose (panels C and D). In the figure, the effect of the substance (DRUG UCR – drug unconditional response) is represented by an increased response level (+) from baseline and the drug-compensatory CR (DRUG CR – drug conditional response) is represented by a decreased response level (−) in the opposite direction of the DRUG UCR. Figure 8.1 aims to illustrate that the effect of the substance depends on the interaction of the two types of responses that occur, the effects of one being opposite to the effects of the other.

Panel A shows the effect of the substance in the occasion of its first administration. In this case, the substance is not conditioned or associated with stimuli or environmental cues that precede its intake –the substance then has a full effect. The positive curve (+) represents the effect of the substance that increases until its peak and decreases according to the substance's pharmacokinetics due to the time elapsed since its ingestion. Panel B shows that, when there is an increase in the frequency of administration of the substance, and the ingestion response becomes conditioned by environmental stimuli, such ingestion of the substance is no longer accompanied just by pharmacological URs itself, it is then followed by drug-compensatory CRs, represented by the negative curve (−) in the graph. Panel B also shows that the effect resulting from substance use (UR – represented in hatch) is smaller than the one observed in its first administration because it becomes attenuated by compensatory CR, resulting in the tolerance effect. Panel C demonstrates the interaction between drug UR and compensatory/preparatory CR when there is a history of several substance administration events in a context with the same environmental cues. Drug UR now becomes minimal in the presence of drug CR, demonstrating a high tolerance to the drug. Panel C also illustrates a biphasic effect: a small effect of the substance intake is followed by another effect in the opposite direction of drug UR. As an example, when mice continued to receive morphine doses, they became tolerant to its analgesic effects and started to experience hyperalgesia (Siegel, 1975). This mechanism also explains withdrawal symptoms and active substance-seeking, because a dose that produces minimal effects also produces subsequently compensatory responses, which are themselves aversive to the body. When this happens, substance-seeking would have the function of eliminating withdrawal symptoms caused by the minimum dose. Panel D shows that when the organism is exposed to CSs before ingestion, they produce uncomfortable conditioned preparatory responses through reflex mechanisms, and that, depending on the substance, it elicits tachycardia, sweating, hypoglycemia, changes in breathing and decreased oxygen, among others. This mechanism explains withdrawal, which are symptoms that appear when the body is exposed to stimuli that precede the ingestion of the drug, but without taking it. Let us take as an example a person with heroin use disorder who had its material (spoons, syringes, and lighters) paired with the ingestion of the drug. When coming into contact with these stimuli, compensatory responses –which have the function of homeostasis and serve to protect the organism from the harmful effects of heroin action—end up eliciting aversive symptoms in the absence of the drug, such as hyperthermia, chills, diarrhea, and hyperalgesia. For aversive CRs to be eliminated, the person resorts to substance use, thereby negatively reinforcing drug-seeking (Banaco & Montan, 2018).

Panel D also illustrates that the amount that previously produced positive or negative reinforcing effects now has a minimal effect, which explains why the individual needs to use increasing amounts to experience the reinforcing effects of the substance. This results in a further drug-seeking and an increased dosing, thus establishing a state of dependence (Banaco & Montan, 2018).

According to Banaco and Montan (2018), the action of compensatory CRs may also account for an overdose. In their article, they present a hypothetical case in which an individual always ingests the same dose in the same situations –thus in the presence of the same CSs— and, on the account of that, has already developed tolerance, along with being used to ingesting a known quantity that is sufficient to achieve the intended effect under these conditions. Following the authors' example:

> (…) a cocaine dependent person knows how many "bags" they can sniff to achieve behavioral arousal. As he or she goes to the usual place of consumption (bar, club etc.), their body gradually prepares itself, through anticipatory responses, for the drug to enter the organism, and "craving" increases. However, if cocaine is presented outside their usual consumption environment (for example, in the workplace) which had not been associated with use, the commonly consumed amount will have a much greater effect than the intended familiar one, thus causing overdose with serious risks. This is because the stimuli that compose the work environment do not have the power to elicit the compensatory effects of the drug in anticipation (p. 125).

By understanding the role of compensatory CRs in SUD, we could see that the Pavlovian conditioning theory explains tolerance, withdrawal symptoms, and overdose. We shall now address the role of respondent processes in relapse. Respondent processes in substance use states that compensatory CRs tend not to dissipate over time without extinction. CSs can lose the control over CRs if presented many times without being followed by USs –in this case, the drug. For CSs to lose their ability to elicit CRs, several CS presentations without pairing it with the US (drug) are necessary. This implies that treatments with long abstinence periods in places that have no occurrence of drug CSs fail to extinguish CRs. In other words, if an individual presents compensatory CRs in an environment that has drug cues, removing the individual from this eliciting environment for long "detoxification" periods does not affect the ability of drug CSs to elicit CRs, as the extinction of the CS–US pairing does not occur. If individuals spend long hospitalization periods in rehabilitation clinics, upon returning to their natural environment –previously associated with substance use—they are likely to present compensatory CRs, which can be eliminated through using the substance, thus configuring a relapse (Siegel, 1979).

Even if an individual has been admitted to rehabilitation clinics, several drug CSs may be present in the seclusion environment. For instance, heroin users may require spoons and lighters to administer the substance, which can be found in the hospitalization environment. Even if they elicit withdrawal and craving CRs, they will not be followed by heroin in this setting. Presenting these anticipatory stimuli (spoons and lighters) without pairing them to drug use over time causes them to lose their control over the body that becomes habituated to them (by extinguishing the CS–US pairing), thus ceasing to present withdrawal and craving responses when such stimuli are present. When these individuals return to their natural drug use environment, they are reexposed to another group of stimuli that had not been present in the treatment environment, thus keeping intact those stimuli pairing relations established until the moment before admittance. These can be former user partners or even the room where they used to do drugs at home. All those stimuli would be sufficient to elicit withdrawal or craving CRs, and now these stimuli that were not submitted to the extinction process would cause unpleasant states and drug-seeking responses, and by doing so, drug use (relapse) can help eliminate these aversive states (Banaco & Montan, 2018).

Clinical Implications of Cue Exposure

Findings and theories derived from the literature that investigate the role of respondent conditioning on substance use have influenced clinical practice and research within the field of behavior analysis. In the treatment context, CE is studied and applied within CET. It systematically exposes substance abusers to drug CSs, usually within a clinical setting that prevents its ingestion, thus contributing to the extinction of responses elicited by drug related environmental stimuli. The rationale behind this approach is based on the principles of respondent extinction processes. The classic conditioning literature presents great evidence that repeated exposures to a CS in the absence of the US decreases the strength of CRs and extinguishes its conditioned function, thus returning the CS to a state of neutral stimulus for the target response. The objective is to reduce physiological reactions (compensatory CRs) caused by CSs that are present in real life environments, with the benefit of lowering the discomfort caused by the eliciting stimulus, which, in general, produces craving. It also tends to reduce the subsequent seeking for abusive drug use (now operant), which is ultimately reinforced by the removal or reduction of aversive symptoms present when individuals experience craving (Drummond et al., 1995).

To assess the conditioning properties of stimuli associated with the drug, URs and CRs are deliberately elicited in a controlled environment with the presentation of CSs historically paired with the natural substance use environment. The most commonly collected UR and CR measures are physiological responses –such as heart rate, skin conductance, and temperature—and self-report measures –via questionnaires and analog scales that assess urge ratings for a particular substance (Carter & Tiffany, 1999). CET consists of presenting CSs represented in the form of photos and videos, as well as auditory, in vivo, imaginal, and virtual stimuli (Carter & Tiffany, 1999; Saladin et al., 2006).

Kinds of Cue Exposure

As explained earlier, CE is commonly used as an initial assessment method that investigates the level of dependence by observing cue reactivity and helps the patient to identify high-risk stimuli for relapse. CET, on the other hand, is an intervention method whose goal is to habituate or extinguish CRs. Both consist of presenting CSs with the use of appropriate stimuli that, human subjects, were regularly present either during drug use, preparation, or anticipation of drug intake (Carter & Tiffany, 1999; Saladin et al., 2006).

In the field of substance use, the variety of stimuli conditioned to substance intake and its effect is broad, which makes identifying all CSs an unattainable task. According to Drummond et al. (1995), stimuli that can be paired with the use of substances can be both *exteroceptive* and *interoceptive*. *Exteroceptive stimuli* can include those that are present before ingesting the substance, such as sight, smell, or taste of the alcoholic beverage or cigarette, sight of crack pipe, or crack rock itself. *Exteroceptive stimuli* may also include drug-taking rituals, which involve the preparation or administration of the substance before ingestion; advertisements of legal substances; seeing a place of consumption; listening to a musical stimulus associated with drug use; and temporal stimuli –such as the time of day or day of the week when the episode of drug use usually occurs. *Interoceptive stimuli* range from sensations of the substance entering the body – e.g., passing through the stomach or nasal airways—to the effects of the substance on neuroreceptors. A dose of the substance can also function as an MO and evoke successive self-administration responses. This effect is known as the *priming dose effect*, which can be observed in alcohol users who, after a long period of abstinence, avoid the first sip in order not to evoke further self-administration responses. *Interoceptive stimuli* can also include moods or emotions –such as anger, sadness, or euphoria—and thoughts—such as self-constructed rules about the effects of the substance. Other stimuli that can be considered as interoceptive are withdrawal symptoms that occur a few hours after the effect of the substance in the body ceases and, according to the literature already presented here, leads the individual back into contact with CSs that produce compensatory CRs. Regardless of which of these orders the stimulus belongs –public or private—both exteroceptive and interoceptive stimuli can acquire a function of motivating operation and/or eliciting stimulus, producing effect upon responses at the operant and respondent level.

Given the wide variety and properties of stimuli that are conditioned to substance use, researchers and clinical psychologists use different forms of stimulus exposure in an attempt to access and present them in experimental and clinical settings (Araújo & Lopes, 2013; Monti et al., 2002; Saladin et al., 2006). To assess the level of dependence through cue reactivity and/or the need and choice of therapeutic intervention, stimuli are most commonly presented in the form of photos, videos, audios, in vivo, imaginal, and virtual stimulation (Bordnick et al., 2009; Carter & Tiffany, 1999). Photographic stimuli show two-dimensional images of people using the substance or the image of the substance itself, for example. Video stimuli present images of people performing drug rituals of preparing and administering the substance either in places of use or others that have been related to the effect of the substance. Auditory stimuli present the sound of people talking about the substance, the sound of it being served, prepared, and ingested, or sounds that surround drug use environments (sexual intercourse, for example). In vivo stimulation presents the substance itself or a simulated substance with the same appearance, as well as the material used to administer the drug –which may be glasses or cups with alcohol, paraphernalia kit for smoked drugs containing pipe, lighter, or rolling paper. In in vivo presentations, the individual is asked to handle the material and perform the preparation ritual without using the substance. They are also instructed to smell it and describe its properties that trigger the desire to use it.

Due to the difficulty in accessing and bringing certain stimuli to a clinical setting – such as places or people who are linked to substance use—imaginal stimulation has been used as an alternative to circumvent this obstacle. Patients are asked to close their eyes and imagine situations associated with drug use, such as family conflicts, induction of emotional states, imagine themselves buying the substance from the dealer, or inside a bar or market.

Finally, CE and CET also use virtual stimuli. In this case, the patient is immersed in a three-dimensional virtual environment specially created for this application. The stimulation occurs through the presentation of places where people use substances, virtual manipulation of the substance, and access to situations that present social pressure –such as offers and invitations to use the substance.

Topographies

In the study with psychoactive substances, cue exposure results in reactions that occur at both respondent and operant levels and, among the operant, also at verbal levels. Each of them can be measured by certain instruments that, taken together, form a more comprehensive assessment of the target problem.

As means to assess respondent responses, the effects of CE have been observed through: heart rate, respiration, body temperature (Childress et al., 1988); sweat gland activity (galvanic skin resistance, skin conductance, etc.) (Carter & Tiffany, 1999); salivation (MacKillop & Lisman, 2008); and limbic activation (amygdala, anterior cingulate, temporal pole, hippocampus, and orbitofrontal cortex) (Childress et al., 1999).

We can also find measures of responses at a verbal operant level. Martin et al. (2010) gathered studies that used craving analog scales to obtain verbal reports on private events associated with the predisposition to emit drug-seeking or drug administration. On analog scales, craving levels are scored from 0 to 10, where 0 means "feeling no urge to use substances" and 10 means "extreme urge to use substances." Analog scales are also used to measure self-confidence reports –a term that refers to how much the client estimates the probability of exercising self-control by not using the substance if available. It is assessed on a scale from 0 to 10, where 0 means "feeling not at all confident in remaining abstinent if the drug were available," and 10 means "feeling extremely confident in remaining abstinent if the drug were available."

The authors also present studies that evaluate operant and verbal responses through follow-ups obtained 6–12 months after participants were submitted to CET. They assessed use reduction, abstinence maintenance, and self-confidence through questionnaires that investigate craving and other response rates during follow-up. They found no evidence to support that the efficacy of CET is superior to other forms of substance use treatment, but it has also not been shown to be ineffective. In fact, subjects who underwent CET showed significant improvement in relation to baseline, although these improvements do not differ from other treatment conditions.

Since some studies showed a craving reduction through extinction techniques in smoking treatments (Park et al., 2014), and few long-term effects in alcohol users (Mellentin et al., 2017), we can conclude that more attention should be given to methodological issues of the interventions and more studies should be designed to address the effects of renewal, spontaneous recovery, and reinstatement of extinct responses, as well as the failure to extinguish the most salient conditioned cues. All these processes would show the limitations of the technique upon the results.

Methodological Issues of CET and Effectiveness Data

Conklin and Tiffany (2002) examined 18 studies on the effectiveness of CET on SUD conducted between 1980 and 2002 and concluded that there was little evidence to support its effectiveness. Other authors identified methodological issues in its application and suggested innovations for the technique through virtual reality, as well as research that considers differences between subjects, and/or the use of pharmacological approaches to increase the impact of CET (Martin et al., 2010). Many researchers, however, argue that CET has the potential to be further studied if new parameters are discovered, for example, number of exposure sessions, use of multiple contexts, if appropriate stimuli are used, or if combined with other types of therapy (Bouton & Ricker, 1994; Cunningham, 1998; Gunther et al., 1998; Havermans & Jansen, 2003; Kim et al., 2015; Monti & Rohsenow, 1999; Rohsenow et al., 2001; Xue et al., 2012).

Conklin and Tiffany (2002) also studied processes that threaten learned extinction and emphasize that, with the study of these phenomena, relapse can be better understood and addressed.

Pavlov (1927), had already described that repeated non-reinforced reexposures to CSs do not break the learned CS–US relation. The initial idea that extinction is "unlearning" a CS–US relationship was then replaced by the notion that extinction never occurs entirely. It replaces a learning experience with a new one, but once a CS–US relationship has been learned, it remains intact. What is observed is that new associations with the original CS can be developed (Conklin & Tiffany, 2002) and can become more prominent than the old ones if more strongly reinforced.

We can also find the description of several factors or processes that threaten the development and maintenance of extinction training acquired during CET. The most important being: the renewal effect, spontaneous recovery, reinstatement, and failing to extinguish the most salient stimuli.

The renewal effect refers to the reappearance of an extinct response in a context different from the one in which the CET occurred. If a CS is paired with a US in context 1 and the same CS is presented and extinguished in context 2, after returning to the original context 1, the extinct response can be renewed (Bouton & Ricker, 1994). Consider a cocaine user who uses drug at home (context A) and receives CET sessions with in vivo stimulation of the kit of drug use in a hospital room (context B). After discharge, when returning home (context A) and being reexposed to the drug kit, he or she relapses, which is called *renewal of response*. Cunningham (1998) suggests that a solution to this problem would be to conduct CET in as many contexts as possible. Animal research found that, when the extinction process is performed in multiple contexts, the effects of renewal are attenuated. Animals that received extinction training in several new contexts and were then tested in the original conditioning context exhibited responses indicating extinction. These studies suggest that extinguishing conditioned responses in multiple contexts increases the generalization of extinction (Chelonis et al., 1999; Gunther et al., 1998). Despite not corroborating with these results, studies with humans have quite inconsistent findings, sometimes showing renewal effects, sometimes not. The fact that some studies demonstrate no renewal effects shows that extinction can generalize to other contexts (Barnier, 2015; Collins & Brandon, 2002; MacKillop & Lisman, 2008; Stasiewicz et al., 2007; Thewissen et al., 2006).

In contrast to the renewal effect –which occurs when changing contexts—spontaneous recovery happens due to the time elapsed between extinction training and reexposure to CS in the very context in which the pairing happened (Conklin & Tiffany, 2002). Therefore, to attenuate the effects of spontaneous recovery, the interval between CET sessions should be spaced, the number of exposure episodes to the stimulus at each session should be reduced, as well as the exposure time between sessions.

The reinstatement of extinct responses occurs when there is reexposure to the US after extinction. Similar to the renewal of response –in which the emergence of extinguished responses occurs in the presence of the CS—the reinstatement of extinguished responses occurs in the presence of the US. Although the reinstatement of responses can be extinguished more quickly with CET, this phenomenon implies that extinguished CSs also regain a function of eliciting responses, even when there is no pairing between US and CS after extinction. In other words, small substance doses reinstate extinguished physiological responses and the eliciting function of CSs for these responses. (from de Wit & Stewart, 1981).

Therefore, when a CS elicits a CR similar to an UR, it can elicit CRs that resemble the effect of the substance itself and promote renewal of self-administration or drug-seeking responses, just as small doses of the substance reinstate self-administration after extinction (de Wit & Stewart, 1981). Individuals may have contact with small doses of the substance indirectly by taking medicine that contains a small amount of the substance or produce analogous effects. For example, an individual with alcohol use disorder who has reached extinction of CRs through CET, and is abstinent for 3 months, free of craving either in the presence or absence of alcohol environmental cues, when in contact with a cough medicine (containing alcohol), may reinstate extinguished responses. Now, when in the presence of alcohol CSs, they may relapse. Any analogous substance to alcohol –such as anxiolytic drugs—may be enough to reinstate extinguished responses as they have similar effects to those of alcohol on the gabaminergic system (Mellentin et al., 2017). Taking into account the effect of reinstatement of responding, we must consider that CET is not recommended for patients whose goal is to reduce alcohol or any other substance intake to a moderate level, but rather to those patients who aim to achieve abstinence.

A promising study outlines a procedure that intervenes on memory reconsolidation (in behavioral terms: responding again to CSs) thus producing an attenuated effect over the reinstatement, renewal, and spontaneous recovery of extinguished responding. Heroin users who had their memory of heroin cues reactivated by CSs 10 min before extinction sessions exhibited a long-lasting learned extinction of diastolic and systolic blood pressure responses. The attenuation of responding was observed when heroin CSs were presented again after 30 days and 6 months (Xue et al., 2012).

There is an implicit assumption in the CET paradigm that CRs either serve as mediators for drug use, or play an important role in the interaction between respondent and operant behaviors. If CRs do play an important role in substance use, extinction-based treatments should be effective to eliminate it. However, substance use also involves operant conditioning in addition to respondent. Not only do drug CSs have an eliciting function, they also evoke operant responses. In other words, they can have an OM function for self-administration of the substance by removing or attenuating aversive CRs. The extinction process may fail to extinguish the control of certain dimensions of the stimulus over respondent responses. This condition would maintain the motivating aspect of establishing the removal of CRs as reinforcing. If this removal consists of being the greatest reinforcer available in the situation, there will be failure to extinguish CRs to stimuli that are not so salient (the new learning), thereby threatening the extinction training. For example, a bottle can have both the function of a CS and an OM. If CET only extinguishes CRs related to the bottle, without the operant response of drinking becoming extinct (due to the positive effects of alcohol being the only alternative for well-being in a social situation), then drinking will remain intact and some stimuli that are still salient in the contingency will continue to have a discriminative function –in our example, the social situation (Conklin & Tiffany, 2002). If the act of drinking is not extinguished or replaced, for example by social skills training, CR extinction is likely to be insufficient to eliminate drinking (Banaco & Montan, 2018).

In the classic conditioning model, CET should result in habituation or extinction of CRs, enough to be generalized to real life environments (Monti et al., 2002).

However, the generalization of extinction may not occur between the CSs used in the treatment and those present in the natural environment (Thewissen et al., 2006; Barnier, 2015; Kim et al., 2015). As a result, the real-life environment may continue to exert control over drug CRs, which determines that operant substance use is negatively reinforced by removing CRs. Social learning theory states that patients must practice coping skills during CET so that they are trained to emit, in the presence of drug CRs, responses that produce consequences that compete with the reinforcing effect of the substance (Rohsenow, Rohsenow et al., 1995). Some studies have isolated CET procedures by focusing on exposure to CSs without developing skills to cope with urges (Park et al., 2014). Other studies performed urge-specific coping skills training combined with CET and observed that the skills taught during CET are correlated with reduced substance use (Marlatt, 1990; Monti et al., 1993; Monti & Rohsenow, 1999; Rohsenow et al., 2001). Therefore, Monti et al. (2002) renders it important to combine CET and urge-specific coping skills training, both for habituation or extinction of CSs and for practicing skills that can be used outside the clinical setting, in an event of renewal, reinstatement, or spontaneous recovery of CRs extinguished during CET.

Current SUD treatments and other therapeutic interventions in general can be unsuccessful as they present methodological issues. Within the model of behavior therapy, sessions usually last around 1 h and focus on the functional analysis of substance use, offering conditions for the client to have contact with the variables that maintain the target behavior in light of the respondent and operant conditioning theory. The use of functional analysis to understand the variables that maintain substance use is indispensable for the development of effective interventions. However, the psychotherapy session can take place in a clinical outpatient setting or inpatient voluntary, involuntary, or compulsory hospitalization. Regardless of the therapeutic setting, the patient is treated in the absence of the substance and its CSs. Marlatt (1995) thus poses the question: if behavioral interventions based on conditioning theory comprise the interaction between stimulus and response, the most obvious question to be asked is: where is the stimulus? If substance use is the target behavior, why are the stimuli conditioned to its use and context absent in SUD treatment? Instead of exposing patients to stimuli conditioned to the context of use in order to prepare them for inevitable situations that elicit and evoke its use outside the clinical context, the individual ends up being treated in the complete absence of any CSs. The clinical setting –especially hospitalization—is rid of any stimuli that signals the presence of the substance, configuring a protective shield, which keeps the patient away from any stimulus that causes "temptation," often referred to as the "forbidden fruit." A patient who is treated in these conditions receives little preparation to face exposure to stimuli outside the clinical context.

Regardless of whether the patient's objective is abstinence or decreased use to a controlled pattern, leaving this client unprepared without previous experiences to any type of stimulus exposure increases the chances of relapse. CET still requires a functional analysis of substance use and must be complementary to other therapeutic approaches, thus preparing the patient to effectively cope with daily reexposures to high-risk situations that can lead to unwanted relapses.

Final Considerations

SUD is a complex phenomenon widely debated in different therapeutic approaches. This chapter addresses the theoretical and empirical bases, as well as possible clinical implications of a model that emphasizes respondent conditioning and its role in substance use and dependence, while also considering the interaction between respondent and operant processes. Pavlovian conditioning and its mechanisms on substance use produce physiological changes (CRs) that can be measured in the presence of CSs even though in the absence of the US (drug). Drug CSs produce CRs that can occur either in the same or in the opposite direction as the effect of the substance (UR). The factors that determine the relationship between CRs and URs are still unknown, but it is already known that they are not determined by the class of the drug. When it occurs in the same direction as URs –that is, the CS produces similar responses to those of the US— the CRs produce motivational states that establish the effect of the substance as a positive reinforcer. When it occurs in its opposite direction, the CS produces aversive physiological states that establish the effect of the substance as a negative reinforcer. Many theorists understand that these aversive physiological states are compensatory CRs that “protect the organism” from the harmful effects of the substance, and that this same compensatory action is responsible for tolerance, withdrawal, craving, and overdose. According to this theory, relapse and active drug-seeking, after long periods of abstinence, have been understood as an effect caused by the reexposure of the individual to drug CSs that have the ability to elicit and evoke responses that increase the motivational state for drug-seeking.

The clinical implications of this theoretical model guide CE studies –a method of assessing responses in the presence of stimuli—and CET studies –an intervention method on drug CRs. CE is a procedure that exposes substance users to a variety of drug cues, while self-report and physiological responses of craving are monitored. CET, however, proposes an intervention whose goal is to extinguish the pairing between CSs to the drug, hence without presenting it as a US, thus avoiding CRs to CSs. The rationale for this approach explains that repeated reexposures to CSs in the absence of substance intake (UR) should eliminate the CRs elicited by CSs, and thus eliminate physiological states that influence active drug-seeking. However, some factors interfere with the generalization of learned extinction and its maintenance over time. Some effects can cause the responses extinguished through CET to return, these being the effects of renewal, reinstatement, and spontaneous recovery of extinguished responses. Failure to extinguish some stimulus properties may also occur, such as motivating aspects that evoke operant responses that are reinforced by the effect of the substance. To prepare individuals for possible reappearances of CRs after treatment, authors have suggested combining CET with urge-specific coping skills training. This combination would allow users to experience the benefits of coping skills when experiencing decreases in drug CRs during its practice, with the aim of generalizing these skills outside the clinical setting. In any case, CET should be conducted in protected environments that can ensure the prevention of substance use between training sessions. In outpatient settings, the patient may suffer relapses between sessions, so the implementation of methods –such as help from the family or a therapeutic monitoring team—can be essential when CET is applied outside the hospital setting.

CET consists of a complementary technique to the clinical practice of behavior analysts who want to intervene on the interaction of respondent and operant processes observed in the acquisition and maintenance of substance use and dependence. Factors that threaten the extinction process should be the focus of researchers who study new parameters of the technique in search of new discoveries, both through controlled observations of applications and experimental studies.

References

Araújo, R. B., & Lopes, A. M. (2013). Tratamento de exposição a estímulos. In R. B. Araújo (Ed.), *Guia de Terapias Cognitivo-Comportamentais para os Transtornos do Exagero: Tratando Pacientes da Vida Real* (pp. 261–281). Sinopsys.

Banaco, R., & Montan, R. (2018). Teoria analítico-comportamental. In N. Zanelatto & R. Laranjeira (Eds.), *O tratamento dà dependência química e as terapias cognitivo-comportamentais: um guia para terapeutas* (2nd ed., pp. 115–132). Artmed.

Barnier, E. M. (2015). *Cannabis cue exposure: A pilot study about extinction contexts* [Thesis in partial fulfilment of the requirements for the Master of Research degree]. Macquarie University.

Bastos, F. I. P. M., Vasconcellos, M. T. L. D., De Boni, R. B., Reis, N. B. D., & Coutinho, C. F. D. S. (2017). *III Levantamento Nacional sobre o uso de drogas pela população brasileira (LENAD)*. Fundação Osvaldo Cruz.

Bordnick, P. S., Copp, H. L., Traylor, A., Graap, K. M., Carter, B. L., Walton, A., & Ferrer, M. (2009). Reactivity to cannabis cues in virtual reality environments. *Journal of Psychoactive Drugs, 41*(2), 105–112. https://doi.org/10.1080/02791072.2009.10399903

Botella, C., Fernández-Álvarez, J., Guillén, V., García-Palacios, A., & Baños, R. (2017). Recent progress in virtual reality exposure therapy for phobias: A systematic review. *Current Psychiatry Reports, 19*(7), 42. https://doi.org/10.1007/s11920-017-0788-4

Bouton, M. E., & Ricker, S. T. (1994). Renewal of extinguished responding in a second context. *Animal Learning & Behavior, 22*(3), 317–324.

Carter, B. L., & Tiffany, S. T. (1999). Meta-analysis of cue-reactivity in addiction research. *Addiction, 94*(3), 327–340.

Chelonis, J. J., Calton, J. L., Hart, J. A., & Schachtman, T. R. (1999). Attenuation of the renewal effect by extinction in multiple contexts. *Learning and Motivation, 30*(1), 1–14. https://doi.org/10.1006/lmot.1998.1022

Childress, A., Ehrman, R., McLellan, A. T., & O'Brien, C. (1988). Conditioned craving and arousal in cocaine addiction: A preliminary report. *NIDA Research Monograph, 81*, 74–80.

Childress, A. R., Mozley, P. D., McElgin, W., Fitzgerald, J., Reivich, M., & O'Brien, C. P. (1999). Limbic activation during cue-induced cocaine craving. *American Journal of Psychiatry, 156*(1), 11–18. https://doi.org/10.1176/ajp.156.1.11

Conklin, C. A., & Tiffany, S. T. (2002). Applying extinction research and theory to cue-exposure addiction treatments. *Addiction, 97*(2), 155–167. https://doi.org/10.1046/j.1360-0443.2002.00014.x

Collins, B. N., & Brandon, T. H. (2002). Effects of extinction context and retrieval cues on alcohol cue reactivity among nonalcoholic drinkers. *Journal of consulting and clinical psychology, 70*(2), 390.

Cunningham, C. L. (1998). Drug conditioning and drug-seeking behavior. In W. T. O'Donohue (Ed.), *Learning and behavior therapy* (pp. 518–544). Allyn & Bacon.

de Wit, H., & Stewart, J. (1981). Reinstatement of cocaine reinforced responding in the rat. *Psychopharmacology, 75*, 134–143. https://doi.org/10.1007/bf00432175

Drummond, D. C., Tiffany, S. T., Glautier, S., & Remington, B. (1995). Cue exposure in understanding and treating addictive behaviours. In D. C. Drummond, S. T. Tiffany, S. Glautier, & B. Remington (Eds.), *Addictive behaviour: Cue exposure theory and practice* (pp. 1–17). Wiley.

DuFrene, T., & Wilson, K. (2012). *The wisdom to know the difference: An acceptance and commitment therapy workbook for overcoming substance abuse*. New Harbinger Publications.

Glautier, S., & Remington, B. (1995). The form of responses to drug cues. In D. C. Drummond, S. T. Tiffany, S. Glautier, & B. Remington (Eds.), *Addictive behaviour: Cue exposure theory and practice* (The Wiley series in clinical psychology) (pp. 21–46). Wiley.

Gunther, L. M., Denniston, J. C., & Miller, R. R. (1998). Conducting exposure treatment in multiple contexts can prevent relapse. *Behaviour Research and Therapy, 36*(1), 75–91. https://doi.org/10.1016/s0005-7967(97)10019-5

Havermans, R. C., & Jansen, A. T. (2003). Increasing the efficacy of cue exposure treatment in preventing relapse of addictive behavior. *Addictive Behaviors, 28*(5), 989–994. https://doi.org/10.1016/s0306-4603(01)00289-1

Higgins, S. T., Heil, S. H., & Sigmon, S. C. (2007). A behavioral approach to the treatment of substance use disorders. In P. Sturmey (Ed.), *Functional analysis in clinical treatment* (pp. 261–282). Academic.

Kim, J. H., Perry, C., Luikinga, S., Zbukvic, I., Brown, R. M., & Lawrence, A. J. (2015). Extinction of a cocaine-taking context that protects against drug-primed reinstatement is dependent on the metabotropic glutamate 5 receptor. *Addiction Biology, 20*(3), 482–489. https://doi.org/10.1111/adb.12142

Lynch, J. J., Fertziger, A. P., Teitelbaum, H. A., Cullen, J. W., & Gantt, W. H. (1973). Pavlovian conditioning of drug reactions: Some implications for problems of drug addiction. *Conditional Reflex: A Pavlovian Journal of Research & Therapy, 8*(4), 211–223.

MacKillop, J., & Lisman, S. A. (2008). Effects of a context shift and multiple context extinction on reactivity to alcohol cues. *Experimental and Clinical Psychopharmacology, 16*(4), 322–331. https://doi.org/10.1037/a0012686

Maples-Keller, J. L., Bunnell, B. E., Kim, S. J., & Rothbaum, B. O. (2017). The use of virtual reality technology in the treatment of anxiety and other psychiatric disorders. *Harvard Review of Psychiatry, 25*(3), 103. https://doi.org/10.1097/2FHRP.0000000000000138

Marlatt, G. A. (1990). Cue exposure and relapse prevention in the treatment of addictive behaviors. *Addictive Behaviors, 15*(4), 395–399. https://doi.org/10.1016/0306-4603(90)90048-3

Marlatt, G. A. (1995). Foreword. In D. C. Drummond, S. T. Tiffany, S. Glautier, & B. Remington (Eds.), *Addictive behaviour: Cue exposure theory and practice* (The Wiley series in clinical psychology). Wiley.

Martin, T., La Rowe, S., & Malcolm, R. J. (2010). Progress in cue exposure therapy for the treatment of addictive disorders: A review update. *The Open Addiction Journal, 3*, 92–101.

McKim, W. A., & Hancock, S. (2012). *Drugs and behavior*. Pearson Australia Pty Limited.

Mellentin, A. I., Skøt, L., Nielsen, B., Schippers, G., Nielsen, A. S., Stenager, E., & Juhl, C. B. (2017). Cue exposure therapy for the treatment of alcohol use disorders: A meta-analytic review. *Clinical Psychology Review*. https://doi.org/10.1016/j.cpr.2017.07.006

Melo, W. V., Baldisserotto, G., & Valdivia, L. (2018). Terapia comportamental dialética nos transtornos por uso de substâncias. In N. A. Zanelatto & R. Laranjeira (Eds.), *O tratamento da dependência química e as terapias cognitivo-comportamentais: um guia para terapeutas*. Artmed.

Michael, J. (1980). The discriminative stimulus or SD. *The Behavior Analyst, 3*(1), 47.

Miguel, A. Q., Madruga, C. S., Cogo-Moreira, H., Yamauchi, R., Simões, V., … Laranjeira, R. R. (2016). Contingency management is effective in promoting abstinence and retention in treatment among crack cocaine users in Brazil: A randomized controlled trial. *Psychology of Addictive Behaviors, 30*(5), 536.

Miller, W. R., & Rollnick, S. (2012). *Motivational interviewing: Helping people change*. Guilford press.

Monti, P. M., & Rohsenow, D. J. (1999). Coping-skills training and cue-exposure therapy in the treatment of alcoholism. *Alcohol Research, 23*(2), 107.

Monti, P. M., Rohsenow, D. J., Rubonis, A. V., Niaura, R. S., Sirota, A. D., Colby, S. M., Goddard, P., & Abrams, D. B. (1993). Cue exposure with coping skills treatment for male alcoholics: A preliminary investigation. *Journal of Consulting and Clinical Psychology, 61*(6), 1011. https://doi.org/10.1037//0022-006x.61.6.1011

Monti, P. M., Kadden, R., Rohsenow, D. J., Cooney, N., & Abrams, D. B. (2002). *Treating alcohol dependence: A coping skills training guide* (2nd ed.). Guilford Press.

Niaura, R. S., Rohsenow, D. J., Binkoff, J. A., Monti, P. M., Pedraza, M., & Abrams, D. B. (1988). Relevance of cue reactivity to understanding alcohol and smoking relapse. *Journal of Abnormal Psychology, 97*(2), 133. https://doi.org/10.1037//0021-843x.97.2.133

Opriş, D., Pintea, S., García-Palacios, A., Botella, C., Szamosközi, Ş., & David, D. (2012). Virtual reality exposure therapy in anxiety disorders: A quantitative meta-analysis. *Depression and Anxiety, 29*(2), 85–93. https://doi.org/10.1002/da.20910

Park, C. B., Choi, J. S., Park, S. M., Lee, J. Y., Jung, H. Y., Seol, J. M., … Kwon, J. S. (2014). Comparison of the effectiveness of virtual cue exposure therapy and cognitive behavioral therapy for nicotine dependence. *Cyberpsychology, Behavior and Social Networking, 17*(4), 262–267.

Pavlov, I. P. (1927). *Conditioned reflexes: An investigation of the physiological activity of the cerebral cortex*. Oxford University Press.

Rohsenow, D. J., Monti, P. M., & Abrams, D. B. (1995). Cue exposure treatment for alcohol dependence. In D. C. Drummond, S. Glautier, B. Remington, & S. Tiffany (Eds.), *Addiction: Cue exposure theory and practice* (pp. 169–196). Wiley.

Rohsenow, D. J., Monti, P. M., Rubonis, A. V., Gulliver, S. B., Colby, S. M., Binkoff, J. A., & Abrams, D. B. (2001). Cue exposure with coping skills training and communication skills training for alcohol dependence: 6-and 12-month outcomes. *Addiction, 96*(8), 1161–1174. https://doi.org/10.1046/j.1360-0443.2001.96811619.x

Saladin, M. E., Brady, K. T., Graap, K., & Rothbaum, B. O. (2006). A preliminary report on the use of virtual reality technology to elicit craving and cue reactivity in cocaine dependent individuals. *Addictive Behaviors, 31*(10), 1881–1894. https://doi.org/10.1016/j.addbeh.2006.01.004

Schwarz, K. S., & Cunningham, C. L. (1990). Conditioned stimulus control of morphine hyperthermia. *Psychopharmacology, 101*(1), 77–84. https://doi.org/10.1007/bf02253722

Siegel, S. (1975). Evidence from rats that morphine tolerance is a learned response. *Journal of Comparative and Physiological Psychology, 89*(5), 498. https://doi.org/10.1037/h0077058

Siegel, S. (1979). The role of conditioning in drug tolerance and addiction. In J. D. Keehn (Ed.), *Psychopathology in animals: Research and clinical implications* (pp. 143–168). Academic.

Siegel, S. (1989). Pharmacological conditioning and drug effects. In *Psychoactive drugs* (pp. 115–180). Humana Press.

Siegel, S., Hinson, R. E., & Krank, M. D. (1978). The role of predrug signals in morphine analgesic tolerance: Support for a Pavlovian conditioning model of tolerance. *Journal of Experimental Psychology: Animal Behavior Processes, 4*(2), 188. https://doi.org/10.1037//0097-7403.4.2.188

Souza, A. A., & Oshiro, C. K. B. (2019). Contribuições da Psicoterapia Analítica Funcional (FAP) no tratamento do Transtorno por Uso de Substâncias (TUS). *Acta Comportamentalia: Revista Latina de Análisis del Comportamiento, 27*(2), 197–213.

Stasiewicz, P. R., Brandon, T. H., & Bradizza, C. M. (2007). Effects of extinction context and retrieval cues on renewal of alcohol-cue reactivity among alcohol-dependent outpatients. *Psychology of Addictive Behaviors, 21*(2), 244–248. https://doi.org/10.1037/0893-164X.21.2.244

Stewart, J., De Wit, H., & Eikelboom, R. (1984). Role of unconditioned and conditioned drug effects in the self-administration of opiates and stimulants. *Psychological Review, 91*(2), 251.

Thewissen, R., Snijders, S. J., Havermans, R. C., van den Hout, M., & Jansen, A. (2006). Renewal of cue-elicited urge to smoke: Implications for cue exposure treatment. *Behaviour Research and Therapy, 44*(10), 1441–1449. https://doi.org/10.1016/j.brat.2005.10.010

Wikler, A. (1948). Recent progress in research on the neurophysiologic basis of morphine addiction. *American Journal of Psychiatry, 105*(5), 329–338. https://doi.org/10.1176/ajp.105.5.329

Xue, Y. X., Luo, Y. X., Wu, P., Shi, H. S., Xue, L. F., Chen, C., Zhu, W. L., Ding, Z. B., Bao, Y. P., Shi, S., Haham, Y., Lu, L., & Epstein, D. H. (2012). A memory retrieval-extinction procedure to prevent drug craving and relapse. *Science, 336*(6078), 241–245. https://doi.org/10.1126/science.1215070

Zanelatto, N. A., & Laranjeira, R. (2018). *O tratamento da dependência química e as terapias cognitivo-comportamentais: um guia para terapeutas*. Artmed Editora.

Chapter 9
Functional Analytic Psychotherapy (FAP) as an Adjunct Treatment to Substance Dependence Cases

Alan Souza Aranha, Claudia Kami Bastos Oshiro, and Elliot Cozzens Wallace

Introduction: Functional Analytic Psychotherapy (FAP)

FAP is a psychotherapy based on the philosophy of radical behaviorism and the conceptual aspects of behavior analysis (Kohlenberg & Tsai, 1991; Skinner, 1945, 1953, 1957, 1974). FAP intends to develop the client's interpersonal repertoire, making them more capable of producing positive reinforcement and eliminating aversive stimuli in its social context. To accomplish this goal, FAP therapists propose that the psychotherapeutic relationship be used as (a) a source of additional information about the client's behaviors and (b) a mechanism for clinical change (Tsai et al., 2009).

The authors of FAP argue that a portion of human suffering occurs as a result of problems in interpersonal repertoire: contact with the social environment evokes problematic patterns of interaction, either with an increase in aversive stimulation density or in the scarcity of positive reinforcers. The individual seeks a psychotherapist in order to receive assistance to feel better and because it is a social relationship, the deficits and excesses presented in the individual's daily life are generalized to the psychotherapeutic relationship. This is the ideal scenario to evaluate the client's repertoire and strengthen more effective behaviors in-session. When the client establishes a healthier relationship with the professional, generalization strategies can be outlined so that the therapeutic progress are transposed to the out-of-session context and the individual establishes healthier relationships with his or her peers (Kohlenberg & Tsai, 1991).

A. S. Aranha (✉) · C. K. B. Oshiro
University of São Paulo, São Paulo, SP, Brazil
e-mail: claudiaoshiro@usp.br

E. C. Wallace
University of Washington, Seattle, WA, USA
e-mail: elliotcw@uw.edu

S. M. Oliani et al. (eds.), *Behavior Analysis and Substance Dependence*,
https://doi.org/10.1007/978-3-030-75961-2_9

There is a classification of possible therapist and client behaviors that occur in an FAP therapy session. Regarding the client's behaviors, the main ones are named *clinically relevant behaviors* (CRBs). A CRB1 is a behavior that occurs in-session, which is functionally similar to the out-of-session problem behavior; CRB2 is a therapeutic progress; and a CRB3 is a verbal report of the client's behavior and the variables of which is a function. The description of the client's own behaviors and the contingencies of reinforcement that control them help the client to emit the skills learned in the presence of the psychotherapist in situations that evoke his or her problem behaviors outside the session (Kohlenberg & Tsai, 1991).

It is important to clarify the relationship between CRBs and out-of-session problem behaviors. Both behaviors are perceived as part of the same *response class,* defined as responses that produce the same consequences, regardless of their form (Catania, 1998/1999). A person can eat using a fork and knife, spoon, or with his hands. All topographies would be in the "lunch" response class, as they produce the "food" consequence. The difficulties of the client must be understood in the same context. The psychotherapist may identify that the client's problem behaviors are associated with the aggressiveness with which he addresses people (e.g., offending, increasing tone of voice), but should not expect the client to emulate similar topographic behaviors in-session (e.g., expressing offenses or increasing tone of voice toward the psychotherapist). Firstly, the therapist should understand the function of the aggressiveness – to cause harm, to draw attention, to avoid – and then hypothesize which responses may contain the same function in therapy. There are several possible topographies to annoy, call attention to, or avoid professional's interventions.

Regarding the therapist's behaviors, the Five Therapeutic Rules are instructions on how the clinician should behave in-session to assist his client. They are a systematization of the functional analysis for the therapeutic relationship (Kohlenberg & Tsai, 1991; Tsai et al., 2009): (1) observe the emission of CRBs, (2) evoke CRBs, (3) contingent responding to CRBs, (4) evaluate the intervention, and (5) program the generalization of behaviors.

Rule 1: The first rule refers to the activity of identifying CRBs (Tsai et al., 2009). In the case conceptualization stage, it consists of the psychotherapist observing and relating the client's behaviors that occur in-session with the problem behaviors that occur outside the session. Briefly, three questions can be raised:

1. How can problem behaviors both described by the client and identified by the therapist be generalized to the context of the session?
2. How do the observed CRBs occur in the client's daily life?
3. What are the functions of these behaviors? Or what are the antecedents and consequences of all the behaviors of the response class, inside and outside the session?

In the intervention, with the knowledge of the function of the CRB1s, Rule 1 proposes to pay attention to the CRBs and to proceed with the other rules. If the professional is not under control of the relevant behaviors of the client that occur in-session (under control of not very relevant behaviors or the topography of the CRBs), he will face challenges in managing them therapeutically.

Rule 2: CRBs may occur in-session due to the social nature of the psychotherapeutic relationship (by processes of generalization and stimulus equivalence). A person who behaves according to the demands of the social group to avoid the negative evaluation (e.g., using a psychoactive substance to not be disapproved), is likely to be under control of the possible negative evaluations that the psychotherapist has about such individual in-session (e.g., following the therapist's requests to change the time of the meeting, agreeing with the therapist's analyses). The professional may also manipulate different events in order to *intentionally* evoke the CRBs, as mands ("could you behave in a certain way?") (Callaghan & Follette, 2008; Vartanian, 2017), structured exercises (Nelson et al., 2016), and free association (Tsai et al., 2012). Rule 2 aims to increase the frequency of CRBs in-session and the number of opportunities to apply the third rule (Vartanian, 2017).

Rule 3: Consistent with an analytic-behavioral model, FAP holds that the behaviors of any individual are selected for their consequences (Skinner, 1953). It is postulated that Rule 3 is the FAP's mechanism of clinical change, the therapist's contingent responding to the client's CRBs. The professional should present aversive consequences to weaken CRB1s (punishment, extinction), but mainly present positive reinforcing consequences to strengthen CRB2s. The available consequences are the therapist's own actions in-session (Kohlenberg & Tsai, 1991).

It is important to stress that the psychotherapist's behaviors are also defined by their functions – their effects on the client's repertoire – and not by their topographies. The inexperienced therapist may praise his client believing that this is a "positive reinforcement" or criticize him to "punish unwanted behavior," but interventions have different functions depending on the history of contingencies of reinforcement and the CRBs identified in case conceptualization. For the individual who expresses feelings of low self-esteem, a compliment can be an aversive stimulus ("my therapist is an actor," "he just wants to please me"). On the other hand, for the person who has a history of family conflicts and social isolation, criticism can have a conditioned reinforcing function by pairing with attention opportunities. The professional's criticism does not decrease the frequency of unwanted behavior, but evokes a chain of discussions and an increase in the frequency of the problematic pattern. It is necessary for the FAP therapist to build intervention strategies that are sensitive to the case conceptualization and to judge its results throughout the therapeutic process.

Rule 4: The only way to know if the case conceptualization was correct and if the intervention had a successful repercussion is to evaluate its effects. This is accomplished in FAP, both by asking the client directly ("what did you feel when I explained it to you?") and by considering the change in CRB frequency. In a research environment, the frequency of CRBs can also be recorded with the *Functional Analytic Psychotherapy Rating Scale* (FAPRS) (Callaghan & Follette, 2008).

Rule 5: CRB2s built in-session should be generalized in the client's out-of-session relationships, the ultimate goal of psychotherapy. Generalization can be facilitated with homework ("you were able to express your opinions to me. What do you think about trying to reproduce this behavior with your husband?") and discussions about the functions of client behavior in-session ("I believe you agree with my analysis of your fear that I will judge you. Is it similar to what you told me about smoking marijuana so no one makes fun of you?"). FAP psychotherapeutic model is summarized in Fig. 9.1.

Other categories of behavior can occur in FAP sessions. For example, throughout the psychotherapeutic process the client will discuss problem behaviors and, progressively, improvement behaviors emitted outside the session (O1 and O2, *outside CRB1s* and *outside CRB2s*). In turn, the therapist will be able to respond to these descriptions (RO1 and RO2, *response to outside CRB1s* and *response to outside CRB2s*). Explanations of other categories can be checked in the FAPRS categorization system (Callaghan & Follette, 2008).

Which clients can benefit from FAP strategies? In the first book published, Kohlenberg and Tsai (1991) argued that interpersonal problems would be the ideal targets of psychotherapy, such as intimacy and personality disorders. Thus, it is possible to find studies discussing the application of FAP to problems in the interpersonal repertoire, such as borderline personality disorder (Oshiro et al., 2012), histrionic personality disorder (Callaghan et al., 2003), oppositional defiant disorder (Xavier, 2018), and social anxiety (Lovo, 2019). In the same period, authors described FAP application for other clinical conditions, such as major depression (Kanter et al., 2006), posttraumatic stress disorder (Lima, 2017), obsessive-compulsive disorder (Vandenberghe, 2007), and panic disorder with agoraphobia (Pezzato et al., 2012). One of the psychiatric conditions studied in recent years was substance dependence, which is discussed in this chapter.

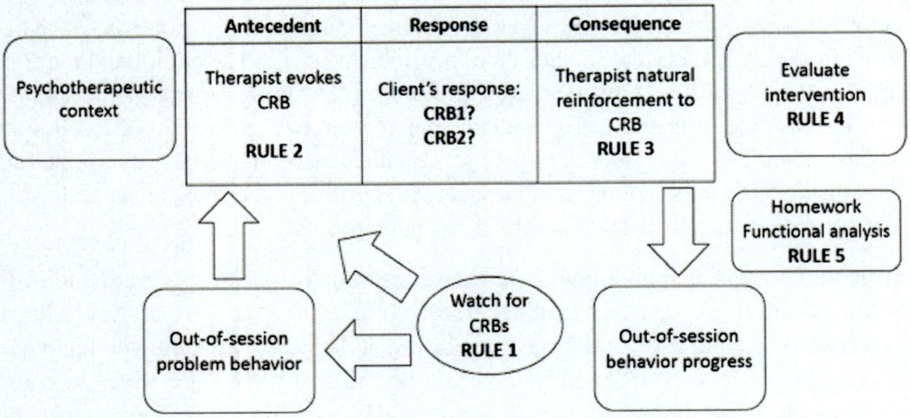

Fig. 9.1 FAP psychotherapeutic model. Adapted from "Psicoterapia Analítica Funcional. Functional Analytic Psychotherapy (FAP)" by Oshiro (2014). *Instituto de Terapia Cognitiva*

Substance Dependence

The psychopathologies described in mental health diagnostic manuals, such as the International Classification of Diseases (WHO, 2018) and the Diagnostic and Statistical Manual of Mental Disorders-5 (APA, 2013), are conceptualized by behavior analysts as respondent and operant responses in the individual's repertoire. These psychopathologies are differentiated from other behaviors only by the harm they cause to the social environment and to the person who behaves (Banaco et al., 2010; Vilas Boas et al., 2012). The analytic-behavioral therapist is interested in describing all the behaviors that contribute to the repertoire classified as psychopathological, identifying the contingencies that maintain these behaviors and proposing strategies to change them (Banaco et al., 2012).

In this regard, it is worth mentioning an example of the functional analysis of depression provided by Ferster (1973). The author described that among the responses that would characterize the depressive pattern, the following stand out: reduction in performance (decrease in the frequency of activities that produce positive reinforcement and eliminate aversive stimulation), excessive ineffective escape behavior (they do not remove aversive stimuli from the environment, keeping the subject in contact with the stimuli), and "bizarre and irrational" behavior (rituals and stereotypes). Contingencies of reinforcement that maintain depression would be difficulties in discriminating the environment (not evoking adequate responses to produce positive reinforcement and eliminate aversive stimulation), unfavorable environment for the development of effective behaviors, reinforcement schemes that require high frequency of responses (leading to extinction and inactivity), changes in the environment (absence of antecedents that evoke the available repertoire), and emotional changes that compete with operants (decreasing access to positive reinforcement). In the light of the above, the main goal of the treatment would be the construction of an appropriate repertory to manipulate the present contingencies, removing the client from the depressed and stereotyped condition. One purpose of psychotherapy would be to refine the verbal description of the client about the environment, improving his discrimination of relevant antecedents that would consequently evoke positive and negative reinforced responses.

In order to understand substance dependence, it is first necessary to operationalize the relationship between the individual and the drug into respondent and operant components. Two important respondent phenomena are the withdrawal syndrome and tolerance. A psychoactive substance has the function of an unconditioned stimulus (US) that elicits two unconditioned responses (UR), its pharmacological effect and the compensatory responses that reestablish the homeostasis of the organism (e.g., when administering heroin, the user feels a decrease in sensitivity to pain and later an exaggerated sensitivity to pain). Friends, places of use, feelings, etc. (NS, neutral stimuli), are paired and acquire conditioned function (CS) for aversive compensatory conditioned responses (CR), the withdrawal. Contact with CS elicits unpleasant physical symptoms and the user experiences craving to use again. When the drug is consumed in the same or similar environments, a new respondent conditioning occurs (US-CS pairing) and, consequently, abstinence syndromes perpetuate over time. Tolerance occurs when the user administers the drug in contact with the previously conditioned CSs and, with the compensatory effects present, the effect of the drug is smaller. The individual begins to demand increasing amounts of the substance to achieve the desired effects (Benvenuti, 2004, 2007; Siegel, 2005).

In an operant contingency, substance consumption is evoked by antecedents (discriminative stimuli and reflexive establishing operations) and selected by consequences (positive and negative reinforcement). In the context of being in a bar with peers (physical and social discriminative stimuli), drinking alcohol can lead to drunkenness (positive pharmacological reinforcement) and group attention (positive social reinforcement). The use of alcohol can also be solitary (besides the pharmacological effect, it can have a conditioned function by pairing between alcohol and social reinforcement). Difficulties that the client experiences and withdrawal syndrome (aversive stimuli as antecedent) may lead him/her to consume substances to temporarily reduce contact with these stimuli (negative reinforcement). Private events such as feelings and thoughts are paired with the original aversive stimuli and begin to evoke escape-avoidance behaviors (conditioned aversive stimuli as antecedents) (Borloti et al., 2015; Higginset al., 2007; Miguel et al., 2015).

Most of those who administer drugs themselves are sporadic or occasional users who do not produce serious consequences for themselves and others (Laranjeira et al., 2014), which is essential to label consumption as psychopathological (Banaco et al., 2010; Vilas Boas et al., 2012) (for a list of consequences of substance abuse, see Tonigan & Miller, 2002). The basic processes explain certain situations where use brings harm. For example, withdrawal syndrome can be a relevant variable for consumption to become harmful; the unpleasant physical symptom evokes escape responses to eliminate such state, negatively reinforcing the use. At the same time, the contact between the substance (US) and the environment (CS) maintains the respondent conditioning and, consequently, the withdrawal on future occasions. The very behavior that removes the syndrome allows it to perpetuate, sustaining the cycle of abuse (Banaco & Montan, 2018). However, it is worth noting that this is only one of the possibilities for a dependent pattern to manifest itself. The existence of the abstinence syndrome is not essential for the use of the substance to become pernicious (APA, 2013; Higgins et al., 2007; Rush et al., 2019).

Researchers study which other possible variables, besides the respondent conditioning associated with escape-avoidance behaviors, influence a portion of the population to develop relevant compulsion (Bernardes, 2008; Garcia-Mijares & Silva, 2006; Heyman, 1996; Wilson & Byrd, 2004). Another critical variable for the development of substance dependence is when a person who exhibits excess behavior under control of short-term consequences at the expense of long-term consequences may experience problems with their consumption (APA, 2013; Higgins et al., 2007; Madden & Bickel, 2010). In a context where the client may emit two responses that produce different reinforcers – smoking marijuana to "relax" or studying for the vestibular at the end of the year – he will probably emit the behavior that produces immediate consequences. Even in contact with aversive consequences (e.g., losing the school year, not starting a professional life), the user will continue to emit short-term responses (e.g., smoking) at the expense of the long term (e.g., studying). Problem-solving (Moos, 2007; Silva & Serra, 2004; Wilson & Byrd, 2004), frustration tolerance (Guilhardi, 2010/2013, 2018; Marlatt & Donovan, 2009), and sensitivity to the consequences that he/she produced to others (Costa & Valerio, 2008; Guilhardi, 2010/2013, 2018) are some repertories that, when little or badly elaborated, can facilitate the progression of the psychopathology.

Both deficits and excesses in the interpersonal repertoire that the client manifests are risk factors that can lead to substance dependence (Aranha & Oshiro, 2019; Marlatt & Donovan, 2009; Wilson & Byrd, 2004). A young person may feel judged by his friends, not have many day-to-day activities, and suffer due to family conflicts. Drug use would decrease his sensitivity to criticism (making him neutral or less aversive), give him something to do when he is idle (e.g., smoking marijuana alone), and guarantee him a tool to forget the problems he experiences at home (e.g., sniffing cocaine and being more under control of pharmacological effects than family contingencies). The reinforcement promoted by the substance strengthens the use behavior and marks the antecedents as evocative stimuli. In situations with similar difficulties, planning, search, and use behaviors occur and are again reinforced. The cycle decreases the space for the client to learn how to deal with the problems and, as a result, makes him/her more and more dependent on the substance (Banaco & Montan, 2018; Holman et al., 2012; Ribeiro & Laranjeira, 2012). Psychotherapeutic intervention focusing on interpersonal repertoire would provide access to new sources of positive social reinforcement (e.g., expressing feelings, creating intimacy), physical reinforcement (e.g., meeting groups with interests in games and sports), and escape-avoidance behaviors (e.g., seeking help, dealing with criticism). The antecedent that evoked unwanted responses will now evoke alternative responses that will be progressively consolidated in the client's repertoire, moving him away from drug use (Aranha & Oshiro, 2019; Gifford et al., 2006; Holman et al., 2012; Rachlin, 1997).

For clients who suffer from withdrawal syndrome, interpersonal intervention promotes important complementary improvements. The same antecedents that evoke the use have conditioned stimuli function (CS) that elicit the syndrome. When the subject is exposed to these stimuli and emits alternative behaviors instead of consuming the substance (US), the process of respondent extinction occurs, making the unpleasant physical symptoms less and less intense (Gifford et al., 2011; Holman et al., 2012).

FAP is a behavioral psychotherapy whose goal is to develop the interpersonal repertoire of clients. It uses the therapeutic relationship as a source of information to perform case conceptualization and as a mechanism for clinical change when the therapist presents differential consequences for relevant behaviors (Tsai et al., 2009). FAP can be used as an adjunct treatment for substance dependence, since there is a chance that substance dependents have deficits and/or excesses in the interpersonal repertoire that inhibit access to reinforcers and keep them in contact with aversive stimulation of social origin. The repertory restriction helps in the installation and progression of dependence (it increases the frequency of substance-consuming behaviors) and intensifies interpersonal problems (it decreases the opportunities for learning effective repertories). When deficits and excesses become generalized in the relationship with the psychotherapist as CRB1s, the psychotherapist can use the FAP to model more effective repertories, the CRB2s. The positive reinforcing consequences not only strengthen the CRB2s but also mark the psychotherapist's discriminative function for these behaviors. By encountering other interpersonal out-of-session relationships, the psychotherapeutic progress becomes generalized, producing new reinforcers. The strengthening of the repertoire broadens the possibilities for the user to recover (Aranha & Oshiro, 2019; Holman et al., 2012). If the client exhibits withdrawal symptoms, the respondent extinction may also occur in-session. The psychotherapist's behaviors have both discriminative and eliciting functions (Kohlenberg & Tsai, 1991), causing the syndrome to continue. When CRB2s are emitted and produce social enforcers and not drugs, there is a break in US-CS conditioning. In addition, the operant generalization of CRBs helps to have a higher frequency of responses that do not result in drug use outside the session and, as a result, a higher likelihood of respondent extinction in the natural environment (Gifford et al., 2011). FAP psychotherapeutic model for substance dependence is summarized in Fig. 9.2.

antecedent	response	consequence
out-of-session social context	1. psychoactive substance abuse	1. pharmacological and social positive and negative reinforcement
	2. interpersonal behavior deficits and excesses	1. social punishment
therapeutic relationship	1. CRB1s	1. extintion, punishment, block avoidance
	2. CRB2s	2. social natural positive reinforcement
out-of-session social context	1. effective interpersonal repertoire	1. reinforcers not related to substances
	2. decrease in behavioral problems and substance abuse	2. absence of consequences

Fig. 9.2 FAP psychotherapeutic model for substance dependence

The Application of FAP to Substance Dependence

Articles related to FAP and substance dependence offer possibilities for the application of psychotherapy to the population. We describe the main studies published, emphasizing the CRBs identified, the proposed interventions, the benefits of applying the FAP within the treatment plan, and the results obtained.

Pedersen et al. (2012) presented a clinical case of a client who met the diagnostic criteria for posttraumatic stress disorder (PTSD), dysthymia, alcohol dependence, bulimic behaviors, and characteristics of dependent personality disorder. PTSD symptoms (traumatic reexperience, hyperexcitability, and avoidance) were related to a history of sexual abuse and a threat to physical integrity. The proposed treatment included two steps. In the first stage, cognitive-behavioral therapy (CBT) for substance dependence, bulimia, and PTSD was conducted, and in the second stage, CBT was added to FAP with a focus on interpersonal difficulties.

The first phase was effective in eliminating bulimic behavior, promoting abstinence from alcohol, and decreasing PTSD symptoms, except for social avoidance behaviors. Deficits in the interpersonal repertoire led the client to isolation and relapse from alcohol use. At this time, researchers chose to add FAP to intervene in the repertory deficits, identifying as CRB1s: difficulty in discriminating the appropriate context to self-disclosure, avoidance behaviors from interpersonal contexts, and not reinforce behaviors of approaching by others. The expected CRB2s were listed as discriminating opportunities to expose oneself emotionally, building intimacy by discussing positive and negative experiences, asking how the client could behave to be more reinforcing, and reinforce the disclosure of others. The goals of promoting CRB2s were to decrease escape behaviors and increase the participant's probability of obtaining social reinforcement. Instruments for PTSD symptoms and interpersonal functioning were used. After 9 months of FAP, results of the instruments ascertained that reexperience and hyperexcitability remained stable; however, the frequency of avoidance behaviors decreased and self-disclosure behaviors increased. A clinical evaluation pointed to increased frequency and effectiveness of social connections, abstinence from alcohol, decreased use of health services, decreased dependence of the therapist, and increased accountability for his choices and well-being (Pedersen et al., 2012).

Since this is not a specific study for substance dependence, Pedersen et al. (2012) did not describe the relationship between interpersonal deficits and alcohol use. It can be conjectured that substance abuse had two functions: in the absence of significant social connections, as a response that produced positive reinforcement stimuli, and, under control of the same history of PTSD symptoms, negatively reinforced escape behavior. The development of the social repertoire increased the positive reinforcers available to the participant, changed the aversive function of social interactions and consequently decreased the frequency of drinking. The FAP strategies were not made explicit, only the CRBs and those that were targeted for intervention.

Paul et al. (1999) conducted a research targeting deviant sexual behavior and substance abuse. The client met the diagnostic criteria for marijuana abuse and exhibitionism. Given that he was exposing himself in public, the judiciary system ordered the client to be submitted to mandatory psychotherapy. Initially, the psychotherapist investigated the sequence of events that led to the sexual pattern; when driving and using marijuana, the client was looking for a woman he considered attractive, which produced in him an intense desire to adopt exhibitionist behavior. After expressing the exhibitionist behavior, he would return to his house, where he would smoke, masturbate, and reminisce the exhibitionism event.

A functional analysis evidenced that deficits in the interpersonal repertoire would be one of the variations for the maintenance of problematic sexual activity and drug abuse. The client experienced anxiety when he was around women (he had never met or had sexual intercourse with one). Exhibitionism ensured access to social enforcers that the client would not otherwise produce, but he needed to consume marijuana so that social disapproval would not inhibit him. The pharmacological effect of the substance also acquired a negative reinforcement function when used in the presence of feelings of loneliness and inadequacy (Paul et al., 1999).

The client became aware that the cycle of dependence and public exposure brought losses in the academic and social areas, besides producing feelings of inadequacy and guilt. Exhibitionist tendencies and impulses became aversive (indicating that the exhibitionist behavior was imminent), but attempts of self-control failed. "Holding on" did not modify the contingencies maintaining the problem behaviors, leading the client to relapse. Due to attempts to control private events, acceptance and commitment therapy (ACT) was proposed (Hayes et al., 2012), with the following purpose: acceptance of sexually deviant thoughts and feelings, reduce the frequency of exhibitionist behavior, reduce the frequency of marijuana use, and increase social connections. Changes in intensity and frequency of impulses related to exhibitionist behavior, episodes of exhibitionism, masturbation, and marijuana use were recorded with self-monitoring, and symptoms of anxiety and depression recorded with standardized inventories. In 6 months of ACT, increased connections with women and decreased social anxiety were observed, but the results for exhibitionism were insufficient. The authors decided to add FAP strategies (Paul et al., 1999).

- **Rule 1:** The therapist identified that *attempts of self-control* outside the session were functionally similar to the avoidance behaviors of *not talking about exhibitionism* in-session, so these were conceptualized as CRB1s. Both were inefficient responses to minimize access to aversive stimulation (*desire to express* exhibitionist behavior and *report the desire* for exhibitionism). The proposed CRB2s were to acknowledge and report feelings, thoughts, and exhibitionist tendencies in-session.
- **Rule 2:** The therapist intentionally evoked self-disclosure about exhibitionism and addiction to marijuana.
- **Rule 3:** The therapist presented verbalizations with possible positive reinforcement function ("I'm feeling closer to you" and "I'm enjoying getting to know you better") contingent the client's self-disclosure. Later, he started to reinforce any self-disclosure. The goal was to improve social skills and increase the prob-

ability that the new repertoire would become generalized in the client's relationships with third parties.

- **Rule 4:** It served the purpose of recognizing the effect of the intervention on the client's repertoire. Upon 1 month of FAP treatment, the client revealed that he was using marijuana on a daily basis and committed to reducing the frequency.
- **Rule 5:** Whenever possible, the therapist would describe the CRB1s in relation to the client's learning history and the parallel between *disclosure oneself in-session* and *accepting private events outside the session*. It was also discussed how smoking marijuana facilitated him to manifest exhibitionist behavior.

As a result, the frequency of exhibitionist urges decreased from an average of four/five impulses to two per week, masturbation decreased from seven to three times per week, with changes in the content of the fantasies (he stopped imagining the exhibitionist behavior), and smoking marijuana decreased from seven to 4 days a week. In the 6-month follow-up, the urges to express exhibitionist behavior occurred twice a month and the use of marijuana once a week. Finally, his stage of anxiety and depression were no longer at the clinical level, there was a possible generalization of CRB2s with a greater social connection in the academic context, and the client began to date a girl.

The study by Paul et al. (1999) demonstrated how the principles of FAP can be included in complex clinical cases involving drug abuse. In the context of clinical private service, clients with severe difficulties and in multiple areas are more the rule than the exception (Kazdin, 2008). FAP was helpful for the therapist identify target behaviors that occurred in-session and intervene on them, producing encouraging results.

Gifford et al. (2011) studied how behavioral therapies could enhance the results of drug treatment for harmful tobacco use. Two groups received 10 weeks of the bupropion antidepressant; however, pre-established ACT and FAP strategies were added to the experimental group. Psychotherapies occurred weekly, with one group meeting and one individual meeting. The ACT intervention consisted of accepting unpleasant physical symptoms (abstinence syndrome) that increased the probability of relapses. The application of FAP aimed to create circumstances within the therapeutic context for unpleasant physical symptoms to be evoked (Rule 2), effective avoidance behaviors under the control of aversive stimulation (asking for help instead of smoking, accepting physical symptoms) to be reinforced in-session (Rule 3), and discussing how tolerating aversive stimulation in-session was functionally similar to tolerating aversive stimulation out-of-session (Rule 5).

The researchers recorded changes throughout the process and in post-treatment. Process measurements were symptoms of nicotine abstinence, mood swings, experiential avoidance, acceptance, and therapeutic relationship; and the outcome records included client satisfaction and objective measurement for nicotine. The data pointed to a higher proportion of abstinence after the intervention and at the 12-month follow-up for the experimental group and that the underlying hypothesized processes (acceptance and therapeutic relationship) were responsible for the change. Such study conducted by Gifford et al. (2011) provided more robust results

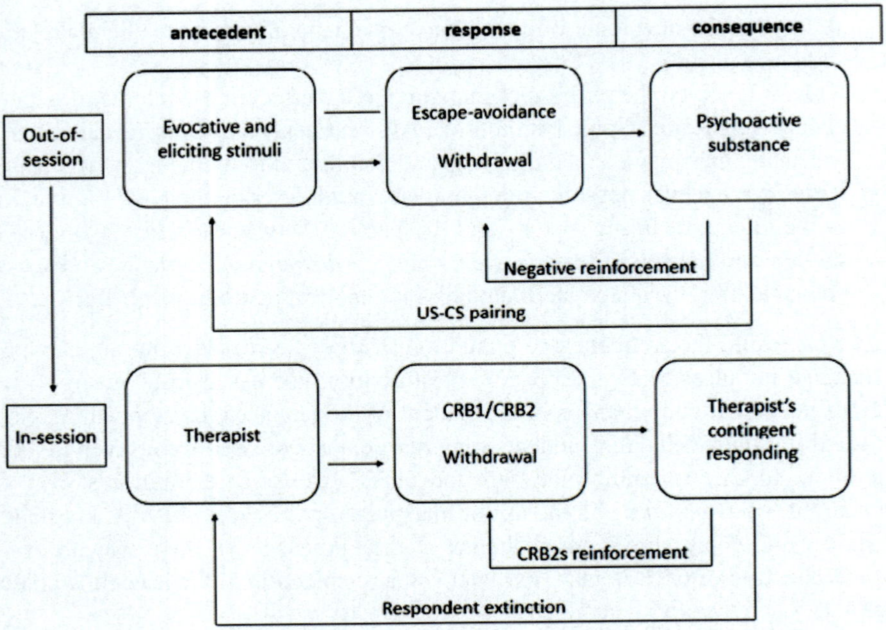

Fig. 9.3 FAP psychotherapeutic model for substance-dependent clients who manifest withdrawal syndrome

on the relationship between interpersonal interventions focusing on the therapeutic relationship and improvement regarding substance consumption. FAP psychotherapeutic model for substance-dependent clients who manifest withdrawal syndrome is summarized in Fig. 9.3.

Holman et al. (2012) conducted a study with the purpose of integrating empirically validated treatments for depression and smoking with FAP strategies. The intervention combined behavioral activation (Martell et al., 2001), smoking cessation (Perkins et al., 2008), and ACT (Hayes et al., 2012). FAP was applied as an opportunity to modeling behaviors that impacted depressed mood and smoking urges; a repertoire that produced positive social reinforcement was incompatible with depressed and nicotine-dependent behaviors. Five participants received 24 sessions of psychotherapy. Self-reported measures for depression, smoking, psychiatric symptoms and interpersonal functioning, and objective measures for nicotine were recorded. The results revealed that four of the five clients were exempt of the diagnostic criteria for major depression, significantly decreased the symptoms manifested, and improved interpersonal functioning. One of the clients had his diagnosis maintained, but his symptoms were moderately decreased and his interpersonal functioning was increased. Three of the five patients abstained from smoking, one presented significant changes (from an average of 13.2 to less than one cigarette a day), and the last patient had moderate changes (a 25–50% decrease in use).

Holman et al. (2012) used a number of pre-established sessions and interventions and only the FAP was conducted ideographically. The advantages of adding FAP to the protocols were (a) to identify problem behaviors that could go unnoticed and not be targets for intervention and (b) to relate them to treatment for nicotine dependence. In addition to the overall results, the researchers presented how the FAP intervention was performed and the possible progress observed.

In the first case example, the therapist identified that the client presented countercontrol behavior when he felt obliged to perform a certain task. The escape function seems to have been learned in a context where trusting someone was followed by punishment. The behavior made treatment difficult, as the client had to adopt the psychotherapist's instructions to stop smoking. It was conceptualized that intimacy avoidance behaviors were CRB1s, while acceptance of support and care were CRB2s. Initially the professional discussed that the client would like to create intimacy with people, but was afraid and ended up preventing this relationship (Rule 5). Later, he actively promoted CRB2s assisting the client to divide the number of cigarettes he would consume during the week (to progressively decrease consumption) and direct recommendations to perform activities for the therapist and not for himself (influencing the client to "do for the other"). As a result, the client complied with part of the smoking cessation protocol and felt that the therapist was "on his side" – a feeling that usually did not emerge in his relationships.

The second client presented difficulty expressing his needs due to the fear of causing conflict or disappointment. Asking for help in difficult situations is a significant behavior in the treatment because the individual ensures access to social reinforcers instead of the pharmacological effects of nicotine. Thus, requests made in-session were considered CRB2s. During one session, the client requested if he could postpone the day of his last cigarette since he had been through a stressful week. Would this be considered an escape behavior to keep smoking (CRB1) or a cry for help (CRB2)? The therapist used the case conceptualization and understood the response as an example of self-knowledge and expression of needs. The professional reinforced the behavior by stating that "the client knew the right moment to stop smoking." As a result, the client quit smoking weeks later and a possible generalization occurred when he was more assertive with his family.

Previous research provided relevant data on the use of FAP for substance dependence, but methodological issues made it impossible to state the exclusive impact of psychotherapy on this population, since it was applied in conjunction with other therapies and there was no record of behaviors in-session (the studies recorded drug abuse and reporting on symptoms). In this regard, Aranha et al. (2020) intended to evaluate the isolated effect of the FAP and its hypothesized mechanism of clinical change (the therapist's contingent response to CRB2s) for substance dependence. A single-case A/A + B quasi-experimental was proposed, where A = analytical-behavioral therapy strategies (Meyer et al., 2010), prioritizing the analysis of external contingencies of reinforcement to the session, and B = FAP, prioritizing the modeling of CRBs. 20 sessions were recorded and transcribed for participant 1 and 18 sessions for participant 2. The FAPRS instrument (Callaghan & Follette, 2008) was applied to categorize the behaviors of two therapist–client dyads into 5 sessions at each stage, and there was record of drug abuse 3 months before and 3 months after the procedure. Clients were assisted at a voluntary admission clinic, which included medical consultations, lectures on chemical dependence, cognitive-behavioral psychotherapy, psychoanalytical group therapy, alcoholic/narcotics anonymous group meetings, family group counseling, and physical exercises. FAP sessions were applied individually, focusing on modeling CRB according to case formulations.

The first participant was diagnosed with alcohol use disorder and sought help for "fights with relatives." In reality, other areas of his life were also affected: unemployment, expulsion from his parents' home, conflicts with his sister and son-in-law, distance from friends, and 20 years without romantic relationships following his divorce. It caught the psychotherapist's attention (Rule 1, observe CRBs) that the client did not express his feelings and opinions (CRB1s). The same behavior occurred with the other professionals ("he is very closed off") and with his daughter ("I would like my father to talk more"). It was hypothesized that the deficit in the repertoire minimized his access to social and emotional reinforcers and increased the alcohol reinforcer value (Heyman, 1996). The therapeutic goals outlined were to express feelings and opinions (CRB2s). The vignette illustrates how the psychotherapist strengthened the client's CRB2s in-session:

T: *And what did you feel at the time?* (Rule 2, intentionally evoking CRBs).
C: *Well, I was very upset with myself, hurt. Just my daughter, who has always fought, is always fighting, always, you know… it's… doing everything for my good, for my well-being… and there comes a point that says, "I got tired. Enough of causing trouble." I have to walk with my own legs, I have to become aware of everything I've done, of all the results I've brought to myself and to people* (CRB2, express feelings and opinions).
T: *Can I say something I feel now?*
C: *You may.*
T: *In these sessions that we're talking, that we've been talking about certain issues, talking about your family, we also talked about certain strategies on not drinking again, we talked about your new house. But it's the first time I feel that you talk with emotion about a subject. I mean, with a very real emotion, a very real emotion… I can feel it, I can feel you talking about the impact that your daughter had telling you "I can't stand it anymore." While you are telling me about it, it is possible to see that impact here in session. You've even changed your countenance a bit* (Rule 3, positively reinforce CRB2).

The second participant was diagnosed with cocaine use disorder and sought hospitalization for the consequences that cocaine and crack caused in his professional routine. A change was identified in the client's pattern of consumption depending on his marital status. When single, (a) he increased drug use and (b) opted to smoke crack over sniffing cocaine. The psychotherapist sought to understand which problems in the interpersonal repertoire decreased the probability that his relationships would remain stable and intensify dependence. He observed that the client was in conflict with professionals at the clinic for not understanding their intentions (for example, resocialization should occur at lunch time with his family, but he should return before night falls. The client was irritated with the imposition). The client had difficulty in establishing relationships between the behavior of others and the contingencies of reinforcement. Functionally similar behavior occurred in-session (CRB1s) when he reported not understanding his spouse's complaints. In fact, the client performed certain tasks at home, ended up going out with friends and overloading his wife. More conflicts were caused and increased the probability of cocaine/crack use. This excerpt exemplifies how the researcher modeled the establishment of more effective relationships between events in-session (CRB2s):

T: *I mean… let's start backwards. What do you think would justify, from a* [professional] *point of view, not letting someone out* [in re-socialization]*? Not that she won't let… she does, but you must to come back. Goes out and return* (Rule 2, intentionally evoking CRBs).
C: *She made this decision because I think it was made in the meeting here, with all the members,* i.e., *the whole team there* (CRB2, the client relates the behavior of the professional with a discussion between professionals).
T: *Maybe* (Rule 3, positively reinforce CRB2).
C: *Then, just like that, it's gone. Then I picked it up and talked like this… I started to think: "the guys are going out so much, not getting in trouble or anything like that," there is a limit, I think, but each case is a case* (CRB2, the client discriminates the individual reasons he can go out to lunch and come back, while other residents can't go out or can go out and come back the other day etc.).
T: *That's it: each case is different, but let's look at what possibly led* [a professional] *to do that. She has a lot of experience* (Rule 3, positively reinforcing the previous behavior and Rule 2, evoking new relationships between events).

The results indicated that the introduction of FAP, specifically the therapist's contingent responding to CRB2s, followed the progress and there was a decrease in substance consumption for both participants. Participant 1, who stayed longer in psychotherapy, obtained maintenance in the frequency of CRB2s and lower rates of drug use in the follow-up. The study provided by Aranha et al. (2020) strengthened data from previous research on the relationship between the FAP intervention and changes in use patterns and, most importantly, explained that the relationship is likely to be achieved due to changes in the frequency of CRBs in-session. For a detailed description of the case conceptualizations, refer to Aranha (2017) and Aranha & Oshiro (2019).

Final Considerations

The goal of this chapter is to describe the FAP model to substance dependence and the evidence of its efficacy and effectiveness. Since substance dependents have difficulties in interpersonal repertoire that increase the frequency of drug use, FAP intends to develop the interpersonal repertoire of clients, using the therapeutic relationship as the main vehicle for change. When the user's problem behaviors become generalized in the session, it is possible to model more effective repertories and, later on, to trace strategies of transposition to the out-of-session context. Interpersonal progress is expected to decrease substance consumption. The description of FAP conceptual framework for addiction and the research data were intended to promote an additional tool for therapists who work with chemical addicts and want to increase the chances of psychotherapeutic success.

References

American Psychiatric Association (APA). (2013). *Diagnostic and statistical manual of mental disorders* (5th ed.). APA. https://doi.org/10.1176/appi.books.9780890425596

Aranha, A. S. (2017). *Delineamento experimental de caso único: A psicoterapia analítica funcional aplicada ao transtorno por uso de substâncias*. Master's thesis. University of São Paulo. https://doi.org/10.11606/D.47.2017.tde-06092017-101420

Aranha, A. S., & Oshiro, C. K. B. (2019). Contribuições da psicoterapia analítica funcional (FAP) no tratamento do transtorno por uso de substâncias (TUS). *Acta Comportamentalia, 27*(2), 197–213.

Aranha, A. S., Oshiro, C. K. B., & Wallace, E. (2020). A single-case quasi-experimental design of functional analytic psychotherapy for substance abuse. *Psicologia: Teoria e Prática, 22*(3), 263–286. https://doi.org/10.5935/1980-6906/psicologia.v22n3p263-286

Banaco, R. A., & Montan, R. N. M. (2018). Terapia analítico-comportamental. In N. A. Zanelatto & R. Laranjeira (Eds.), *O tratamento da dependência química e as terapias cognitivo-comportamentais: Um guia para terapeutas* (2nd ed., pp. 115–132). Artmed.

Banaco, R. A., Zamignani, D. R., & Meyer, S. B. (2010). Função do comportamento e do DSM: Terapeutas analítico-comportamentais discutem a psicopatologia. In E. Z. Tourinho & S. V. Luna (Eds.), *Análise do comportamento: Investigações históricas, conceituais e aplicadas* (pp. 175–191). Roca.

Banaco, R. A., Kovac, R., Martone, R. C., Vermes, J. S., & Zamignani, D. R. (2012). Psicopatologia. In M. M. C. Hübner & M. B. Moreira (Eds.), *Temas clássicos de psicologia sob a ótica da Análise do Comportamento*. Guanabara Koogan.

Benvenuti, M. F. (2004). Condicionamento respondente: Algumas implicações para o desenvolvimento de tolerância, síndrome de abstinência e overdose. In C. N. Abreu & H. J. Guilhardi (Eds.), *Terapia comportamental e cognitivo-comportamental: Práticas clínicas* (pp. 186–193). Roca.

Benvenuti, M. F. (2007). Uso de drogas, recaída e o papel do condicionamento respondente: Possibilidades do trabalho do psicólogo em ambiente natural. In D. R. Zamignani, R. Kovac, & J. S. Vermes (Eds.), *A clínica de portas abertas: Experiências e fundamentação do acompanhamento terapêutico e da prática em ambiente extraconsultório* (pp. 307–327). Esetec.

Bernardes, A. M. T. (2008). *Relação entre enriquecimento ambiental na auto-administração oral de álcool em ratos*. Master's thesis. University of São Paulo. https://doi.org/10.11606/D.47.2008.tde-05062008-172705

Borloti, E. B., Haydu, V. B., & Machado, A. R. (2015). Crack: Análise comportamental e exemplos das funções da dependência. *Acta Comportamentalia, 23*(3), 323–338.

Callaghan, G. M., & Follette, W. C. (2008). FAPRS manual: Manual for the functional analytic psychotherapy rating scale. *The Behavior Analyst Today, 9*(1), 57–97. https://doi.org/10.1037/h0100649

Callaghan, G. M., Summers, C. J., & Weidman, M. (2003). The treatment of histrionic and narcissistic personality disorder behaviors: A single-subject demonstration of clinical effectiveness using functional analytic psychotherapy. *Journal of Contemporary Psychotherapy, 33*, 321–339. https://doi.org/10.1023/B:JOCP.0000004502.55597.81

Catania, A. C. (1999). *Aprendizagem: Comportamento, linguagem e cognição* (4th ed.) (D. G. de Souza, Trad.). Artmed. (Original work published in 1998).

Costa, J. B. P., & Valerio, N. I. (2008). Transtorno de personalidade anti-social e transtornos por uso de substâncias: Caracterização, comorbidades e desafios ao tratamento. *Temas em Psicologia, 16*(1), 119–132.

Ferster, C. B. (1973). A functional analysis of depression. *American Psychologist, 28*(10), 857–870. https://doi.org/10.1037/h0035605

Garcia-Mijares, M., & Silva, M. T. A. (2006). Dependência de drogas. *Psicologia USP, 17*(4), 213–240.

Gifford, E. V., Ritsher, J. B., McKellar, J. D., & Moos, R. H. (2006). Acceptance and relationship context: A model of substance use disorder treatment outcome. *Addiction, 101*(8), 1167–1177. https://doi.org/10.1111/j.1360-0443.2006.01506.x

Gifford, E. V., Kohlenberg, B. S., Hayes, S. C., Pierson, H. M., Piasecki, M. P., Antonnucio, D. O., & Palm, K. M. (2011). Does acceptance and relationship focused behavior therapy contribute to bupropion outcomes? A randomized controlled trial of functional analytic psychotherapy and acceptance and commitment therapy for smoking cessation. *Behavior Therapy, 42*, 700–715. https://doi.org/10.1016/j.beth.2011.03.002

Guilhardi, H. J. (2013). Alcoolismo: Conceitos da análise do comportamento para superação. *Instituto de Terapia por Contingências de Reforçamento.* (Original work published in 2010). Retrieved from http://itcrcampinas.com.br/txt/alcoolismo.pdf

Guilhardi, H. J. (2018). Mais do bom não faz bem: Problemas do reforço livre. *Revista Brasileira de Análise do Comportamento, 14*(2), 171–190. https://doi.org/10.18542/rebac.v14i2.7537

Hayes, S. C., Strosahl, K. D., & Wilson, K. G. (2012). *Acceptance and commitment therapy: The process and practice of mindful change* (2nd ed.). Guilford Press.

Heyman, G. (1996). Resolving the contradictions of addiction. *Behavioral and Brain Sciences, 19*(4), 561–574. https://doi.org/10.1017/S0140525X00042990

Higgins, S. T., Heil, S. H., & Sigmon, S. C. (2007). A behavioral approach to the treatment of substance use disorders. In E. P. Sturmey (Ed.), *Functional analysis in clinical treatment* (pp. 261–282). Elsevier. https://doi.org/10.1016/B978-012372544-8/50015-X

Holman, G., Kohlenberg, R. J., Tsai, M., Haworth, K., Jacobson, E., & Liu, S. (2012). Functional analytic psychotherapy is a framework for implementing evidence-based practices: The example of integrated smoking cessation and depression treatment. *International Journal of Behavioral Consultation and Therapy, 7*, 58–62. https://doi.org/10.1037/h0100938

Kanter, J. W., Landes, S. J., Busch, A. M., Rusch, L. C., Brown, K. R., Baruch, D. E., & Holman, G. I. (2006). The effect of contingent reinforcement on target variables in outpatient psychotherapy for depression: An investigation of functional analytic psychotherapy. *Journal of Applied Behavior Analysis, 29*, 463–467. https://doi.org/10.1901/jaba.2006.21-06

Kazdin, A. E. (2008). Evidence-based treatment and practice: New opportunities to bridge clinical research and practice, enhance the knowledge base, and improve patient care. *American Psychologist, 63*(3), 146–159. https://doi.org/10.1037/0003-066X.63.3.146

Kohlenberg, R. J., & Tsai, M. (1991). *Functional analytic psychotherapy: A guide for creating intense and curative therapeutic relationships*. Plenum.

Laranjeira, R. et al. (Orgs.) (2014). *II Levantamento nacional de álcool e drogas (LENAD) –2012*. São Paulo: INPAD.

Lima, G. O. (2017). *Psicoterapia analítica funcional como tratamento do transtorno de estresse pós-traumático: Delineamento experimental de caso único*. Master's thesis. University of São Paulo. https://doi.org/10.11606/D.47.2018.tde-06022018-162328

Lovo, A. R. B. R. (2019). *Psicoterapia analítica funcional como tratamento do transtorno de ansiedade social*. Master's thesis. University of São Paulo. https://doi.org/10.11606/D.47.2019.tde-12112019-110625

Madden, G. J., & Bickel, W. K. (2010). *Impulsivity: The behavioral and neurological science of discounting*. APA. https://doi.org/10.1037/12069-000

Marlatt, G. A., & Donovan, D. M. (Orgs.). (2009). *Prevenção de recaída: Estratégia de manutenção no tratamento de comportamentos adictivos* (2nd ed.). Artmed.

Martell, C. R., Addis, M. E., & Jacobson, N. S. (2001). *Depression in context: Strategies for guided action*. WW Norton & Co..

Meyer, S. B., Del Prette, G., Zamignani, D. R., Banaco, R. A., Neno, S., & Tourinho, E. Z. (2010). Análise do Comportamento e Terapia Analítico-Comportamental. In E. Z. Tourinho & S. V. Luna (Eds.), *Análise do comportamento: Investigações históricas, conceituais e aplicadas* (pp. 153–174). Roca.

Miguel, A. D. Q. C., Yamauchi, R., Simões, V., da Silva, C. J., & Laranjeira, R. R. (2015). From theory to treatment: Understanding addiction from an operant behavioral perspective. *Journal of Modern Education Review, 5*(8), 778–787. https://doi.org/10.15341/jmer(2155-7993)/08.05.2015/006

Moos, R. H. (2007). Theory-based active ingredients of effective treatments for substance use disorders. *Drug and Alcohol Dependence, 88*(2–3), 109–121. https://doi.org/10.1016/j.drugalcdep.2006.10.010

Nelson, K. M., Yang, J. P., Maliken, A. C., Tsai, M., & Kohlenberg, R. J. (2016). Introduction to using structured evocative activities in functional analytic psychotherapy. *Cognitive and Behavioral Practice, 23*(4), 459–463. https://doi.org/10.1016/j.cbpra.2013.12.009

Oshiro, C. K. B. (2014). Psicoterapia analítica funcional. Functional Analytic Psychotherapy (FAP). In *Especialização em Terapia Cognitiva*. São Paulo: Instituto de Terapia Cognitiva.

Oshiro, C. K. B., Kanter, J. W., & Meyer, S. B. (2012). A single-case experimental demonstration of functional analytic psychotherapy with two clients with severe interpersonal problems. *International Journal of Behavioral Consultation and Therapy, 7*, 111–116. https://doi.org/10.1037/h0100945

Paul, R. H., Marx, B. P., & Orsillo, S. M. (1999). Acceptance-based psychotherapy in the treatment of an adjudicated exhibitionist: A case example. *Behavior Therapy, 30*, 149–162. https://doi.org/10.1016/S0005-7894(99)80051-3

Pedersen, E. R., Callaghan, G. M., Prins, A., Nguyen, H., & Tsai, M. (2012). Functional analytic psychotherapy as an adjunct to cognitive-behavioral treatments for posttraumatic stress disorder: Theory and application in a single case design. *International Journal of Behavioral Consultation and Therapy, 7*(2–3), 125–134. https://doi.org/10.1037/h0100947

Perkins, K. A., Conklin, C. A., & Levine, M. D. (2008). *Practical clinical guidebooks series. Cognitive-behavioral therapy for smoking cessation: A practical guidebook to the most effective treatments*. Routledge/Taylor & Francis Group.

Pezzato, F. A., Brandão, A. S., & Oshiro, C. K. B. (2012). Intervenção baseada na psicoterapia analítica funcional em um caso de transtorno de pânico com agorafobia. *Revista Brasileira de Terapia Comportamental e Cognitiva, 14*(1), 74–84. https://doi.org/10.31505/rbtcc.v14i1.495

Rachlin, H. (1997). Four teleological theories of addiction. *Psychonomic Bulletin & Review, 4*(4), 462–473. https://doi.org/10.3758/BF03214335

Ribeiro, M., & Laranjeira, R.. (Orgs.) (2012). *O tratamento do usuário de crack* (2nd ed.). Artmed.

Rush, B., Tremblay, J., & Brown, D. (2019). Development of a needs-based planning model to estimate required capacity of a substance use treatment system. *Journal of Studies on Alcohol and Drugs, s18*, 51–63. https://doi.org/10.15288/jsads.2019.s18.51

Siegel, S. (2005). Drug tolerance, drug addiction, and drug anticipation. *Current Directions in Psychological Science, 14*(6), 296–300. https://doi.org/10.1111/j.0963-7214.2005.00384.x

Silva, C. J., & Serra, A. M. (2004). Terapias cognitiva e cognitivo-comportamental em dependência química. *Revista Brasileira de Psiquiatria, 26*(1), 33–39. https://doi.org/10.1590/S1516-44462004000500009

Skinner, B. F. (1945). The operational analysis of psychological terms. *Psychological Review, 52*(5), 270–277. https://doi.org/10.1037/h0062535

Skinner, B. F. (1953). *Science and human behavior*. Macmillan.

Skinner, B. F. (1957). *Century psychology series. Verbal behavior*. Appleton-Century-Crofts. https://doi.org/10.1037/11256-000

Skinner, B. F. (1974). *About behaviorism*. Alfred A. Knopf.

Tonigan, J. S., & Miller, W. R. (2002). The inventory of drug use consequences (InDUC): Test-retest stability and sensitivity to detect change. *Psychology of Addictive ehaviors, 16*(2), 165–168. https://doi.org/10.1037/0893-164X.16.2.165

Tsai, M., Kohlenberg, R. J., Kanter, J. W., Kohlenberg, B., Follette, W. C., & Callaghan, G. M. (2009). *A guide to functional analytic psychotherapy: Awareness, courage, love and behaviorism*. Springer. https://doi.org/10.1007/978-0-387-09787-9

Tsai, M., Kohlenberg, R. J., Kanter, J. W., Holman, G. I., & Loudon, M. P. (2012). *The CBT distinctive features series. Functional analytic psychotherapy: Distinctive features*. Routledge/Taylor & Francis Group.

Vandenberghe, L. (2007). Functional analytic psychotherapy and the treatment of obsessive compulsive disorder. *Counseling Psychology Quarterly, 20*, 105–114. https://doi.org/10.1080/09515070701197479

Vartanian, J. F. (2017). *Efeitos da evocação sobre os comportamentos clinicamente relevantes na psicoterapia analítica funcional*. Master's thesis. University of São Paulo. https://doi.org/10.11606/D.47.2017.tde-26092017-110243

Vilas Boas, D. L. O., Banaco, R. A., & Borges, N. B. (2012). Discussões da análise do comportamento acerca dos transtornos psiquiátricos. In N. B. Borges & F. A. Cassas (Eds.), *Clínica analítico-comportamental: Aspectos teóricos e práticos* (pp. 95–101). Artmed.

Wilson, K. G., & Byrd, M. R. (2004). ACT for substance abuse and dependence. In S. Hayes & K. D. Strosahl (Eds.), *A practical guide to acceptance and commitment therapy* (pp. 153–184). Springer. https://doi.org/10.1007/978-0-387-23369-7_7

World Health Organization. (2018). *International classification of diseases and related health problems* (11th ed.). Recuperado de. https://icd.who.int/browse11/l-m/en

Xavier, R. N. (2018). *Eficácia da psicoterapia analítica funcional para o transtorno de oposição desafiante: Experimento de caso único*. Doctoral thesis. University of São Paulo. https://doi.org/10.11606/T.47.2018.tde-04072018-154838

Chapter 10
Dialectical Behavioral Therapy (DBT) for Substance Use Associated with Borderline Personality Disorder

Jan Luiz Leonardi and Dan Josua

Introduction

Dialectical behavioral therapy (DBT) is an approach based on behavior analysis, the dialectical philosophy, and Zen practice. First developed by Marsha Linehan to treat patients with suicidal and self-injury behaviors, DBT has been recognized as a gold-standard treatment for borderline personality disorder (BPD) and more recently extended to other clinical conditions such as eating disorders, substance use, major depression, and adherence to medical treatments, in addition to being adapted to children and adolescents with severe behavioral issues (Lungu & Linehan, 2016).

Soon after the first randomized clinical trial for patients with BPD, (Linehan et al., 1991), Linehan began adapting DBT for a population at greater risk of early death – patients with BPD and substance use (Linehan et al., 1999) followed by BPD and opioid addiction comorbidities (Linehan et al., 2002). Thus, incorporating procedures aimed at better attending people with substance use-related disorders has been a priority in the development of DBT for at least 20 years. Such adaptation is essential as the double diagnosis of substance use disorder and BPD ranks among the most common in the field of mental health (Dimeff & Linehan, 2008).

To serve this population, addiction-oriented procedures retrieved from other empirically sustained interventions were added to DBT's standard therapeutic structure. Thus, while keeping forms and functions of traditional treatment, DBT for substance abuse disorder (DBT-SUD) has introduced procedures (such as toxicological tests) and synthetized strategies from other well-established intervention models (e.g., treatments focused both on damage control and withdrawal symptoms) (Axelrod, 2018).

As such, to better explain DBT-SUD, we must first describe an overview of standard DBT – background and rationale underlying its structure, as well as its

J. L. Leonardi (✉) · D. Josua
Instituto de Psicologia Baseada em Evidências, São Paulo, SP, Brazil

S. M. Oliani et al. (eds.), *Behavior Analysis and Substance Dependence*,
https://doi.org/10.1007/978-3-030-75961-2_10

necessary adjustments for understanding and treating behavioral addictions. After this introduction, we proceed to describe mechanisms specifically added to deal with substance use disorders.

History and Philosophical Framework of DBT

DBT can be considered the product of the difficulties experienced by its developer in applying standard behavioral therapy with patients suffering from chronic suicidal ideation, multiple diagnosis, and severely impaired behavioral control (Miga et al., 2018). When successful, DBT helps building a valuable life from the dialectical balance between two fundamental opposites – the principles of acceptance and change (Dimeff & Linehan, 2008).

To ensure such balance, strategies from Zen Buddhism and humane psychological traditions were added to behavioral therapy (Linehan, 1993). By observing the effects of these oscillations –essential for effective therapeutic processes—as well as swings between extreme behaviors of patients diagnosed with BPD, Linehan noticed that understanding the dialectical philosophy and its therapeutic implications derived from this philosophy would be fundamental to ensure the efficacy of DBT. To her words:

> The tensions that I experienced during therapy; the need to move, to balance or synthesis with this patient population; and the treatment strategies reminiscent of paradoxical techniques that seemed a necessary adjunct to standard behavioral techniques –all these led me to the study of dialectical philosophy as a possible organizing theory or point of view. (Linehan, 1993, p. 30)

The dialectic philosophy, as understood by DBT, comprehends three fundamental treatment-orienting principles. The *wholeness and interrelatedness principle* states that the parts and the whole evolve from their mutual transaction, having a covariant development. Such a concept relates to Skinner's view on the interaction between individual and environment, as represented by his famous quote "Men act upon the world, and change it, and are changed in turn by the consequences of their action" (Skinner, 1957/1992, p. 1).

The *polarity principle* states that seemingly opposite concepts can in fact represent two sides of the same coin. Thus, behaviors that seem dysfunctional at first glance have an important function in extreme living conditions. To Linehan's (1993) words, "It was turning this idea around 'contradictions within wisdom' to 'wisdom within contradictions'—that led me to a number of decisions about the form of DBT" (p. 33).

Finally – and possibly the most intuitive of all principles—the *continuous change* states that the nature of reality itself is marked by inconstancy and novelty, not repetition. This idea can be best summarized by Heraclitus of Ephesus' famous aphorism: "no man ever steps in the same river twice, for it's not the same river and he's not the same man."

Therefore, we must understand that the dialectic philosophy influences DBT both as a way of viewing the world and as a form of dialogue. In addition to adopting such principles, DBT therapists must be clear on the role of their therapeutic stance in ensuring the conversion of these opposites –thesis and antithesis—into a new synthesis. Thus, conflicts brought to session by BPD patients can be faced not entirely as setbacks, but rather as opportunities to build a new reality (i.e., a synthesis).

The Biosocial Model: Central DBT Theoretical Postulate

DBT has a central role in understanding that underneath the chaotic behaviors of individuals with BPD lies their difficulty in finding an intermediate pathway between over and underregulating emotional responses. (Axelrod, 2018; Koerner, 2012; Linehan, 1993, 2015). The same can be argued about suicidal (Linehan, 2015) and substance use behaviors (Dimeff & Linehan, 2008) in the same population. It is particularly interesting to note how the urgency in attenuating negative feelings and low perseverance were highly predictive of BPD characteristics associated to alcohol abuse (Hahn et al., 2016), which suggests the relevance of emotional dysregulation in the genesis of these disorders. Thus, seemingly chaotic behaviors observed in these patients may be understood as disorganized efforts in controlling their emotional suffering.

For this reason, as means to understand the biosocial model and emotional dysregulation, we must first understand DBT's definition of emotion itself. According to Linehan (2015), "are brief, involuntary, full-system, patterned responses to internal and external stimuli" (p. 6). Like some other authors (e.g., Ekman, 2004), DBT emphasizes that emotions are determined by their survival role in evolutionary history and, as such, contains typical action patterns. To wit, emotions are as transcultural as their evoking conditions, and their expression follows a predetermined pattern. The rage we feel when witnessing a threat to someone we love is therefore universally expressed through the same physiological responses and possibilities of action –muscle tension and increased chances of behaving aggressively (damage oriented).

An emotion is the result of the interaction between six subsystems: (1) emotional vulnerability factors; (2) internal and external events that serve as emotional cues (e.g., prompting events) (3) appraisal and interpretations of cues; (4) emotional response tendencies (including physiological, cognitive, experiential responses, and action urges); (5) nonverbal and verbal expressive responses and actions; and (6) after-effects of the initial emotion (Linehan, 2015).

An example can better illustrate the interactions between these subsystems. Imagine that, after a night of excessive drinking, John wakes up feeling nauseated and hungover (1). When he walks into his living room, he catches sight of a pile of beer bottles and food leftovers spread on the floor (2 – external event). He beholds what he reckons to be chaos around him (3). His heart races and he hunches into a defeat body posture (4). He starts to walk towards his bed (5 – nonverbal response) and to think his life is broken beyond repair (5 – verbal behavior). Finally, he lies in bed feeling exhausted and helpless (6), further nourishing the cycle of neither coping nor changing.

DBT sees emotion as the interaction between this complex group of responses, not being isolated in any of those points. In turn, emotional dysregulation is essentially characterized by five factors: (1) proneness to experiencing emotions more intensely; (2) difficulty regulating impulsive behaviors related to strong emotions; (3) difficulty regulating arousal involved in the emotional episode; (4) difficulty to act according to their objectives and values when said action differs from the behavioral inclination evoked by the emotion; and (5) difficulty paying attention to anything other than the emotion-triggering event (Linehan, 2015). Pervasive emotional dysregulation in turn is the inability to regulate emotions in a broad range of situations –a global pattern of emotional dysregulation that may lead to multiple problem-behaviors such as suicide, self-injury, and substance abuse (Koerner, 2012).

Notably, the effects that emotions have over behavior are universal –not exclusive to individuals with emotional regulation deficits. For instance, after waking up late and rushing to a meeting, most people speed in traffic, feel more frustrated with slow drivers, and presume the number of red lights in their way will be higher than normal. In other words, what defines a person with emotional dysregulation is not the effect of emotions over behavior, but the intensity and frequency in which it occurs, as well as an increased difficulty in acting upon emotional urges (Linehan, 1993).

Thus, the biosocial model proposed by Linehan (1993) consists of the theoretical background to describe the possible origins of such emotional regulation deficit. It also helps to promote a scientific understanding of the phenomenon, guide the treatment, and generate compassion (Linehan, 2015). The biosocial model posits that pervasive emotional dysregulation experienced by individuals with BPD stems from the interaction between a biological vulnerability and an invalidating environment. Here is a description of the two poles in this proposal:

The BIO in Biosocial

A good review of the evidence on biological vulnerability in the development of BPD –as proposed by Linehan—can be found in Crowell et al. (2009). In sum, they consist of[1]: genetic influence such as 5-HTT s/s, the TPH-1 gene, and the 5-HT receptor gene, DAT-1; abnormalities in cerebral systems (5-HT, DA, HHA axis); and a neuro limbic disorder. It is also worth noting that substance use disorder is considered to be 30–80%.

[1] 5-HT stands for serotonin; 5-HTT for serotonin transporter; TPH-1 for tryptophan hydroxylase 1; DA for dopamine; DAT-1 for dopamine transporter 1; HHA, hypothalamus-hypophysis-adrenal.

In addition to genetics, such vulnerability may stem from intrauterine factors, physical damage to the nervous central system, or even premature learning during brain development (Linehan, 1993). Thus, impulsivity-related genes to early traumas can alter a person's neurophysiological structure, leaving them more sensitive to emotional stimuli. In practice, this vulnerability is demonstrated in three ways of responding. According to Koerner (2012, p. 5):

> First, people prone to emotion dysregulation react immediately and at low thresholds (high sensitivity). Second, they experience and express emotion intensely (high reactivity), and this high arousal dysregulates cognitive processes too. Third, they experience a long-lasting arousal (slow return to baseline).

In other words, people with pervasive emotional dysregulation feel at lower thresholds, for longer periods of time, and more intensely. Not surprisingly, the environment fails to understand their suffering, which leads to invalidation. Metaphorically, this sensitivity to stimuli that evokes such emotions can be understood similarly to skin burns. Just as pouring warm water onto an intact skin triggers a much different reaction to that provoked by the same water onto a skin with third-degree burn injuries, a person with this biological fragility can respond much more intensely than people with an intact emotional skin.

The SOCIAL in Biosocial: The Invalidating Environment

Invalidating environment is an expression created by Linehan (1993) to designate a social group that is unable to recognize individuals' expressions of covert experiences as natural outcomes of their life trajectory and genetic constitution. In this kind of environment, such expressions are regarded as inappropriate, wrong, or pathological. They also tend to be diminished, mocked, ignored, or neglected. In the words of the author:

> Invalidation has two primary characteristics. First, it tells the individual that she is wrong in both her description and her analyses of her own experiences, particularly in her views of what is causing her own emotions, beliefs, and actions. Second, it attributes her experiences to socially unacceptable characteristics or personality traits (Linehan, 1993, p. 49–50).

When this form of communication is the general rule, individuals struggle to map the world based on covert experiences. For DBT, emotions should serve as a compass that help us interpret the world around us –all in all, they select stimuli that stand out and increase the likelihood of this event being recorded in the future (Barrett, 2017). When an experience is labeled as an unacceptable character trait, individuals lose their ability to learn from these responses. People raised in a chronically invalidating environment thus start questioning their natural emotional experiences, developing more rigid behavioral patterns instead (Koerner, 2012).

The invalidating environment can render people phobic of their own emotional responses, thus worsening the problem in an attempt to escape "bad feelings." As the environment fails to teach emotional regulation and forces people to extreme behaviors, individuals start to escalate expressions. For instance, instead of verbalizing their suffering or feelings of invalidation once more, they start engaging in self-harm – such as cutting themselves – which may initially result in care, attention, etc. When self-injury stops generating the same effects, they start making suicide threats, which may ultimately result in an actual suicide attempt. Vicious escape patterns are thus consolidated, which lead to an oscillation between attempts to eliminate emotional responses (an unreachable goal) and extreme responses (intense and inexorable emotional crises) (Linehan, 1993).

In this context, substance abuse often appears as an attempt at emotional regulation, in the absence of more skilled means of dealing with emotions. Therefore, the function of therapy in DBT is both to block harmful emotional regulation strategies (e.g., excessive alcohol intake) and to teach skills that can fulfill the same regulatory function without the harmful side effects of the old pattern (e.g., emotional regulation skills from DBT; cf. Linehan, 2015).

The Interaction Between BIO and SOCIAL

Linehan's model regards the biological and social as systems in constant interaction, so that the fragility on one side causes vulnerability on the other and vice versa. Thus, an environment of extreme invalidation –where signs of child abuse are ignored, for example—can alter a person's neurological structure so that, throughout life, they become more sensitive to emotion-evoking stimuli. The same is true the other way around: children with greater sensitivity have more difficulty having their reactions validated, precisely because they differ from the norm of a particular family. Thus, children who are so sensitive as to feel "pain in the eyelashes" when anxious struggle more to have their pain validated than those who simply say they are afraid, swallow hard, and manage to get on with their day.

Whichever side the problem begins (so to speak), the question becomes important when an interaction between the social and the biological fields starts generating a dysfunctional emotional regulation. In these cases, such interaction results in people who failed to learn healthy self-regulation and self-care skills. Classic BPD patients may present behaviors such as self-injury, while others start abusing substances as means of emotional regulation, leading to a BPD plus substance use disorder comorbidity. In this context, therapy plays the role of both reaching a commitment to end harmful behavioral patterns and ensuring that the individual learns new, more skillful, and relevant means to be used for the rest of their lives.

Structure of DBT-SUD

DBT states that the intervention process must serve five functions: improve the patient's motivation to remain in treatment and perform behavioral changes; promote the acquisition and strengthening of new behaviors; ensure the generalization of these behaviors for relevant life contexts; help patients restructure their daily environment so that it favors their progress; encourage the therapist to provide the best possible intervention (Koerner, 2012; Linehan, 2015).

In standard DBT, each function is addressed by at least one form of intervention, namely individual psychotherapy, skills training, telephone consultancy, and consultancy between therapists. Importantly, forms of intervention can be adapted depending on the implementation setting, but all functions must be present (Dimeff & Koerner, 2007).

In the case of substance use, new elements have been added to each form. To improve patients' motivation to stay on treatment and make behavioral changes, DBT-SUD includes new commitment strategies, such as scheduling regular phone calls to check on the patient's well-being and meeting friends and/or family members to find and convince patients to return to treatment if contacted by the therapist. As means to promote the acquisition and strengthening of new behaviors, skills training includes specific content focused on substance dependence –such as dialectical abstinence and the notion of *clear mind* (explained in further sections). In the case of generalization of new behaviors to relevant contexts, DBT-SUD emphasizes that the patient must be able to use new skills, even under substance effects –often when most needed. To help the patient restructure their environment and sustain their progress, DBT-SUD addresses the need of burning bridges and building new ones, as well as the importance of community reinforcement. Finally, the consultancy meeting –aimed at monitoring the therapist's compliance to treatment and motivation (cf. Sayrs & Linehan, 2019)— has been provenly fundamental, since DBT-SUD patients commonly miss sessions, abandon therapy, and relapse to substance use, which often render professionals frustrated (Axelrod, 2018).

DBT traditionally ranks behaviors hierarchically (based on the therapist–patient dyad) to determine the intervention sequence (cf. Linehan, 1993, 2015). This helps to organize each session and the whole therapeutic process (especially important in cases of multiple problems), as well as to determine behaviors subject to daily monitoring throughout therapy (see below). This ranking is also important given that substance intake can have different purposes and implications. For example, substance use as a suicide attempt differs from the one that jeopardizes the effectiveness and continuity of treatment, or even the one that severely impairs the patient's quality of life but neither brings risks nor interferes with the therapeutic process. Thus, these uses must be ranked according to their associated risks – in the examples here, a suicide attempt ranks higher in priority than uses that simply affect life quality – which can be left for a more advanced moment in therapy.

The pretreatment phase constitutes the starting point, in which both therapist and patient agree on a structure and outline a treatment plan –which starts to be implemented more avidly on the next stage. Thus, both in standard and DBT-SUD, pretreatment serves to: increase the patient's motivation; establish a 1-year psychotherapy agreement; provide relevant psychoeducation to the case (which includes presenting the biosocial model); explain how DBT works; and rank target behaviors hierarchically from most to least severe (Linehan, 1993). Once these goals are met, the patient can proceed to therapy itself, which begins at Stage 1 (described below) and follow a sequence that is not necessarily linear –going back to previous stages is common practice according to the requirements of the case.

Stage 1 of standard DBT contains behaviors that (1) put the patient's life at risk, such as suicidal actions, self-injury, and suicidal ideation; (2) interfere with the therapeutic process, such as being late or absent, overlooking therapeutic tasks; (3) cause severe losses to the patient's life quality; and (4) constitute essential but absent components of the patient's repertoire (severe behavioral deficits).

In Stage 1 of DBT-SUD, therapists must pay attention to possible life-threatening uses of the substance, such as those involving a clear suicidal intention, an ambivalent possibility of death by overdose (even with no noticeable suicidal intent), intended bodily harm (e.g., drinking with liver disease to cause further damage), and an imminent risk according to medical evidence (e.g., doing cocaine when having a severe heart disease). The therapist must then prioritize behaviors that interfere with therapy, which includes substance use events that limit the patient's ability to participate or benefit from treatment –e.g., missing sessions, being unable to learn due to intoxication, or even running the risk of arrestment due to drug use during probation. Next on the list are behaviors that cause severe losses to the patient's life quality. Here, DBT-SUD employs subcategories, namely discontinue substance use, decrease physical and emotional discomforts associated with withdrawal, reduce cravings and substance-seeking, eliminate options (burn bridges), decrease contact with triggers, approach stimuli whose avoidance would only be superficially safe, and increase community reinforcement (Axelrod, 2018; Dimeff & Linehan, 2008).

Finally, therapy must move to further, less-complex treatment stages. Thorough descriptions of these stages can be found in standard-DBT chapters and textbooks (e.g., Koerner, 2012; Leonardi, 2018; Linehan, 1993). They are not addressed here as they should only be implemented after reaching stable substance use rates, therefore not consisting of DBT-SUD stages themselves.

Behaviors that were chosen and ranked in Stage 1 are then registered by the patient on a daily card that must be examined at the beginning of each individual therapy session. Roughly speaking, the card contains action tendencies on a scale from 0 to 5, actions that occurred, use of trained DBT skills, among other relevant information. It is traditionally filled in pencil or pen on a standardized printed sheet (see Linehan, 2015, p. 73), but some therapists have replaced this format with cell phone applications.

Intervention Strategies: Acceptance, Change, and Dialectics

DBT strategies are sorted into three paradigms: acceptance, change, and dialectics. For Swenson (2016), effective DBT conduct can be described as the dance between these three elements –most resourceful therapists would have the ability to navigate between the principles of acceptance and mindfulness (and the Zen tradition), change techniques from behavior therapy, and the dialectic philosophy.

Within acceptance, the main intervention techniques are (1) *mindfulness* –intentionally and effectively observing, describing, and participating in a single activity at the present time, free of judgment (Linehan, 2015); (2) *radical acceptance* –experiencing a situation in its entirety without attempting to modify it; and (3) *validation* stating that the way a person behaves, thinks, and feels is coherent and justified (Koerner, 2012; Linehan, 1997). Validating includes paying attention to what the patient is talking about, asking questions that facilitate the continuation of the report, demonstrating an understanding of their experiences, acknowledging their feelings, thoughts, and behaviors as an effect of their biology, their interaction history with the world, and their current context.

Linehan (1997) ranks validation strategies into six different levels and argues that simply acknowledging the magnitude of the problem can be insufficient or, at times, iatrogenic. Therefore, following validation strategies, the therapist must then move towards the change paradigm and actively seek solutions to the problem. In other words, as noted by Swenson (2016), the dance between paradigms is essential and the excessive permanence in one can configure a risk for a satisfactory therapeutic development.

In the change paradigm, the therapist performs a chain analysis of the target behavior –a step-by-step functional analysis of events that have occurred and elements that are subject to intervention (see Fig. 10.1). In brief terms, a chain analysis first requires an objective and accurate description of the behavior (e.g., snorting 5 g of cocaine in the bathroom at home). Then it specifies events that preceded and followed its occurrence, namely (1) *triggering event* – the initial stimulus that led to the behavior; (2) *vulnerability factors* –conditions of the organism that modulate the evocative power of the triggering event, such as pain, illness, sleep deprivation, hangover, hunger, malnutrition, and stress; (3) *links* –events that occurred between the trigger and behavior, which may be the patient's actions, thoughts, sensations and emotions, and/or environmental events, including other people's actions; and (4) *positive and negative consequences of the behavior*, indicating whether they are short-, medium-, or long term and the hypothetical behavioral processes (positive reinforcement, negative reinforcement, intermittent reinforcement, punishment, and extinction). For an in-depth look at the chain analysis protocol, see Rizvi and Ritschel (2014) and Rizvi (2019).

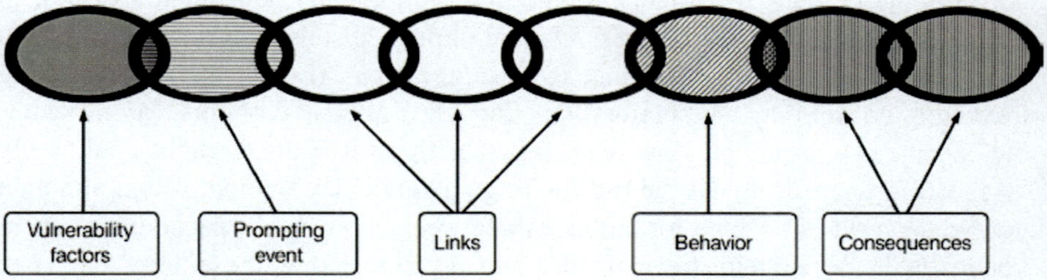

Fig. 10.1 Graphic representation of chain analysis

After concluding the chain analysis, the therapist and the patient proceed to planning and implementing the intervention – phase called *solution analysis*. As explained by Heard and Swales (2015), the first step consists of selecting elements from the chain analysis that needs to be modified according to how strongly and frequently they exert control over the behavior as well as how difficult it is to change it. Next, therapist and client name as many forms as possible to interrupt the occurrence of problem behaviors and achieve their goals; at this point, feasibility, pros/cons, and potential success of the solutions should not be considered. This second step involves the therapist proposing specific intervention procedures for the selected element of the chain, both those imported from behavior and cognitive-behavioral therapies as well as those developed by DBT itself. Implementing such procedures must be done with guidance, in which the therapist (1) explains how it works and how it can contribute to achieving a certain objective, (2) provides relevant theoretical background, (3) specifies the course of action, and (4) describes possible side effects.

That done, the therapist–patient dyad seeks to evaluate the effectiveness of the proposed solutions by analyzing each one's obstacles (repertoire deficit, other chain elements, logistics), pros and cons, and possible outcomes. Whenever possible, chosen solutions should be trained or tested in session, so that the patient is better prepared to use it in other contexts. Finally, patients implement solutions in their daily context and, after reported in session, therapists must evaluate the patient's experience, give positive feedback, refine its implementation, and value the attempt – regardless of its effectiveness. For a more in-depth analysis of solutions and various interventions aimed at each chain element, see Heard and Swales (2015).

Such step-by-step description of the intervention can give the false impression of simplicity or mechanism. Interventions with patients who present multiple diagnoses and substance abuse rarely take such a linear course. On the contrary, the dance between the paradigms of acceptance and change are expected to occasionally occur during chain and solution analyses.

In addition, before implementing solutions, the patient must be provenly motivated to adhere to a certain therapeutic objective (e.g., lower cocaine use to zero), abide by a specific procedure, or commit to the entire treatment plan (Koerner, 2012). As a recognition of the importance and difficulty to produce such motivation, Linehan (1993) included commitment strategies drawn from the cognitive-behavioral tradition and social psychology research. Some consist of interventions with curious names such as *door in the face*, *foot in the door*, and *devil's advocate*. An example consists of connecting current commitments with previous ones, in which the therapist recalls a successful commitment episode in the patient's life and links it with the possibility of change in the current context. If a patient who is being treated for cocaine says something like "Enough, I'm done with this! My life without cocaine is unbearable! I'm doing some and that's it!", the therapist could reply "It recently seemed impossible for you to go a single day without using, although you've been rid of cocaine for the past three weeks now. Let's rescue the moment you made the decision to stop and what helped you to endure those times and try to remake your commitment."

Finally, in the dialectical paradigm, the therapist aims to balance the need for acceptance and change to coexist both in the life and the treatment of patients with chaotic lives. From a dialectical point of view, the therapist embraces the notion of polarities and sees them as opportunities rather than obstacles to find syntheses in the therapeutic process (Koerner, 2012). The dialectical posture allows flexibility when facing common clashes in psychotherapy. Particularly relevant for DBT-SUD is the idea of dialectical abstinence (explained in more detail below), which proposes that abstinence and compassion for those who have returned are possible.

In addition, dialectics appears as a series of strategies on how the therapist can handle the steadiness of the process and ensure movement. These strategies have thought-provoking names and often try to convey the notion that tying with only one side of the truth is unnecessary. In this sense, a strategy called *entering the paradox* has remarkable effects, in which the patient is invited to experience the idea that some dilemmas cannot be solved (Koerner, 2012). For example, the therapist genuinely cares for a patient and, at the same time, is paid to care (and, to some extent, becomes less concerned once the payment ceases). Another interesting strategy is the idea of *making lemons into lemonade*, which proposes that some bitter situations in life can be reversed into something as refreshing as possible. This is the case of a patient who hates a colleague from skills training while also needs to exercise his or her ability of not judging (mindfulness). The complete skills list can be found in DBT textbooks (cf. Koerner, 2012; Linehan, 1993).

DBT-SUD-Specific Strategies

Although DBT-SUD is part of a therapeutic effort that falls within the scope of standard DBT, some specific strategies have been developed to assist the population that (also) suffers from substance use disorder. Like other DBT concepts, this skill set can be remembered by its acronym DCBA – dialectical abstinence, clear mind and community reinforcement, burning bridges and building bridges, alternate rebellion, and adaptive denial.

Dialectical Abstinence

As Linehan (2015) explains, dialectical abstinence is a relapse prevention strategy that integrates the goal of total abstinence whenever one is suffering from withdrawal symptoms (even for a short time) and adequate damage control at each relapse. Here, the patient is instructed and encouraged to (1) establish a solid commitment to abstinence, (2) plan how to remain abstinent, and (3) manage relapses to avoid getting worse. Some examples of absenteeism and relapse management involve calling the therapist –or other people who can be of help—, writing down the pros and cons of using the substance; eliminating rules like "I've already done drugs today, so I'm not abstinent anymore and it doesn't matter whether I do more or not"; renew the commitment to total abstinence –telling themselves this was the last time they relapsed; etc.

Clear Mind

Linehan adopted and adapted several techniques from his experience with Zen Buddhism (Koerner, 2012; Swenson, 2016), among which stands the notion of three states of mind, namely the *rational*, *emotional*, and *wise mind*. According to Linehan (2015), DBT-based treatment fundamentally includes helping patients to get out of severe oscillations between the emotional, excessively impulsive, and immediate mind and the rational, excessively cold, and calculating mind. Thus, there would be a third state of mind, inherent to any human being (and more than the mere intersection between *emotional* and *rational* mind) that would allow a response that is both adapted to life situations and faithful to one's values. Linehan calls this a *wise mind* and argues that accessing this type of functioning is essential, as it favors good decision-making by ensuring that such a process is both intuitive, immediate, and aligned with important long-term values (Linehan, 1993). For DBT-SUD and other addictive behaviors, Linehan (2015) developed similar concepts, called *addict mind*, *clean mind,* and *clear mind*.

The *addict mind* is a state in which the individual is dominated by addiction, so that behaviors, thoughts, and emotions are focused on consuming the substance. In this context, the individual exhibits behaviors such as glamorizing the drug, stealing to finance their addiction, buying paraphernalia, and, of course, using the drug. In addition, the *addict mind* involves thoughts such as "I am not a drug addict" or "no problem if I do drugs only once a week," as well as the urgency to eliminate craving sensations, such as dysphoria, jittering, sweating, and body temperature changes. In a nutshell, the addicted mind makes the patient willing to do anything for one dose.

Individuals with a *clean mind* present seemingly irrelevant behaviors that had previously led to substance use (e.g., going out with the same friends, to the same type of party where it occurred), in addition to keeping paraphernalia, lowering or interrupting medication, and abandoning treatment. This state of mind also involves thoughts such as "I am healed" and "I can solve my own problems," associated with a sense of control and invincibility. In short, patients with *clean minds* risk overlooking the dangers of having a relapse when seeing themselves immune to the temptation of consuming the substance.

The *clear mind* – intervention goal—is the synthesis of the dialectical tension between *addict* and *clean mind*. In this state, individuals can and should enjoy the success of their abstinence, but also accept the possibility of a relapse and thus make plans for when feeling compelled to use the drug. In the words of Linehan (2015):

> Overcoming addiction is like fighting a long war against urges to engage in the addictive behavior. The urges win a battle when you end up doing the addictive behavior, and you win when, despite the urges' attacks on you, you don't do the addictive behavior. Clean mind is

> forgetting the war once a few battles are over, it's thinking that because you've repelled the urges a few times, they will not come back, or that if they do come back, they will be easy to repel. When you are in clean mind, you don't prepare for battle, and your defenses are down. Urges can catch you unprepared and win. Addict mind is like being under siege by the urges and believing that you can never repel them again. When you are in addict mind, you don't remember your victories; when you are defeated, you don't regroup and fight back. Clear mind is remembering both your victories and your defeats, fighting with all your might, and staying prepared for battle even when you are experiencing no urges. (Linehan, 2015 p. 483)

Community Reinforcement

Based on the concept of operant behavior (cf. Skinner, 1938/1991) –in which subsequent events can retroact and alter the individual's behavior in the future—community reinforcement (cf. Meyers & Smith, 1995) aims to strengthen behaviors that are alternative and/or incompatible with drug use, such as spending time with non-addicts, playing sports, trying new activities, going to the movies, listening to music, reading, learning a new language, and structuring a career.

A central aspect of community reinforcement refers to behavioral experiments on abstinence. Based on the premise that full abstinence can be difficult to achieve and increase the chances of treatment dropout, the therapist encourages short abstinence periods. After the client having spent 2 days without using the drug, the therapist has the role of valuing this achievement and encouraging gradually longer periods. In parallel, the patient can engage in various pleasurable activities while abstinent, which can only occur when not under the effect of the substance.

Burning Bridges and Building New Ones

As explained by Linehan (2015), burning bridges corresponds to all behaviors that patients exhibit to eliminate any stimuli involved in substance consumption from their lives. The goal is for the patient to get rid of phone numbers, e-mail addresses, and other contact information of drug dealers or friends who contribute to drug use, as well as clothing and household items associated with the substance and drug use paraphernalia (syringe, herb grinder, lighter), among others. The point is to destroy anything that makes addictive behaviors more likely.

In turn, building new bridges is the strategy of creating images and smells as vividly as possible to compete with the stimuli involved in a craving episode. Roughly speaking, the idea is to distract the patient from the sensations, images, and smells related to addiction and thus lessen the urge to consume the substance.

Alternative Rebellion and Adaptive Denial

If addictive behavior is intended to express revolt, disobedience, or insubordination to a person or society, other behaviors can be used as substitutes. *Alternative rebellion* aims to meet the need patients have to rebel without affecting their life quality by engaging in activities –as suggested by Linehan (2015)—such as shave the hair off, dye the hair an extravagant color, make a tattoo, expose unpopular opinions, give an honest rather than a polite answer, wear clothes inside out, wear shoes from different pairs, print a social criticism message on a t-shirt, and post a world view on a blog or Facebook feed.

Adaptive denial, on the other hand, can be understood as a "mental vacation" for logical arguments concerning the risk of using the substance. By adopting this strategy, patients force themselves to say they are not going to do the drug now – even when the impulse is particularly high. In the words of Linehan (2015), "Adaptive denial' refers to adamantly convincing yourself that you don't want to engage in the addictive behavior when an urge hits, or that the addictive behavior is not a possibility." (p. 490). Thus, patients are invited to engage in another task such as counting coins in a glass jar while repeating to themselves "I need to count these 10-cent coins." Alternatively, they can simply commit to not using the drug for 5 min and then extending this period for another minutes, and so on.

Patient Consultancy Vs. Environmental Intervention

In addition to DCBA skills, an important adaptation of DBT-SUD concerns the relationship between *patient consultancy* versus *environmental intervention*. Standard DBT emphasizes the need for the patient to independently produce important consequences. Thus, direct interventions made by the therapist in the client's environment are an exception. Conversely, due to the frequency with which addicts omit information on their substance use, DBT-SUD uses toxicological tests –such as urine tests and breathalyzers—which are common in empirically supported treatments for substance use. In other words, while standard DBT therapists emphasize patient consultancy, DBT-SUD favors environmental intervention.

A Brief Clinical Example

The patient – Bia (fictitious name)—came to the clinic without a diagnosis but little analysis was necessary to assess the severity of the case. Both shallow (more recent) and deeper (slightly older) scars on her arms pointlessly tried to hide behind skull tattoos. The blunt speech hid a den of anger and resentment towards her parents who "could never understand her".

Since she was little, she felt different, more sensitive than other people. Even before she turned 10, she experienced violent anxiety episodes before going to sleep. The parents, facing their daughter's increased sensitivity, simply told her to stop with the nonsense and go to sleep. Her talking about her childhood seemed almost like a literal description of Linehan's (1993) biosocial model.

During her adolescence and early adulthood, her emotional dysregulation crises worsened, and she began a cycle of self-harm combined with alcohol abuse. The relief brought by alcohol intake and self-injuries in her arms gradually demanded larger doses and deeper perforations. By the age of 25, alcohol use had already extended to cocaine followed by crack –self-harm, although without a suicidal intent, had already taken her to the hospital twice.

It took just over a month of work (and psychiatric care assistance) for target behaviors to be established in collaboration with the therapist – zeroing the use of crack, cocaine, and self-harm, as well as not consuming alcohol for at least 6 months. As the use of crack was uncontrolled and put her physical integrity at risk (spending days "lost" in the city's biggest community of crack addicts called *Cracolândia*), this was ranked as the highest behavior in the hierarchy, followed by self-harm, and then by cocaine and alcohol. The latter was important mainly for constituting a frequent link preceding her crack relapses, as revealed by chain analyses.

However, at the beginning of treatment Stage 1, Bia realized the size of her challenge, especially in abandoning substance dependence. She asked to be admitted to a rehabilitation clinic to earn (in her words) "a breather." At that moment, it was essential to validate her sense of helplessness – as she really seemed to lack the tools to solve the problem—and the desperation to find herself trapped in a self-destructive cycle.

During rehab, it was essential to take advantage of her free time to ensure that she continued with her skills training. Interestingly, a series of chain analyzes showed that cocaine use was particularly associated with the presence of a specific friend. When talking about the ability to "burn bridges to build new ones," Bia promptly offered to completely suspend contact with this friend at least during the first year.

However, several other concepts were still challenging. She found it especially difficult to tolerate mindfulness exercises, since it seemed unbearable to endure the bodily sensations linked to the process of doing less busy activities –such as observing her own breathing. The notion of clear mind or dialectical abstinence, on the other hand, seemed particularly difficult to achieve in the rehabilitation environment. Within the security of hospital gates, the idea of relapsing into drug use seemed exceptionally distant.

Thus, not surprisingly, the first post-hospitalization session was marked by a relapse. After being contacted by the psychiatrist to arrange the first urine test – scheduled as a routine – Bia performed a quick mental calculation and realized she only had that day to do crack without getting caught by the test. In this session's chain analysis, the doctor's message was understood as the triggering event, while all the movement between the mental calculation and crack use (about an hour later) were marked as links. The target behavior (or problem) was the drug use itself. The reinforcing consequences are linked to all the chemical effects of the drug in her body. However, we must also highlight delayed (aversive) consequences –in particular, the remorse, feeling of incompetence, and boyfriend's disapproval (with whom she lived).

In this context, it is essential to establish a list of solutions to prevent this chain of events from reoccurring by first scheduling test intervals without this window of opportunity for use. Then, enabling her to talk to the psychiatrist so that these intervals could be adjusted (in this scenario, interpersonal effectiveness skills, with emphasis on patient consultancy, were particularly important). Other solutions – DBT skills that Bia had trained during hospitalization – were discussed, such as the importance of knowing how to get distracted and waiting for emotions to fade, known in DBT as the ACCEPTS skills and emotional mindfulness.

Treating patients like Bia – with multiple diagnoses and a lifelong suffering – is certainly never simple or linear. Nevertheless, it is essential to note how DBT-SUD can help to structure the treatment to prevent the therapist from sinking into the client's ocean of difficulties. If, on the one hand, the ups and downs are expected, on the other, it is essential to always be prepared to deal with inevitable relapses and, above all, restructure both the treatment and the motivation of the patient (and therapist) involved in this type of psychopathology.

Final Considerations

This chapter described the adaptation of DBT by Linehan and collaborators for the comorbidity of substance use and borderline personality disorder (titled DBT-SUD). We briefly presented the central principles of DBT and detail the elements that constitute DBT-SUD, both from the perspective of theory (biosocial model) and clinical practice (treatment stages, intervention techniques, and specific strategies for addictive behaviors).

Finally, we must note that, although DBT-SUD may be effective for substance use disorder without the presence of BPD, it may not be advantageous when compared to other substance use interventions with empirical support that tend to be more direct and require fewer implementation resources. In addition, the focus on chronic emotional dysregulation as the underlying process that drives substance use in DBT-SUD may not be widely applicable to individuals who only suffer from SUD. On the other hand, DBT-SUD could be justified for individuals with SUD and other comorbidities marked by emotional dysregulation.

References

Axelrod, S. R. (2018). Dialectical behaviour therapy for substance use disorders. In E. M. A. Swales (Org.), *The Oxford handbook of dialectical behaviour therapy*. Oxford University Press.

Barrett, L. F. (2017). *How emotions are made: The secret life of the brain*. Houghton Mifflin Harcourt.

Crowell, S. E., Beauchaine, T. P., & Linehan, M. M. (2009). A biosocial developmental model of borderline personality: Elaborating and extending Linehan's theory. *Psychological Bulletin, 135*, 495–510. https://doi.org/10.1037/a0015616

Dimeff, L. A., & Koerner, K. E. (2007). *Dialectical behavior therapy in clinical practice: Applications across disorders and settings*. Guilford Press.

Dimeff, L. A., & Linehan, M. M. (2008). Dialectical behavior therapy for substance abusers. *Addiction Science & Clinical Practice, 4*, 39–47.

Ekman, P. (2004). *Emotions revealed*. Phoenix.

Hahn, A. M., Simons, R. M., & Hahn, C. K. (2016). Five factors of impulsivity: Unique pathways to borderline and antisocial personality features and subsequent alcohol problems. *Personality and Individual Differences, 99*, 313–319.

Heard, H. L., & Swales, M. A. (2015). *Changing behavior in DBT: Problem solving in action*. The Guilford Press. https://doi.org/10.1016/j.paid.2016.05.035

Koerner, K. (2012). *Doing dialectical behavior therapy: A practical guide*. The Guilford Press.

Leonardi, J. L. (2018). A Terapia Comportamental Dialética (DBT). In A. E. A. Antúnez & G. Safra (Eds.), *Psicologia clínica: da graduação à pós-graduação* (pp. 95–103). Atheneu.

Linehan, M. M. (1993). *Cognitive-behavioral treatment of borderline personality disorder*. The Guilford Press.

Linehan, M. M. (1997). Validation and psychotherapy. In A. C. Bohart & L. S. Greenberg (Eds.), *Empathy reconsidered: New directions in psychotherapy* (pp. 353–392). American Psychological Association.

Linehan, M. M. (2015). *DBT skills training manual*. The Guilford Press.

Linehan, M. M., Armstrong, H. E., Allmon, D., & Heard, H. L. (1991). Cognitive-behavioral treatment of chronically parasuicidal borderline patients. *Archives of General Psychiatry, 48*, 1060–1064. https://doi.org/10.1001/archpsyc.1991.01810360024003

Linehan, M. M., Schmidt, H., Dimeff, L. A., Craft, J. C., Kanter, J., & Comtois, K. A. (1999). Dialectical behavior therapy for patients with borderline personality disorder and drug-dependence. *The American Journal on Addictions, 8*, 279–292. https://doi.org/10.1080/105504999305686

Linehan, M. M., Dimeff, L. A., Reynolds, S. K., Comtois, K. A., Welch, S. S., Heagerty, P., & Kivlahan, D. R. (2002). Dialectical behavior therapy versus comprehensive validation therapy plus 12-step for the treatment of opioid dependent women meeting criteria for borderline personality disorder. *Drug and Alcohol Dependence, 67*, 13–26. https://doi.org/10.1016/s0376-8716(02)00011-x

Lungu, A., & Linehan, M. M. (2016). Dialectical behavior therapy: A comprehensive multi- and transdiagnostic intervention. In C. M. Nezu & A. M. Nezu (Eds.), *The Oxford handbook of cognitive and behavioral therapies* (pp. 200–214). Oxford University Press.

Meyers, R. J., & Smith, J. E. (1995). *Clinical guide to alcohol treatment: The community reinforcement approach*. Guilford Press.

Miga, E. M., Neacsiu, A. D., Lungu, A., Heard, H. L., & Dimeff, L. A. (2018). Dialectical behaviour therapy from 1991-2015: What do we know about clinical efficacy and research quality? In M. A. Swales (Ed.), *The Oxford handbook of dialectical behaviour therapy*. Oxford University Press.

Rizvi, S. L. (2019). *Chain analysis in dialectical behavior therapy*. The Guilford Press.

Rizvi, S. L., & Ritschel, L. A. (2014). Mastering the art of chain analysis in dialectical behavior therapy. *Cognitive and Behavioral Practice, 21*, 335–349. https://doi.org/10.1016/j.cbpra.2013.09.002

Sayrs, J. H., & Linehan, M. M. (2019). *DBT teams: Development and practice*. Guilford Press.

Skinner, B. F. (1991). *The behavior of organisms: An experimental analysis*. Copley.

Skinner, B. F. (1992). *Verbal behavior*. Copley Publishing Group. (Original work published in 1957).

Swenson, C. R. (2016). *DBT principles in action: Acceptance, change, and dialectics*. The Guilford Press.

Chapter 11
Contributions of Acceptance and Commitment Therapy (ACT) with an Emphasis on Values and Committed Actions in the Treatment of Substance Dependence

Rafael R. de Q. Balbi Neto and Simone Martin Oliani

Introduction

Acceptance and Commitment Therapy, with the abbreviation ACT, is a therapeutic approach currently recognized as empirically grounded for the treatment of some mental disorders, according to the Society of Clinical Psychology – also known as Division 12 of the American Psychological Association (APA). The main disorders treated with ACT are Depression, Mixed Anxiety Disorders, Obsessive-Compulsive Disorder, Psychotic Disorders, and it is recognized for the treatment of Chronic Pain (APA, 2016). On the topic of Substance Use Disorder (SUD), there are empirically based treatments for the use of alcohol, cocaine, and tobacco, the Contingency Management (as described in Chap. 7 of this book), also proposed by APA (2016), being among them.

ACT is relevant in the treatment of substance dependence for two reasons: (a) anxiety and depression comorbidities are frequent; and (b) ACT can enhance the effects of other treatments, such as Contingency Management. Comorbidity rates in SUD and mood disorders are very high, reaching 20.13%, with Major Depressive Disorder being the most frequent, present in approximately 15% of patients diagnosed with SUD. Anxiety disorders are close to 18% of all the people diagnosed with SUD, with Specific Phobia being the most frequent disorder, present in about 11% of cases (Grant et al., 2006). In addition, recent studies developed in Brazil (e.g., Silveira et al., 2018; Silva et al., 2018) point out that Mental Disorders are more prevalent in users of psychoactive substances (PAS) than in the general

R. R. d. Q. Balbi Neto (✉)
Universidade Federal do Espírito Santo, Vitória, ES, Brazil

S. M. Oliani
Centro Integrado de Neuropsiquiatria e Psicologia Comportamental (CINP), Londrina, PR, Brazil

S. M. Oliani et al. (eds.), *Behavior Analysis and Substance Dependence*,
https://doi.org/10.1007/978-3-030-75961-2_11

population, and that patients with Depression or Schizophrenia are more likely to develop SUD.

Although there is a lack of research that recognizes ACT as an empirically based treatment for SUD, A-Tjak, Davis, Morina, Powers, Smits, and Emmelkamp (2015), in a review, concluded that "ACT is more effective than treatment as usual or placebo and that ACT may be as effective in treating anxiety disorders, depression, addiction, and somatic health problems as established psychological interventions" (p. 30). Furthermore, according to Stotts and Northrup (2015), studies on ACT and DBT (Dialectical Behavior Therapy, presented in Chap. 10 of this book), carried out in different populations, have shown that these types of interventions are promising for the treatment of SUD regarding the use of various substances such as: opiates, methamphetamine, multiple substances and within varied environments, namely: prisons, methadone clinics, residential, and outpatient treatment.

A reference article was published by Hayes, Wilson, Gifford, Bissett, Piasecki, and Batten (2004). They compared the treatment as methadone-only use with the treatment of methadone combination with 16 weeks of Twelve Step Facilitation Therapy (TSF) or Acceptance and Commitment Therapy (ACT) in an efficacy study with opiate addicts who abuse substances and who continued to use PAS while on methadone treatment. The results showed that treatment with ACT led to a reduced drug use. Hayes et al. suggested that both ACT and TSF should be focused on further studies to assess effectiveness as a resource that makes it possible to reduce the harmful use of psychoactive substances (PAS).

Subsequent studies (e.g., Stotts et al., 2009, 2012) have shown positive results in the treatment of opiate addiction with ACT and DBT. Another example is the study by Luoma et al. (2008), in which ACT was used in a 6-hour workshop to reduce self-stigma in 88 patients with SUD. The results showed medium to large effects on many variables in the post-treatment, signaling the relevance of ACT as a complementary treatment for SUD, which in turn may reduce the risk of relapse.

ACT can also enhance the effects of other treatments, such as Motivational Interviewing and Relapse Prevention Therapy, as proposed in the work Mindfulness-based sobriety: a clinician's treatment guide for addiction recovery using relapse prevention therapy, acceptance and commitment therapy, and motivational interviewing (Turner et al., 2014) and Mindfulness-based relapse prevention for addictive behaviors: A clinician's guide (Bowen et al., 2011). Likewise, ACT therapeutic processes, such as Mindfulness, can collaborate with the treatment of SUD, which can be observed in different studies (e.g., Witkiewitz et al., 2013; Wupperman et al., 2015) regarding substance dependence.

In this chapter, a description of ACT based on the principles of Behavior Analysis will be presented, explaining briefly its processes. Afterward, some aspects of ACT that may contribute to the treatment of substance use disorder will be specified. Finally, a description of two techniques related to the therapeutic process of Committed Actions will be presented, which demonstrate the relationship of four processes, Mindfulness, Acceptance, Disclosure, and Contextual Self, the applicability to Values and Committed Actions with a valuable life and without drug abuse.

Principles of Behavior Analysis in Explaining ACT

The first book that presents ACT in a systematic way is "Acceptance and Commitment Therapy: An experimental approach to behavior change" (Hayes et al., 1999). When read by behavior analysts in Brazil, it raised doubts as to whether ACT would be based on Behavior Analysis. This doubt may have been minimized with the publication of the article "Acceptance and Commitment Therapy: Is it a Cognitive Intervention Proposal?" (Costa, 2012). Costa (p. 117) stated that ACT is a "therapeutic model completely compatible with Skinner's Radical Behaviorism and Behavior Analysis". In 2014, ABPMC (Brazilian Association of Psychology and Behavioral Medicine) recognized the book "Acceptance and commitment therapy: An experimental approach to behavior change" (Hayes et al., 1999) as a source of guidance for the analyst's work and considered valid by ABPMC (2014), as well as publications on Relational Frames Theory (RFT), which supports a large part of the interventions in ACT. Given the documents, it is suggested that ACT is a proposal primarily based on Behavior Analysis.

ACT Processes

ACT proposes six therapeutic processes, called Acceptance, Cognitive Defusion, Mindfulness, Dimensions of the Self, Values, and Committed Actions. Each of these therapeutic processes develops different skills in clients so that the result is an increase in Psychological Flexibility. The term Psychological Flexibility is related to the ability to experience difficult thoughts and emotions, being able to perceive oneself within this process and still walk in the direction of what really matters to build in life, connected with one's values, guiding one's actions to live a meaningful life. This term proved to be of little use in practice, as apparently, it is of little to no interest for clients to know if they are developing "Psychological Flexibility". On the other hand, the term can be useful from a theoretical point of view, for example, in researches such as that of Kashdan and Rottenberg (2010), which correlates Health with Psychological Flexibility.

ACT is a very different proposal from anything that clients have ever known in western culture, so it is important to prepare them for the processes of ACT (especially Acceptance and Disclosure). The therapist must assist the client in assuming that in order to learn something new it is necessary to put aside what has been done to deal with negative thoughts and feelings so far, at least, for a while. This preparation in ACT is called Creative Helplessness (or Creative Despair), and it can be done in several ways, like the Creative Desperation Exercise (Saban, 2015) or the Man in the Hole metaphor (translated by Saban 2011).

To understand Acceptance and Defusion, it is important to understand the concept of "experiential avoidance" of ACT. We take the following point of view, invariably, human beings are faced with events and/or stimuli during life, which can produce "negative feelings" and "negative thoughts", such as aversive contexts of different types. "Negative feelings" can be identified as being the feelings considered as having aversive characteristics to Western culture, like sadness, fear, anger, disgust, frustration and its variations, such as anxiety, disappointment, guilt, distrust, despair, irritation, annoyance, loneliness, and shame. "Negative thoughts" are covert verbal behaviors that produce negative feelings through different types of relational processes (literalness, assessment, reason-giving), as proposed by Hayes et al., 2011), as "something of bad will happen" (literalness, treating thoughts as if they were facts), "I am a failure" (assessment, treating evaluations as descriptions), "I use drugs, because I feel cracked and addicted" (reason-giving, feelings, and labels that cause/justify actions).

Cognitive fusion is defined as one of three relational processes: literalness, assessment, and reason-giving. In turn, from an analytical-behavioral point of view, it can be said that clients with SUD generally say they use a certain substance to evade or to escape from negative internal experiences (feelings or thoughts), that is, they report avoidance of verbal or emotional covert behaviors, which is characterized as being a negatively reinforced behavior.

Substance use often momentarily relieves the "emotional pain" described by clients, but reinforces the covert operant behavior and the aversive emotional or verbal response. The operant behavior returns strengthened for a short period, with greater frequency and/or magnitude of response, as it was negatively reinforced with the end of aversive stimulation. And in general, it is again "controlled" by users with a more intense substance use, which strengthens or develops addiction. ACT Acceptance processes train skills in clients to better deal with negative feelings arising from life facts which have no solution or that there is nothing more to be done. Defusion processes help the client to develop skills to better deal with negative thoughts, which are not functional.

Mindfulness processes seek to help clients stay more connected to the present, in the here and now, in a more flexible way. The term mindfulness is difficult to translate, even more to find a technical word that defines it. In Behavior Analysis, the proposal is to analyze functionally and not be under control of the topography and, to facilitate, we will then describe the behavioral processes that are present in this proposal. It is being present in the present moment. Discriminating both internal and external stimuli. Observing thoughts without judgment or avoidance. Accepting feelings and its respondents as such (Tsai et al., 2009).

The skills developed with mindfulness practices work as support for the other therapeutic processes, since all processes occur in the here-now. Being mindful – in touch with the here-now – is very advantageous for clients who spend a lot of time thinking about the future, popularly called "suffering by anticipation" or the past that cannot be changed in the present. In ACT, the past is considered to be gone forever, the future has not yet happened, and behaviors regarding the past and future occur in the present. As a result, concerns about the future and anxieties about the past have much less effect on clients. Substance users report difficulty sleeping due to "accelerated thinking", in general, mindfulness practices help to "slow thoughts down", which makes sleeping easier. As a therapist, some care must be taken to train mindfulness after doing Creative Helplessness, as clients can use mindfulness practices with the same function as using substances, that is, to evade aversive covert experiences.

The Dimensions of Self processes develop abilities to see oneself from various perspectives, favoring the development of seeing the world in a more flexible way. As in Radical Behaviorism, in ACT it is understood that clients can assume three dimensions about themselves: The conceptual I (conceptual self), procedural I (procedural self), and contextual I (contextual self). The conceptual self is developed based on the properties of the overt responses that clients emit in a verbal community, that is, it is the result of the process of forming the concept of the self ("me"). The conceptual self process produces labels and adjectives about itself, such as "calm", "aggressive", "peaceful", and "tough". The processes of the conceptual I are excessively reinforced in Western culture, in such a way that it seems to be the only possibility of concept of the self. The conceptual self perspective is not a problem in itself, but the inflexibility in this dimension.

The procedural self is the "self" that emits operant or respondent responses, in the here-now. Being mindful becomes very relevant to notice the procedural self. As clients train this new perspective of themselves, they begin to notice that they are more than the labels they receive from themselves and others, and that they are also the repertoire they show in the present moment. Behavioral therapies in the second generation already proposed, directly or indirectly, the training of the procedural self, which makes the dimensions of the self more flexible (Wolpe, 1978; Sampaio & Roncati, 2012).

The contextual self is a much more refined perspective of oneself, as it consists of noticing that there is a contextual "self" for the occurrence of concepts and processes. This proposal appears only in third-generation behavioral therapies. The conceptual and procedural self are contained within the contextual self, since the formation of the concept of the self and the emission/elicitation of responses take place in a certain context. When trained in the contextual perspective, clients begin to "perceive that they perceive", to "notice that they notice". Noticing is a process that takes place in an "I" context, where one can notice that one is noticing. Working with the dimensions of the self with clients results in a higher flexibility, as a repertoire addition in the development of perception skills regarding the perspective of oneself. Like Mindfulness processes, the Dimensions of the Self support other therapeutic processes.

Values in ACT are defined as "consequences verbally constructed from continuous, dynamic and evolving activities, which establish predominant reinforcements for these activities that are intrinsic to the engagement in the valued behavioral pattern itself" (Wilson & DuFrene, 2009, p. 66). To complement this definition, it can be said that values in ACT are arbitrarily reinforced sets of verbal abstractions of positive reinforcing response classes, that is, verbal abstractions that have been arbitrarily reinforced within a verbal community, which constitute values when together. In other words, values are sets of qualities of actions, whether broad or specific. The greater the amount of abstractions in a value, the broader the value becomes, such as the values "family" or "work". On the other hand, values consisting of few abstractions are more specific, such as “intimacy”, which can be contained in broad values such as “family” and/or “work”, given its specificity.

It is important to highlight that, in the therapeutic process, the client will clarify the values that he or she already has, which were acquired throughout one’s history of reinforcement in life. There is no way to teach the client values in a therapeutic process, since this is absolutely contingent, that is, the client learns about values, not about having or not having values, in the therapeutic process.

The process of Committed Actions begins after working on some process of clarifying Values. Clients will not be able to choose Committed Actions if they aren’t clear enough about their own values. Committed Actions are operant responses related to the clients’ values, that is, abstractions, which define Values, also present in Committed Actions. By definition, Committed Actions do not function as Experiential Avoidance, so behavioral responses with an escape function are not Committed Actions functionally. They are also characterized by producing positive feelings in clients, such as: satisfaction, joy, pride, tranquility, hope, even in the face of high response costs, which includes facing aversive stimuli. The positive feelings produced by Committed Actions are indicative of the occurrence of positive reinforcement. For example, for a client with the value of “paternity”, even if unmotivated, “playing with the child” is a Committed action, when the result is the production of satisfaction (positive feeling).

Negative feelings can be produced by the lack of Committed Actions, in general, by a state of deprivation, which increases the value of reinforcement. In this case, Committed Actions do not have an escape function, and are, in fact, the only way to eliminate the negative feeling (covert aversive stimulus).

Notice that negative feelings can come from three factors: (1) events in clients’ lives with no possibility of control; (2) negative thoughts with the function of Cognitive Fusion (literalness, evaluation, and reason-giving); and (3) behavioral deficit (lack of Committed Actions). Acceptance deals with factor 1, Defusion with 2, and Values combined with Committed Actions with 3. Realize that behavioral excesses are produced with the function of Experiential Avoidance, responses with the function of escaping feelings and negative thoughts. For example, when a client uses substances to eliminate negative feelings or thoughts.

ACT processes are grouped in pairs, Acceptance and Defusion are processes of opening, Mindfulness and the Dimensions of the Self are processes of centering, Values and Committed Actions are processes of engagement. Clients diagnosed with mood disorders, anxiety, and obsessive-compulsive disorder, usually have more difficulty opening up, that is, a great deal of difficulty to deal with negative thoughts and/or feelings, suggesting processes of opening as the beginning of treatment (Acceptance and Defusion), going through processes of centering and afterward of engagement. On the other hand, clients with impulse, eating and substance use disorders have more problems related to impulsivity and compulsiveness than problems related to the opening processes, that is, dealing with negative thinking and feeling, which suggests the beginning of treatment by engagement processes (Values and Committed Actions).

With the client's engagement in the therapeutic process and having worked on Acceptance, Defusion, Being Present and the Dimensions of the Self, the therapist will work on clarifying the client's values (processes of Values), it becomes appropriate to apply techniques to identify and organize Committed Actions. Below is the description of two very useful strategies, the **Action Scanner** and the ACT Matrix.

ACT Practical Applications with Committed Actions

Some books are reading suggestions to deepen the theoretical and applied knowledge of ACT, such as "Introduction to acceptance and commitment therapy" (Saban, 2011) in which there is a translation of ACT intervention metaphors and techniques proposed by Hayes et al. (1999), which won a second edition in 2011 (Hayes et al., 2011) and without forgetting the material called "Working on Values - For a Life with More Meaning and Purpose" (Voguel, 2019).

Action Scanner

After some therapeutic process with Values, it becomes interesting to apply the Action Scanner, especially after filling out instruments, such as the Values Narrative Form and Valued Living Questionnaire-2, as explained by Hayes et al. (2011), or another instrument with a list of values.

The Action Scanner (Appendix 1) has three columns. At the top of the first column is the title "Start…", at the top of the second "Stop…", and the third "Continue…". The second column is divided in half, creating an untitled space underneath, a neutral space that serves to make observations or to be filled with information that did not fit in the other columns (including the second one).

Ask clients to write observable actions in the three columns as a basis for each of the values he or she attaches some importance to. Although clients can start with any of the three columns, in general, it is more interesting to start with the first one, as they will write about reinforcing actions that are in deficit. Customers with SUD have more difficulty identifying behavioral deficits, in this sense, helping them dealing with it becomes more interesting and reinforcing for them than dealing with excesses, such as the use of PAS.

The values that guide the completion of the Action Scanner are present in the instruments that clients have already filled in, such as Values Narrative Form, Valued Life Questionnaire-2, or another instrument, such as Family, Marriage/Intimate Relationship, Maternity/Paternity, Friendship/Life Social, Work, Education/Training, Recreation/Fun, Spirituality, Community Life, and Body Self Care. They can follow the order of the values on the instrument or choose the order itself. In the case of choosing the order itself, it is interesting to write it down on the instrument (Values Narrative Form and/or Valued Life Questionnaire-2), as they fill out the

Action Scanner, in order not to get lost in filling it out. Notice that clients need to describe the action in a way they do not depend on another instrument to understand it. For example, the client starts describing actions related to marriage and writes "being affectionate", the therapist may ask "being affectionate to everyone or only in marriage?" If the client's response is "with everyone", the description of the action "being affectionate" is correct; on the other hand, if the client's response is "only in marriage", the description of the action "being affectionate" needs to be more specific, being changed to "being affectionate in marriage" or "with the wife".

Notice that it makes no sense to write actions of values that clients do not care about, that is, values that are meaningless to them, even if they have value for society, such as spirituality and/or maternity/paternity. In addition, it is important to help identify preferentially observable actions – overt behavior, since the covert behaviors will be handled, in large part, through Acceptance and Disclosure processes. A strategy to help clients stay focused on observable behavior is to ask them to write it down on the instrument behaviors that can be filmed (Polk et al., 2016).

In the third column, "Continue ...", there are many actions, as clients perform many actions they wish to maintain. In order to increase the efficiency of the intervention, ask clients to write preferentially observable actions that they have been trying to do lately, which is the ones where there is a response cost. Actions that are already on "autopilot", called unconscious operants, which require little or no effort, that is, with low response costs, do not need to be included in the "Continue…" list.

It is advantageous to write in the three columns everything that clients consider important for a "life change", such as a brainstorm, without judgment, regardless of the priority or viability of the actions. There is no limit to the number of actions to be written, offer a second sheet, if applicable, even though most clients use only 1 sheet. The Action Scanner makes it clear what needs to be done by the client, and the instrument organizes the action planning in a more concrete way, according to the clients' own report. In addition, it serves as a preparation for the application of the Likegram.

Likegram

The classical Likegram (Andrade, 1999) consists of four areas in which clients write down actions. The areas have the following headings "I like and do it", "I don't like and do it", "I like and don't do it", and "I don't like and don't do it". The variable "like"/"don't like" refers to the production of positive (in the "like") or negative/absent ("don't like") emotions, and the variable "I do"/"I don't" refers to the occurrence of the action or not, lately, in the client's life. The Likegram in this format can create more problems than solutions for clients and therapists: (1) it allows the entry of reinforcing actions ("like") in different categories at the same time, such as "drug use" in "like and do" and "don't like and do", which produces more conflict for the client; (2) the client may reach the conclusion that he or she needs to do what he or she "likes" regardless of the delayed aversive consequences, since it is the only variable of analysis to emit the behavior or not, such as "eating too much sweet/salt/fat", "being aggressive" or "using drugs", and (3) the category "don't like and don't do" can be filled with a multitude of actions without any therapeutic objective, which greatly reduces the efficiency of the therapeutic process.

In view of the previous Likegram limitations and problems, the ACT Likegram (which could also be called Likegram of Committed Actions) was created, which introduces another variable, "It is Important"/"It is not Important" based on the ACT Values proposal. As a result, the ACT Likegram (Appendix 2) has six areas for listing actions: (1) "like and do it because it is important", (2) "I want to, but I don't do it (or avoid it), because it isn't important", (3) "I don't like it but I do it, because it is important", (4) "I like it but I don't do it, even if it's important", (5) "I do it because I like it (or relieves me), but I shouldn't do it, because it is not important", and (6) "I don't like it and I don't do it, but I should do it, because it is important". Notice that category 2 "like" is represented by "I want", an easier way for the category to be understood by clients, also called the "avoided temptations" category. In the way the categories of the ACT Likegram were described, it is understood that the arbitrarily applied relational response emerges, that the client needs to prioritize what is "important" over what he or she "likes" and "is not important", as proposed by ACT.

Notice that the action the client "doesn't like" and "is not important" does not exist, they are literally dysfunctional or maladaptive behaviors. If at any time they exist, it makes no sense to talk about them anymore, as they no longer have reinforcing properties. The ACT Likegram has six categories and not eight. It is recommended to apply the Action Scanner before applying the ACT Likegram, even with asymptomatic clients and with good self-knowledge, such as psychologists.

Ask clients to classify the actions listed on the Action Scanner on the ACT Likegram, which is not about filling in one category followed by the other, but rather framing the actions already listed in one of the six categories, with which some categories may remain blank.

Take advantage of this moment of transcribing the Action Scanner to the ACT Likegram to refine the description of the actions, when applicable. "Generic actions", which describe many actions, can be subdivided to improve the description, such as "taking care of health" can be subdivided into "doing therapy", "using medication correctly", "following the diet", "doing physical exercise" and "Do routine exams" . In addition, instruct clients to write actions in the affirmative, for example, instead of "not being aggressive" (or "Stop being aggressive"), writing "be kind and affectionate".

Some clients write many actions on the Action Scanner, either using 2 sheets, or compressing the writing on the edges of the sheet. In some rarer cases, they use 2 sheets, as they write in very large letters. With that, in both cases, an alternative 2-sheet format is recommended for the ACT Likegram (Appendix 3), providing extra space for clients to write. If you start with the 1-sheet format, it is very difficult to insert a second sheet, that is, when in doubt it is advised to use the alternative 2-sheet format in Appendix 3.

One of the therapist's tasks is to help the client notice that he or she perform actions that he or she "likes" (or relieves) and that are not important, that is, there are short-term reinforcing behaviors that produce delayed aversive stimuli, such as "using drugs" or "be aggressive". In general, it is difficult for clients to assume that they perform actions that "they don't like and are important" or that they "enjoy (or relieve) and are not important". Remember that it is always possible to use the instruments previously applied (Narrative Form of Values and/or Valued Life Questionnaire-2) whenever the doubt arises whether a particular action is important to the client or not.

Final Considerations

ACT becomes relevant in the treatment of substance-dependent clients for two reasons: (1) anxiety and depression comorbidities are frequent; and (2) ACT can enhance the effects of other treatments for SUD, such as Contingency Management. Research with ACT and SUD has shown promise as an effective intervention for substance-dependent clients, as it favors dealing with their experiential avoidance when seeking to avoid suffering and the search for immediate pleasure with the consumption of PAS, especially with the process of Acceptance and Defusion. The processes of Mindfulness, the Dimensions of the Self, Values, and Committed Actions help to engage the therapeutic program and build a hierarchy of values and actions with a more meaningful life for the client.

Appendices

Appendix 1 – Action Scanner

Action Scanner

Start...	Stop...	Continue...

Appendix 2 – ACT Likegram

ACT Likegram

I LIKE AND I DO IT, BECAUSE IT'S IMPORTANT J	I WANT BUT I DON'T DO IT (or AVOID IT) BECAUSE IT'S NOT IMPORTANT J	I LIKE AND I DO IT BECAUSE IT'S IMPORTANT J
I LIKE AND I DON'T DO IT, EVEN BEING IMPORTANT L	I DO IT, BECAUSE I LIKE IT (OR RELIEVES ME) BUT I SHOULDN'T DO IT L	I DON'T LIKE IT AND I DON'T DO IT, BUT I SHOULD DO IT BECAUSE IT'S IMPORTANT L

Appendix 3 – ACT Likegram

ACT Likegram J

I LIKE AND I DO IT, BECAUSE IT'S IMPORTANT J	I WANT TO BUT I DON'T DO IT (or AVOID IT), BECAUSE IT'S NOT IMPORTANT J	I DON'T LIKE IT AND I DO IT, BECAUSE IT'S IMPORTANT J

Appendix 3 – ACT Likegram – Part 2

ACT Likegram

I LIKE IT AND I DON'T DO IT, EVEN BEING IMPORTANT L	I DO IT, BECAUSE I LIKE IT (OR RELIEVES ME) BUT I SHOULDN'T DO IT, BECAUSE IT'S NOT IMPORTANT L	I DON'T LIKE IT AND I DON'T DO IT, BUT I SHOULD BECAUSE IT'S IMPORTANT L

References

American Psychological Association (APA). (2016). *Treatments | Society of Clinical Psychology* [online]. Retrieved from https://www.div12.org/treatments/

Andrade, S. G. (1999). *Teoria e prática de dinâmica de grupo: jogos e exercícios*. Casa do Psicólogo.

Associação Brasileira de Psicologia e Medicina Comportamental (ABPMC). (2014). *Regulamento do trabalho de acreditação de analistas de comportamento a ser realizado pela Associação Brasileira de Psicologia e Medicina Comportamental – ABPMC*. ABPMC.

A-tjak, J. G., Davis, M. L., Morina, N., Powers, M. B., Smits, J. A., & Emmelkamp, P. M. (2015). A meta-analysis of the efficacy of acceptance and commitment therapy for clinically relevant mental and physical health problems. *Psychotherapy and Psychosomatics, 84*(1), 30–36. https://doi.org/10.1159/000365764

Bowen, S., Chawla, N., & Marlatt, G. A. (2011). *Mindfulness-based relapse prevention for addictive behaviors: A clinician's guide*. Guilford Press.

Costa, N. (2012). Terapia de Aceitação e Compromisso: É uma Proposta de Intervenção Cognitivista? *Perspectivas em Análise do Comportamento, 3*(2), 117–126.

Grant, B. F., Stinson, F. S., Dawson, D. A., Chou, S. P., Dufour, M. C., Compton, W., Pickering, R. P., & Kaplan, K. (2006). Prevalence and co-occurrence of substance use disorders and independent mood and anxiety disorders: Results from the National Epidemiologic Survey on alcohol and related conditions. *Alcohol Research and Health, 29*, 107–120. https://doi.org/10.1001/archpsyc.61.8.807

Hayes, S. C., Strosahl, K. D., & Wilson, K. G. (1999). *Acceptance and commitment therapy: An experimental approach to behavior change*. Guilford Press.

Hayes, S., Wilson, K., Gifford, E., Bissett, R., Piasecki, M., Batten, S., Byrd, M., & Gregg, J. (2004). A preliminary trial of twelve-step facilitation and acceptance and commitment therapy with polysubstance-abusing methadone-maintained opiate addicts. *Behavior Therapy, 35*(4), 667–688. https://doi.org/10.1016/S0005-7894(04)80014-5

Hayes, S. C., Strosahl, K. D., & Wilson, K. G. (2011). *Acceptance and commitment therapy: The process and practice of mindful change*. Guilford Press.

Kashdan, T. B., & Rottenberg, J. (2010). Psychological flexibility as a fundamental aspect of health. *Clinical Psychology Review, 30*(7), 865–878. https://doi.org/10.1016/j.cpr.2010.03.001

Luoma, J. B., Kohlenberg, B. S., Hayes, S. C., Bunting, K., & Rye, A. K. (2008). Reducing self-stigma in substance abuse through acceptance and commitment therapy: Model, manual development, and pilot outcomes. *Addiction Research & Theory, 16*(2), 149–165. https://doi.org/10.1080/16066350701850295

Polk, K. L., Schoendorff, B., Webster, M., & Olaz, F. O. (2016). *The essential guide to the ACT matrix: A step-by-step approach to using the ACT matrix model in clinical practice*. New Harbinger Publications.

Saban, M. T. (2011). *Introdução à terapia de aceitação e compromisso*. ESETec.

Saban, M. T. (2015). O Que é Terapia de Aceitação e Compromisso. In P. L. Santos, J. P. Gouveia, & M. D. S. Oliveira (Eds.), *Terapias comportamentais de terceira geração: guia para profissionais* (pp. 179–216). Sinopsys.

Sampaio, T. P. A., & Roncati, A. C. K. P. (2012). Algumas técnicas tradicionalmente utilizadas na clínica comportamental. In N. B. Borges & F. A. Cassas (Eds.), *Clínica analítico-comportamental: aspectos teóricos e práticos*. Porto Alegre.

Silva, D. A. S., de Oliveira, N. R., & Graça, M. S. (2018). A relação entre transtornos mentais e o uso de substâncias psicoativas. *Ciência (In) Cena Bahia, 1*(6), 38–50.

Silveira, K. L., de Oliveira, M. M., & Alves, P. F. (2018). Transtornos psiquiátricos menores em usuários de substâncias psicoativas. *SMAD Revista Eletrônica Saúde Mental Álcool e Drogas (Brazilian Edition), 14*(1), 28–36.

Stotts, A. L., & Northrup, T. F. (2015). The promise of third-wave behavioral therapies in the treatment of substance use disorders. *Current Opinion in Psychology, 2*, 75–81. https://doi.org/10.1016/j.copsyc.2014.12.028

Stotts, A. L., Masuda, A., & Wilson, K. (2009). Using acceptance and commitment therapy during methadone dose reduction: Rationale, treatment description, and a case report. *Cognitive and Behavioral Practice, 16*(2), 205–213. https://doi.org/10.1016/j.cbpra.2008.08.003

Stotts, A. L., Green, C., Masuda, A., Grabowski, J., Wilson, K., Northrup, T. F., Moeller, F. G., & Schmitz, J. M. (2012). A stage I pilot study of acceptance and commitment therapy for methadone detoxification. *Drug and Alcohol Dependence, 125*(3), 215–222. https://doi.org/10.1016/j.drugalcdep.2012.02.015

Tsai, M., Kohlenberg, R. J., Kanter, J., Kohlenberg, B., Follette, W., & Callaghan, G. (2009). *A guide to functional analytic psychotherapy: Awareness, courage, love and behaviorism*. Springer.

Turner, N., Welches, P., & Conti, S. (2014). *Mindfulness-based sobriety: A clinician's treatment guide for addiction recovery using relapse prevention therapy, acceptance and commitment therapy, and motivational interviewing*. New Harbinger Publications.

Voguel, K. (2019). *Trabalhando Valores - Por Uma Vida Com Mais Significado e Propósito*. Conscientia Editora.

Wilson, K. G., & DuFrene, T. (2009). *Mindfulness for two: An acceptance and commitment therapy approach to mindfulness in psychotherapy*. New Harbinger.

Witkiewitz, K., Bowen, S., Douglas, H., & Hsu, S. H. (2013). Mindfulness-based relapse prevention for substance craving. *Addictive Behaviors, 38*(2), 1563–1571. https://doi.org/10.1016/j.addbeh.2012.04.001

Wolpe, J. (1978). *Prática da terapia comportamental*. Brasiliense. (Original work published in 1973).

Wupperman, P., Cohen, M. G., Haller, D. L., Flom, P., Litt, L. C., & Rounsaville, B. J. (2015). Mindfulness and modification therapy for behavioral dysregulation: A comparison trial focused on substance use and aggression. *Journal of Clinical Psychology, 71*(10), 964–978. https://doi.org/10.1002/jclp.22213

Chapter 12
Therapy by Contingencies of Reinforcement (TCR) and Substance Dependence: A Clinical Case Presentation

Alan Souza Aranha, Luciana Pellizzaro Naine, and Claudia Kami Bastos Oshiro

Introduction

Therapy by Contingencies of Reinforcement (TCR) is a psychotherapy systematized, developed, and implanted by Guilhardi in 2004,[1] but its development began in the 1970s with the opening of the first behavioral therapy clinic in Brazil (Guilhardi, 2003; Leonardi, 2015). TCR is fully committed to Behavioral Science (BS): the philosophy of Radical Behaviorism (RB) (Skinner, 1945), the research methodology (Andery, 2010), the concepts (Catania, 1998/1999) of *Experimental Behavioral Analysis (*EBA), and *Applied Behavioral Analysis* (ABA) (*Journal of the Experimental Analysis of Behavior*, available at https://onlinelibrary.wiley.com/journal/19383711 and *Journal of Applied Behavior Analysis*, available at https://onlinelibrary.wiley.com/journal/19383703), and procedures of behavior modification technologically described with the possibility of replication (Baer et al., 1968) and based on experimental evidence demonstrated by BS. The foundation of TCR is that the psychotherapist is interested in all the client's manifestations – thoughts, emotions, behaviors, delusions, dreams, etc. – but in order to deal with these phenomena, he identifies and alters the contingencies of reinforcement (CR) of which such phenomena are a function. Thus, "TCR" is a descriptive name of the psychotherapist's work (Guilhardi, 2004). Substance abuse, substance dependence (APA, 1994), and substance use disorders (APA, 2013) are labels that refer to a behavior pattern of the individual who self-minister PAS regardless of the harm that

[1] See also Martin and Pear (2009).

A. S. Aranha (✉) · C. K. B. Oshiro
University of São Paulo, São Paulo, SP, Brazil

L. P. Naine
Institute of Therapy by Contingencies of Reinforcement, Campinas, SP, Brazil

S. M. Oliani et al. (eds.), *Behavior Analysis and Substance Dependence*,
https://doi.org/10.1007/978-3-030-75961-2_12

consumption causes. Diagnostic manuals (APA, 2013) are proposed to describe phenotypes[2] ("craving or strong desire or need to use drugs") and molecular contingencies ("the daily activities of the individual revolve around the substance") that facilitate communication among mental health professionals, but do not allow the identification of the maintaining variables, nor the fundamentals of the evaluation and intervention of a particular client. The TCR proposes to use the laws of BS and knowledge about the effects of PAS to conceptualize and treat individualized cases involving drug consumption. The goal of this chapter is to present the psychotherapeutic model of TCR, the reasoning of TCR when applied to drug abuse cases, and to exemplify with a clinical case.

Psychotherapeutic Model of Therapy by Contingencies of Reinforcement (TCR)

The psychotherapeutic model of TCR can be illustrated when the client seeks help. The client's behavioral repertoire – the set of possible actions in all the contexts in which he lives – is selected in his genetic and environmental history. The repertory that has been built up over time comes into contact with the CRs and, if insufficient, leads to a scarcity of positive reinforcers and/or generates aversive stimulation. The products of the contingencies are felt by the client as suffering, although in general, he is not aware of why he suffers and attributes his pains to spurious causes. When unable to alter the pain on his own, the available escape behavior is to seek the help of a psychotherapist who, theoretically, is trained for such activity. Client and psychotherapist work together to analyze and modify the problem in which the former finds himself (Guilhardi, 2004; Skinner, 1953).

The contingencies of reinforcement therapist respond to three variables in his clinical work: his genetic and environmental history as a person, his theoretical and practical training as a professional, and to the behaviors, verbal and non-verbal, inside and outside the session, of the client and the people involved in the case (Guilhardi, 2004). These sources of information allow the psychotherapist to investigate and identify, on the one hand, the deficits and excesses (Kanfer & Saslow, 1976) that prevent the client from producing positive reinforcement and/or eliminating short- and long-term aversive stimuli for himself and ideally for others (Ferster,

[2] The TCR adopts the term phenotype to illustrate that a response can have the same appearance (phenotype) but different functions. For example, the running response may have, for one person, the function of escape, while for another person the function of chasing. In this example, responses with the same phenotype are different behaviors. On the other hand, responses with different phenotypes may have the same function. For example, crying and swearing are responses with different phenotypes that can have the function of avoiding or escaping punishment. The word topography comes from the Latin *topic,* meaning place. The term "topography" has been used to refer to where the response was emitted and not the form of the response. There is a topography for bar pressure (a single place, the bar on the wall), but several pressure phenotypes (pressing with one or two legs).

1972) and, on the other hand, the CRs of which the deficits and excesses are a function.

TCR begins the psychotherapeutic process by identifying several classes of difficulties that the client exhibits, both in the complaints he brings and in those perceived by the psychotherapist. The psychotherapist does not work with the complaint itself, but seeks to identify the functional difficulties (of which the complaint is one among several) faced by the client in his problem, conceptualizes them behaviorally and works with the current CRs that determine them. A client could seek psychotherapy complaining of "feeling angry" and "being unemployed". The psychotherapist identifies, however, that the client has several other difficulties: he is overweight (likely the product of eating improperly and not exercising often), resides with his parents, and smokes cigarettes. Below we exemplify some of the questions that the psychotherapist could ask on each topic.

(a) How does the anger (that the client says he feels) manifest itself? What types of CRs are related to anger? What is the client's history that is most likely to be related to feelings of anger? Which events have acquired an evocative aversive function for anger? What other feelings can be identified in the client's accounts and related to the CRs in which he or she is involved?
(b) What types of CRs might be related to the difficulty of employment? What has the client done to get a job? What might he have done that was insufficient to keep the job he already had? What could he have done that was crucial to being unemployed? Is this difficulty related to the former (anger)? In what way?
(c) How does the client feel about the weight? What kind of difficulties faced by the client can be related to being overweight? Does the client assign an aversive function to being overweight? What is the eating routine? Has he eaten better in the past? Does the client enjoy physical exercises? If he does, why doesn't he do any? If not, what does he think about sports? What doesn't he like about them? Are there any limitations that prevent him from exercising? Does being overweight limit his daily routine? What limitations are related to him feeling angry?
(d) Has the client always lived with his parents? Has he had an experience living alone, with colleagues or affective and sexual partners? If so, what were the difficulties? How about the positive points? If not, what does he think about leaving home? Has he been able to do so? How does he feel far from his parents? What do parents feel about their children's presence at home? What do the client's age and the fact of being with his parents mean? How does the client feel about his or her parents? How does it feel to live with them? Does living with the parents indicate difficulties in interaction and social living? May social difficulties, if any, have to do with not keeping the job? Are social difficulties related to the difficulties of getting another job? And with anger?
(e) On average, how many cigarettes do the clients smoke per day? Does the pattern change depending on the day? Does he present any health problems? Does he have health concerns? What is the client's goal when smoking? Does the client intend to quit smoking? Can he restrain himself when he cannot smoke

on a particular occasion? Who buys the cigarettes? How did he start smoking? Has he already tried other substances? Does he still use them? Why does he use them? Why doesn't he use them? Does he present self-control in some context? Does smoking relate to anger, family, weight or unemployment?

The relevant behavioral deficits and excesses, in the sense of producing the difficulties presented by the client, are investigated and hypotheses are made on the occurring CRs. It is the professional's responsibility, not the client's, to find evidence for the hypotheses that have been formulated. By questioning "how do you feel about smoking?", the client can answer "pleasure". It is known that positive reinforcing consequences strengthen the response that produced them and generate feelings of pleasure and satisfaction (Skinner, 1986), but it should not be concluded that this is a positive reinforcing contingency – there are several possible stimulus control that would evoke the verbal response "pleasure" (Skinner, 1957). We seek behaviors, thoughts, feelings, and contingencies that strengthen or weaken our hypotheses (Guilhardi, 2007) because they are compatible or incompatible with the client's reports: When he tell us that he smokes to "get satisfaction", we evaluate whether the context is aversive; if he says he smokes because of withdrawal symptoms, he should be able to describe the body states and CRs that elicit the states; when he says he smokes to get over his girlfriend, he must discriminate what his girlfriend does that is aversive to him and how he could interact with her in a way that eliminates or minimizes aversive conditions. The professional's investigation leads to new client reports that work as discriminative stimuli (SD) for other hypotheses: smoking to "get satisfaction" suggests a deficit in the repertoire to produce positive reinforcers; not discriminating the variables on which smoking is a function may indicate deficit in the self-knowledge; smoking cigarettes "to get distracted" from the partner may reveal deficits in the escape-avoidance and countercontrol repertoire. The investigative process develops hypotheses about CRs and, additionally, how they interrelate.

After performing molecular contingency analysis, the psychotherapist will be able to group the identified behaviors into response classes, that is, phenotypically distinct responses that produce the same effects on the environment and are controlled by the same classes of antecedent stimuli (Catania, 1998/1999). Although physically different, getting irritated and smoking cigarettes can temporarily eliminate girlfriend behaviors that are aversive to the client. He may feel irritated and yell at her, which causes her to stop talking, or he may move away from his girlfriend to go to the smoking area. In both possibilities, he could be being negatively reinforced and feeling relieved by the removal of the aversive contingency. We would no longer say that the client gets angry or smokes, but rather that he ineffectually avoids his partner's aversive behavior. The accumulation of observations and information alters or broadens the psychotherapist's analysis: staying at home without looking for a job and residing with parents can also be escape-avoidance behaviors of the difficulties you would encounter in interpersonal relationships (e.g., discussing with the boss, dialoguing with peers). The psychotherapist should infer and seek clues if he gets angry, smoking, not looking for a job, and living with the parents are responses from the same or different classes. The analysis of molar contingencies reveals how the client behaves in various areas, such as family, affective, professional, friendships, etc., making it easier to predict the client's behavior in the future and elucidating clinical priorities, i.e., where to start the intervention.

Although people's repertoire is the result of interactions with the environment since birth (in the past), problem behaviors are controlled by CRs that operate exclusively in the present, and the only way to change them is by proposing interventions in the present. The professional performs an arbitrary cutout of the life of the assisted to understand it and infers the CRs that control certain behaviors. If the intervention–based on inference–works, the investigation is suspended. However, if the intervention is partially or null successful, the psychotherapist will have to re-evaluate the case conceptualization. One form of reassessment is the investigation of the history of contingencies of reinforcement (HCR). Samples of HCR (arbitrary, such as current CRs) may suggest how the events acquired the stimulus functions and how behavioral patterns were developed (Guilhardi, 2010a). In the smoking example given above, assuming that the psychotherapist inferred that smoking was a possible escape from his girlfriend, the professional might ask himself: what led the girlfriend's behavior to be aversive to the client? And how was the pattern of smoking to escape installed? What was the origin of the difficulties of dialogue in aversive social interactions, in order to reach a more harmonious relationship? The answers can be found in the deepening of HCR.

It is important to point out that two clients respond in different ways to the same CRs (the partner could have a neutral function, a positive reinforcement function, the avoidance could be different, the response evoked could be of countercontrol, etc.), not because the CRs evoke different responses in human beings (which would nullify the laws of BS), but because other CRs (identified or not) are interacting with the analyzed CR. It is concluded that even if a set of equal contingencies act on the behavior of two people, the exposure to multiple known and unknown CR in HCR generated unique people and, consequently, with different psychological treatment needs (Guilhardi, 2010a). Two clients classified as "depressive" do not need the same care, just as two clients classified as "obsessive-compulsive" are not necessarily in negative reinforcement contingencies. It is necessary to evaluate what has been classified as "depression" and "obsessive-compulsive disorder" in the case of clients, i.e., to obtain information on the phenotypes and functions of behaviors that are emitted or no longer emitted that allow their classification as corresponding to the diagnostic criteria of depression and obsessive-compulsive disorder.

All the psychotherapist's interventions must be under control of the conceptual framework and experimental rigor of BS (Baer et al., 1968). TCR is not eclectic to these characteristics because it is based on the research methodology and scientific foundations of the Natural Sciences; monistic conception of human being; behavior as organism-environment interaction, which is instrumented in the form of CRs; adoption of the basic attitudes of Science (empiricism, experimental manipulation, parsimony, etc.); rejection of the mechanistic causal model and adherence to the Darwinian model of selection by consequences. Problem behavior is reduced by applying techniques to weaken its emission and, simultaneously, installation of desired behavioral repertoires, which are incompatible or alternative to the unwanted. The emphasis of the intervention is on the set of procedures aimed at building desired behaviors (Guilhardi, 2004).

It is essential that the psychotherapeutic procedures are constructed in an individualized manner and that the contact of the psychotherapist with techniques already used (e.g., in the reading of books and articles, in the exposition of clinical cases) serve as SDs to expand the professional repertoire and increase control over relevant aspects of the cases and not for replication based on phenotypic, protocol, or pre-established CR criteria (Guilhardi, 1988). This would put the psychotherapist under control of rules and make him less sensitive to the CRs present in the therapeutic relationship.

Finally, the psychotherapeutic process will be insufficient without the proper generalization of progress (Baer et al., 1968) and this must be programmed by the psychotherapist. Desired behaviors installed in the clinical setting should be generalized to three areas: 1) other behavioral classes, so that the client's development is amplified in multiple areas of his life; 2) diverse daily environments (home, school, work, leisure, social interactions) and not restricted to progress in the therapeutic context; and 3) changes should be lasting and extend over time. Only when the client demonstrates that he has incorporated the three areas of generalization into his repertoire will the intervention have been successful.

Substance Dependence

Substance dependence is the usual nomenclature for problems with consumption of PAS (Diehl et al., 2011), with the main characteristic being the pattern of drug use despite the adverse consequences that the use causes. The health area usually uses the diagnostic criteria of the Diagnostic and Statistical Manual of Mental Disorders (DSM) as a reference because, although they do not describe the etiology of the problem, they facilitate communication between professionals. In its fifth and latest edition (APA, 2013), the manual performs the diagnosis of Substance Use Disorder (SUD) depending on the number of criteria identified in the client over a 12-month period. Two or three criteria suggest a mild disorder, four or five a moderate disorder, and six or more severe. The diagnostic criteria are shown in Table 12.1.

The TCR does not use the diagnostic criteria of manuals for assessing substance dependence (in fact, any behavior classified as psychopathological) because it considers them phenotypic ("unsuccessful efforts to control use") or molecular ("use resulting in failure to play important roles at work") and does not specifically refer to any individual. People classified with SUD, like any client, have a wide repertoire, with functionally different behaviors, and we should interpret them individually in the light of BS. The difference is the inclusion of the behavior of consuming PAS in the psychotherapist's analysis, but the analysis is not restricted to this behavior.

Table 12.1 Diagnostic criteria for substance use disorder

A. A problematic pattern of substance use, leading to clinically significant impairment or distress, as manifested by at least two of the following criteria, occurring within a 12-month period:
Impaired control
(1) The substance is often consumed in larger amounts or over a longer period than was intended.
(2) There is a persistent desire or unsuccessful effort to cut down or control use.
(3) A great deal of time is spent in activities necessary to obtain, use or recover from their effects.
(4) Craving, or a strong desire or urge to use drugs.
Social impairment
(5) Recurrent use resulting in failure to fulfill major role obligations at work, school, or home.
(6) Continued use despite having persistent or recurrent social or interpersonal problems caused or exacerbated by their effects.
(7) Important social, occupational, or recreational activities are given up or reduced because of use.
Risky use
(8) Recurrent use in situations in which it is physically hazardous.
(9) Use is continued despite knowledge of having a persistent or recurrent physical or psychological problem that is likely to have been caused or exacerbated by use.
Pharmacological criteria
(10) Tolerance, as defined by either of the following:
(a) A need for markedly increased amounts of substance to achieve intoxication or desired effect.
(b) A markedly diminished effect with continued use of the same amount of drug.
(11) Abstinence, as manifested by either of the following:
(a) Characteristic abstinence syndrome for specific substance.
(b) Substance is taken to relieve or avoid withdrawal symptoms.

Source: Adapted from "Diagnostic and Statistical Manual of Mental Disorders" (APA, 2013, p. 491)

The behaviors of thinking about, "feeling like", planning the purchase, seeking and consuming PAS are conceptualized as a set of respondents and operants who respond to the laws of BS, adding the specificities of the stimulus functions of PAS (the TCR defends that the respondent-operant distinction is purely didactic and that in real life behaviors always occur inseparably). In respondent relationships, PAS have the function of unconditioned stimuli, which elicit two types of unconditioned responses: the pharmacological effects of the substance (e.g., cocaine makes the user feel "energized" and "euphoric") and the compensatory effects linked to the body's homeostasis (e.g., in abstinence cocaine leads to fatigue and depression). The neutral stimuli (e.g., money) that are paired with the drug become conditioned stimuli that elicit the aversive compensatory effects, which we call withdrawal syndrome (it is worth remembering that the withdrawal is not essential for a compulsive pattern to occur). Consumption in contact with conditioned stimuli increases the compensatory effects leading to tolerance, i.e., the need for a greater volume of substance to experience the same effect (Benvenuti, 2004).

Consuming SPAs are operants controlled by antecedents and consequents. The reinforcing consequences are the pharmacological effect of the substance (e.g., drinking beer and being "cheerful"), social reinforcers (e.g., approval of a group), and conditioned reinforcers (e.g., when the substance is initially neutral or aversive and becomes reinforcing by pairing with social reinforcers). Consuming substances can also be maintained by negative reinforcement (e.g., removal of withdrawal and other aversive CRs). The antecedents are SDs and pre-aversive stimuli related to consequences (e.g., places of use and conflicts, respectively) (Miguel et al., 2015).

It is essential to know the characteristics of PAS that differentiate them from other environmental stimuli. Skinner (1989) conceptualized them as anomalous reinforcers stimuli that differ from primary reinforcers. Some distinct characteristics of PAS are the immediacy and magnitude of the effect (no event produces such intense changes in the body), the low cost of response to intoxication (e.g., the effort to become a skilled sportsman is superior to the ritual of crack, but with a less intense effect), the lack of satiation mechanisms (e.g., the first chocolate is delicious, but the tenth is aversive. The tenth zip of cocaine may be less reinforcing than the first, but not aversive to the point of the user giving up on aspirating it), the aversion to deprivation (abstinence syndrome) and deleterious alterations in the nervous system of the organism (Garcia-Mijares & Silva, 2006; Heyman, 1996).

Having said that, what is the psychotherapeutic process of TCR with clients who consume SPA? As advocated throughout the text, the inquiry is wrong to suggest that there is *a type of abusive client* or *a pattern of substance dependence* and contingencies of reinforcement therapists should explain what they do with these cases. TCR does not use pre-defined protocols and techniques, but works with concepts derived from BS to assess idiosyncratic affective and behavioral problems. It is possible that the clients have some similarity in the complaints and difficulties that bring them to clinic; however, homogeneity in the evaluation and treatment is not justified. For example, two clients seek psychotherapeutic assistance and present "alcohol and cocaine consumption". The psychotherapist could raise the following questions:

1. Did they seek help because they considered consumption problematic? Or did they look for other reasons and the psychotherapist identified the consumption? If they are worried about how often they are using PAS, what consequences are aversive and have motivated them to seek psychotherapy?
2. What are the functions of consumption? What are the maintenance consequences? What are the expected consequences? What are the antecedents that evoke the use of the substances?
3. What are the HCR that have installed the patterns of drug abuse? Which CR have made individuals vulnerable to the pharmacological effects of drugs? Which CR led to a preference for one drug or another?
4. What are the behavioral deficits and excesses related to drug use? What are the behavioral deficits and excesses in the clients' global repertoire?
5. What are the family members' behaviors toward consumption? What about other customer behaviors? Do they support treatment or not? How do they support it? What are the rules and self-rules about user behavior?

6. Do clients want to stop using drugs? Decrease the consumption? Interrupt a type of substance? Interrupt for a period of time? In the psychotherapist's evaluation, should they stop, decrease, continue or interrupt? Why?
7. What is the academic background of the clients? Work? Housing? Spouse? Children? Income? Plans? Resources to be treated?

By answering these questions (and many others), the psychotherapist will realize the clients are different and they only resemble each other superficially. Although they have in common the consumption of PAS (even if they are identical drugs), the way each one has interacted with the physical and social environment since birth, the HCR with the substance until now and the CRs in the areas of family, affective, professional relationships, etc., are unique. Thus, the professional will use the philosophical and conceptual aspects that govern human behavior (the laws of BS, these are the same for all of us), taking into consideration the specificities of PAS (briefly described in the chapter, however not exhaustively) to understand the learning history (unique to each client) that built them in a way that led to the abusive consumption of PAS, maintained the functions of the stimuli and their behavioral repertoires over time and led them to psychotherapy.

It is worth highlighting the importance of HCR to understand why a minority of people use PAS and experience serious problems, such as those found in rehabilitation clinics and psychosocial care centers. The moderate individual may drink alcohol on Saturday and "waste" Sunday with the hangover, but will probably be under the control of the likely punishments, such as not working, if they risk getting drunk during the week. The individual considered "dependent" can drink every day and lose his job, not try to relocate to the job market and start living on the street. It is essential to analyze which CRs affect different people and lead them to problematic consumption. The man who does not abstain from consuming crack in order to find a job the next day may respond excessively under control of immediate consequences; the woman that does not respond to the probable punishments of drunk driving may be insensitive to the natural aversive consequences; the person who consumes despite the family fighting and her child being hurt may be insensitive to the social consequences (Aranha & Oshiro, 2017). The reasons of exemplified clients to respond in a certain way to present CRs are specified in their HCR.

As described in the previous section, the TCR intervention aims to increase the frequency of desired behaviors (primarily) by applying procedures for installing and strengthening the repertoire, and to decrease the frequency of problem behaviors by applying weakening techniques (Guilhardi, 2004). The psychotherapist must directly attack the respondents and operants of drug use: make the user aware of his physical and psychological condition, identify the CRs that maintain the consumption and change them in the desired direction, develop alternative and incompatible behaviors that produce positive reinforcers and eliminate aversive stimuli without relation to drugs, become sensitive to other reinforcements possibilities, etc. (Guilhardi, 2010a, b/2013). The therapist by contingencies of reinforcement, as with any client, also evaluates the CRs *related to* the problems identified, in this case the self-administration of PAS: the characteristics exemplified in the previous paragraph, such as impulsiveness and insensitivity to social and natural consequences. And, in addition, the professional evaluates other comprehensive repertories that *have no clear relation* with consumption: the client is a human being with a history, difficulties, values, and dreams of his own before a drug user.

The programming for generalizations of psychotherapeutic advances with substance dependents involves at least three groups of procedures: 1) systematic counseling of the user's family (Hunt & Azrin, 1973). This social and affective microcosm is important in the process of generalizing progress in particular because it has almost always participated (consistently or not) in the initiation and development of the process of substance dependence; 2) techniques of self-control (Harris & Miller, 1990) and self-knowledge (Sobell et al., 1976). It is not enough for the other person to participate, without the necessary and proper responsibility and engagement of the user; and 3) therapeutic companions who can use fading, modeling procedures, etc., so that the behaviors are emitted and strengthened in the natural environment (Balvedi, 2003).

Below, we illustrate the psychotherapeutic process of TCR with PAS with a clinical case. As previously mentioned, it is hoped that the case concept and psychotherapeutic strategies are not replicated as indiscriminate techniques (Guilhardi, 1998), but serve as SDs to enrich the repertoire of the psychotherapist in the very cases he/she attends. We suggest reading Guilhardi (2010/2013) as an additional source of SD for better observation of clients involved with PAS.

Clinical Case

Client Identification

Mélvio[34] (29) was the youngest son of Jesus (70) and Pureza (70), and brother of Ivo (39). He began several undergraduate[5] courses, concluding none. When he sought psychotherapy, he was unemployed and participating in several selection processes and, after three weeks, he obtained a position in a technology company. He was in a stable relationship with Raissa (28).

[3] All the names used in this chapter are fictitious.

[4] Production of the text began after the client signed the Free and Informed Consent (TCLE).

[5] Information which compromises the confidentiality of the client and the persons involved has been omitted.

Complaint

After collecting preliminary information, the psychotherapist asked why Mélvio sought psychological care and he replied: "*I came because I have horrible anxiety attacks. I have been panicking for years. I feel that I'm going to die, that my veins are clogging up and I'm going to have a heart attack*". The client sought psychiatric and psychotherapeutic treatment previously, but was unsuccessful – the anxiety crises have continued over time. The first crisis had occurred six years before psychotherapy began, when he became unemployed. Mélvio had obtained a position in a multinational company and, when talking to his superiors, he had the "impression" that they "liked him". In the same week, at a *happy hour* after work, the client got drunk and offered cocaine to his bosses. He was fired the next day.

The psychotherapist was brought under control of drug use and advanced the questions in this direction. The client reported, "*I was two people. From Friday to Sunday only parties, but during the week I was good. I had two personalities and I didn't even think about it, but then you start to see yourself with time to think and then you get depressed* (...) *the personality that is not nice... I drink and send messages* (laughs), *I snort cocaine, I make a mess, I go after women*". The client has not established any relation between anxiety complaints and the consumption of alcohol and cocaine.

In addition, Mélvio's verbalizations had as main themes anxiety complaints, drug use, and interpersonal behavior with bosses. The following questions (private responses) sought to explain the functions of such behaviors by the psychotherapist:

Anxiety: what *exactly* was the anxiety he experienced? If the term "anxiety" is being used correctly by Mélvio, which aversive stimuli would he be responding to? Did the first anxiety crisis occur after being unemployed? Did the other crises occur in similar contexts? Or different contexts?

Realizing the bosses liked him and offering drugs: how did the client "realize" the bosses "liked him" in so little time? What did the bosses do? Does the client believe other people like him too? Even if the bosses had identified with the new employee, why did Mélvio believe using drugs with his superiors would be something reinforcing for them? Did he think about the possible consequences of his behavior on the bosses and their future in the company?

Drug use: what is the client's use pattern? That is, how many times a week does he use it? In what quantity? What contexts evoke consumption? What are the maintaining consequences?

The psychotherapist was also under control of other variables besides anxiety, interpersonal relationship, and drug use of the client that could give "tips" on the target contingencies of reinforcement:

Age of parents and difference from his sibling: the client's parents conceived him over 40 years old and 10 years after the birth of his brother. What led them to this? Was it a conscious decision or did they not use contraceptive methods?

What are the rules and self-rules about having and raising children? How has the behavior of parents affected and continues to affect Mélvio's repertoire?

Undergraduate courses: What led the client to attend colleges and not complete them? Did he choose the courses or was he forced to take them? Forced by whom? If so, what were the criteria used?

Unemployment: How did he lose his job in the other times? Was it because of his own behavior or not? What is his professional repertoire like when he is employed?

Affective Relationship: How long has he been with Raissa? What is the relationship like? Does the girlfriend's behavior influence in any way the difficulties presented?

Behavioral excesses that produced social and physical risks: Were drug use and offering drugs at work (leading to dismissal) the only reckless behaviors the client emitted? Would the different behaviors have the same function? Did he emit risky behaviors? Which ones?

The contingencies of reinforcement therapist identifies, in the verbal and nonverbal behavior of the client and the people relevant to the psychotherapeutic process, inside and outside the session, as many deficits, excesses, and desired behaviors as possible. It raises hypotheses about the contingencies that control the behaviors, looks for information that validates or refutes its hypotheses, and groups the various behaviors into response classes. Knowledge of the client's behavioral patterns in multiple contexts and the interactions of the present contingencies enable the creation of psychotherapeutic goals (where one wants to go) and procedures that attack the target contingencies (how to get there) (Guilhardi, 2004).

Behavioral Characterization of the Client's Difficulties

Initially, five main difficulties were identified in the client's repertoire. The session vignettes illustrate the problem behaviors occurring in different contexts. Because it is the same client, it is expected the examples contain overlapping, i.e., the verbalizations demonstrate more than one difficulty.

1. Excessive behavior under the control of immediate positive reinforcers to the detriment of delayed aversive consequences.

   Examples of verbalizations:

Food: "*I eat too much, I drink*", "*I ate too much yesterday. A lot. I overate. Then I can't sleep because I'm feeling sick.*"

Finance: "*I spend a lot. I have to work to pay for my stuff. I have bad credit. I don't have a credit card. Raíssa lends it to me. If I get unemployed… I don't even want to think about it!*"

Alcohol and drugs: "*I drink reasonably. I drink a lot. I don't have a drinking problem. If I decide to stop during the week, I can*".

The psychotherapist identified that a significant portion of Mélvio's repertoire was under control of immediate reinforcing consequences, despite putting Mélvio's social and physical integrity at risk. He frequented nightclubs until dawn, spent too much money, and drove in such a way as to cause automobile accidents. Specifically in relation to alcohol and cocaine, with the course of the sessions he admitted that, after starting the consumption, he felt difficulty in interrupting it. In this way, he used primarily on weekends (Friday, Saturday, and Sunday) to avoid professional problems (working under the influence of drugs, being fired). To be able to use on workdays, he prepared himself to mitigate the damage (e.g., work in *home office*).

2. Excessive countercontrol behavior in contingencies which would not have immediate reinforcing consequences.

   Examples of verbalizations:

Psychiatrist: "*Yesterday I had a crisis, I called him* [psychiatrist] *and he didn't answer me. I'm not going there anymore, because I think that is inattention*".
Girlfriend: [when girlfriend tried to break up] "*you wanted to break up. When we're not together, you won't know where I am either anyway*".
Psychotherapist: "I *don't agree very much* [with the psychotherapist's analysis], *I thought about not coming anymore, because I think the Behavior Analysis is shallow. This thing of "I did this" or "I didn't do that", I don't think it works very much. I want to understand in depth, it's not deep*".

Mélvio was emitted countercontrol behaviors with an aversive function to others when the social environment did not reinforce his behavior in the way he expected. At the beginning of psychotherapy, the psychiatric medication did not ease the anxiety, which led the client to change professionals. The new doctor managed anxiety attacks by responding quickly to Mélvio's messages; however, as a result of the symptoms decreasing, he started not to respond frequently. Frustrated, Mélvio reported thinking of giving up treatment, despite the stability of his condition. He also considered giving up when he was told to stop drinking and when his suggestions about changing his medication were not heard. The same difficulty occurred in the intimate relationship. When Raíssa said she would like to break up the relationship, claiming she could no longer cope with her boyfriend's relapses and behavior problems, and did not reconsider breaking up despite Mélvio's requests, the client behaved in ways previously described as aversive by her partner, going out to drink without telling her and disappearing for long periods.

Such behavior also occurred in the psychotherapeutic relationship. In a session in which they were analyzing how his girlfriend felt about the client's behavior, Mélvio said he disagreed with the professional's interpretation of the situation. In the next session, he suggested to interrupt the psychotherapy. It is possible that this attempt to negatively punish the professional's behavior was another example of the countercontrol commonly emitted by Mélvio in interpersonal relationships.

3. Excessive feelings and behaviors of distorted self-esteem and self-confidence.

   Examples of verbalizations:

Musical performances: "*When I go up on stage, I kick ass. The crowd raves.*"
Physical: "*I'm fat. I have to lose weight. If I get thin, I'll be unbeatable. I don't know if I'd end up with Raíssa then.*"
Professional: "*I wonder how they see me? I'm well rated. The s*** is when I have to explain myself. I didn't finish college.*"

The client was under the control of self-rules that described components of his self-esteem and self-confidence in a disproportionate fashion in relation to the contingencies, despite the social deterioration that following the self-rules causes. The client concluded "*I'm the best, that's why I'm adored,*" disconnected from what he did and the moment he did it. Playing in his band was "*being the best*" (independent of people liking the music), he thinks that he was able to date the girl he wanted (unaware of the determinants that would lead his partner to feel attracted to him) and, in the work context, he reported being a good professional independent of what the bosses thought of him (not having finished college could change the boss's opinion, despite this, he believed he was good "*even so*" and it was "*the boss who wasn't seeing him right*").

4. Deficit in responding discriminatively under the control of contingencies that affected third parties.

   Examples of verbalizations:

Girlfriend: "*if I don't want to go out with her* [girlfriend], *she understands well:* [and tells me] *'go drink and come back'. She knows I don't like to get stuck at home*".
Mom: "*I didn't go to the hospital to see my mother, I needed to clear my head because the week was heavy and I went to the bar*".
Colleague at work: "*He came for an internship and I taught him everything. Now he got the job, he goes out for happy hour and doesn't invite me. He created his own gang and I'm out of the group.*

The client did not consider how his behavior would affect people's feelings and behaviors. He would rather go to the bar than stay with his girlfriend who was sad at home, or visit his mother who was in a serious health condition at the hospital. In addition, Mélvio also showed difficulty in analyzing the CRs that controlled the behavior of others. He usually expected the other to behave in a reinforcing way (strengthening the friendship, for example), even if the previous interactions did not justify such a relationship. For example, he helped a colleague at work – only once – and felt angry when he found out he hadn't been invited for the night out.

5. Deficit in the repertoire to identify and describe the contingencies that controlled bodily states with aversive function.

   Examples of verbalizations:

Anxiety: "*the crisis comes from nowhere*", "*just like that: 'I'm fine'. Then my heart begins to tachycardize*", "*am I going to die? My fingers are numb, my chest fails. I think it's because I had rib at lunch and I feel my veins clogging up.*"

The client reported chest pains, numbness, and fear of dying during the sessions and by *WhatsApp* messages. At certain times, he did not relate anxiety to environmental events, and at others, he related to immediate events disconnected from HCR and present CR.

Desired Behavior

In psychotherapy, Mélvio behaved with cordial phenotype, assiduity, and interactions with possible positive reinforcement function for the psychotherapist. In the professional context, he responded discriminatively to the stimuli to perform the work activities with good performance. With friends, he had a repertoire of subjects related to history, music, and general knowledge.

History of Contingencies of Reinforcement (HCR) and Behavioral Conceptualization

The behavior of family members is relevant to understand how the events acquired the stimulus functions and how the client's learned his behavioral patterns (Guilhardi, 2010a). Jesus and Pureza celebrated when Mélvio was born. The client said "*the expectation was that I would be a great man*". Pureza suffered several miscarriages between the birth of his brother Ivo and the client (that is why Mélvio was born later). The previous losses made the parents sensitive to aversive stimulation that came in contact with their son's behavior (other variables in the parents' HCR must have contributed to the high sensitivity to Mélvio, however it would be necessary to evaluate them), making free reinforcement (noncontingent reinforcement) the most important CRs in Mélvio's childhood. Free reinforcement occurs when a stimulus with a reinforcement function (a stimulus with properties of strengthen responses that produces it and elicit pleasant feelings) is presented independently of the subject's behavior (Guilhardi, 2018). Mélvio was exposed concomitantly to four classes of CRs:

(a) Mélvio received social and tangible reinforcements that were not contingent on pre-established desired behaviors (the relationship of the parents with Ivo was different, strengthening the hypothesis that there was a change, at least partial, in the parents' repertoire with Mélvio's birth). The client could go out with friends and earned objects of interest regardless of what he was doing: "*the relationship* [with parents] *is very good. They gave everything to me*";
(b) Mélvio received contingent tangible reinforcements upon requests (mands), such as money and travel: "*nobody in the family had what I had. I was the first to travel*";

(c) When he emitted behaviors under the control of immediate reinforcers, but which produced aversive consequences for others, there was a scarcity of social aversive consequences (and eventually positive reinforcers in the form of attention and concern). One year, Mélvio did not attend Jesus' birthday: "*I apologized. He did not say anything. The next year he says: 'take care, beware!'. Nobody says anything. Everything is 'under the carpet' in my house*";
(d) When he emitted behavior under the control of immediate reinforcers that produced aversive consequences for itself, there was a lack of presentation of social aversive consequences (e.g., he was not censored), and on the other hand, he was protected against aversive consequences. In a situation where he had crashed his car, "*he* [father] *was very worried and said that the most important thing is my health*".

The contingencies of reinforcement in this period of Mélvio's history are shown in Table 12.2.

Table 12.2 Contingencies of reinforcement at Mélvio's HCR. In the first two, positive reinforcement is released freely or contingently on mands. In the latter two, the behavior produces aversive consequences for himself and others, but the verbal community reduce or eliminates stimulation

Antecedents	Responses	Consequences	
Family environment *Discriminative stimuli*: Permission to behave in any way Melvio wishes ("What are you gonna do today, son?" "what do you want from us?")	Absence of pre-selected behavior by parents (emission of any behavior)	Short term	Long term
		Positive reinforcers: Social (family): Praise (e.g., "you're the man"), money, concert, tours	Absence of consequences
	Mands (e.g., "I want to go to the show", "I want a guitar")	*Positive reinforcers*: Access to shows, items of interest, money, trips	Absence of consequences
	Behavior that would produce reinforcers for Melvio and aversive stimulation for others (e.g., going out with friends and not going to Dad's birthday)	*Positive reinforcers*: Social contact	*Possible positive punishment*: Father gets hurt *Positive reinforcement*: Father says "*the important thing is the son being well*"
	Behaviors that produced short-term reinforcers and long-term aversive stimuli (e.g., run with the car)	*Positive reinforcers*: Automatic reinforcers, unconditioned and conditioned reinforcers (e.g., speed, social approval for risky behavior)	*Possible positive punishment*: Automobile accident *Negative reinforcement*: The father removes the aversive stimuli from the environment, takes care of Melvio, asks if he is safe

The behavioral results of the contingencies in Mélvio's repertoire were:

Superstitious Behavior Mélvio began to establish superstitious relationships between his behavior and the events of the environment that followed. The parents released reinforcers and eliminated aversive stimulation regardless of how the client behaved (Guilhardi, 2018), facilitating the formulation of self-rules like "*regardless of what I do, they like me*" (specifically on social reinforcers, the client said the father was the most affectionate figure, while the mother was distant: "*she is depressive. It gives me a bad time to stay close*"). The self-rule is superstitious in the sense that does not apply to all of Mélvio's interpersonal relationships – not everyone would like him or protect him regardless of how he behaved.

Feelings of Self-confidence Restricted to the Family Environment Feelings of self-confidence emerge when an individual emits a response that produces positive reinforcers or eliminates aversive stimuli (Guilhardi, 2002). The person feels that they have a repertory available to produce what they want. Mélvio went through a history in which *asking for reinforcers* was strengthened by his parents, but they did not necessarily manipulate CRs that built behaviors that, if emitted, would result in the expected consequences. In this way, self-confidence became circumscribed to the social environment in which Mélvio was. Close to the family, he feels he "*can have it all*" (I desire everything and I feel I can have it, because someone will give it to me); "*far from the family, I feel insecurity*". The passage elucidates the feelings of low self-confidence when Mélvio was away from his family: [therapist asks what will happen when his parents pass away] "*When I have a problem, my father is there* (…) *I always wanted to be independent, not to become a beggar. I put my life in them* [parents]".

Distorted Feelings of Self-esteem Long-lasting feelings of self-esteem occur when the subject a) has developed feelings and behaviors of self-confidence, i.e., has a repertoire to produce positive reinforcers and eliminate aversive stimulation without help from others and b) has access to noncontingent social reinforcers to any pre-established behavior by the community (Guilhardi, 2002). The exposure to both CRs guarantees the affective and behavioral health of the individual: self-confidence without self-esteem generates a competent human in the activities, but who does not feel the affection and consideration of the other; self-esteem without self-confidence generates an insecure or unprepared arrogant when away from the group (Guilhardi, 2018). Mélvio was exposed to free reinforcements that produced distorted feelings of self-esteem, because without the adequate repertoire of self-confidence, he was dependent on the other to feel loved. Despite reporting that "I am the man", he felt bothered when his mother did not pay attention to him (as previously mentioned, "*it's a bad thing to stay close, she's depressive*") and, in the adult stage, when his friends did not recognize him. He felt special without realizing that when the agency releasing reinforcements was not present, he was no longer special.

Sensoriality Because the parents arranged reinforcements unrelated to their children's actions, Mélvio was not strongly deprived or aversively stimulated, becoming little sensitive to certain types of reinforcements (there were no establishing operations that updated the reinforcement function of some events). Thus, there were restricted possible reinforcements Mélvio could respond to in the future. An HCR without important establishing operations (EO) tends to create individuals that are sensitive to reinforcers related to bodily sensations (drugs, fear, danger) (Skinner, 1975). Mélvio, therefore, was more likely to respond to intense reinforcers that would guarantee him some immediate sensation (alienated from the fact that it could be harmful in the medium-long term).

TCR makes a distinction between sensorality and sensitive feeling behavior (Guilhardi, 2012). Sensoriality behavior refers to respondent and operant responses elicited and evoked by antecedents, mediated by the sense organs (hearing, sight, etc.) and which are maintained by the consequences they produce for the subject who emits them and not by the consequences they produce in others. The antecedents and consequences must be present, making the control immediate and direct. For example, a client could steal money from the family to buy drugs, regardless of whether the parents are upset ("I spend all my money, I need to get more"). The parents' sadness would only be aversive if it bothered the client ("I have to find a way for them to stop bothering me"). Sensitive behavior is not elicited and evoked by antecedent stimuli, but by the function that the verbal community attributes to the stimuli and is maintained by the functions the consequences have for the other, not for the one who emits the behavior. The antecedents and consequences do not necessarily need to be present, being conditional signs satisfactory. For example, by manifesting withdrawal, a client could feel guilty before trying to steal his parents ("I can't steal money again, I'll hurt my parents") and eliminate what is aversive to them ("I need to recover, not for myself, but so that my father and mother stop suffering").

Imprudence We call "courageous" behavior likely to produce reinforcers and aversives when the subject has a repertoire to handle aversives (e.g., a radical sport) and "reckless" when they produce reinforcers and aversives, but without the ability to handle the risks or they are disproportionate (e.g., betting all savings on roulette) (Skinner, 1989). Mélvio emitted behaviors that produced punishments attenuated by his parents. This meant that the antecedents of the behaviors did not acquire discriminative stimulus functions for punishment (SDp), because there was no respondent pairing between the behaviors, the environment, and the aversive stimuli. Mélvio started not to discriminate pre-aversive stimuli, did not learn effective escape-avoidance behaviors, and maintained the emission of reckless behaviors.

Impulsivity and Low Frustration Tolerance Mélvio had access to reinforcers because he "existed" and when he asked for them, without having to behave to produce them. In a constructive social environment, the CRs are programmed so that responses produce gradually delayed consequences, with some response cost, in intermittent reinforcement schedules, with mild aversive consequences, creating behavioral persistence and frustration tolerance (Guilhardi, 2019). The result of this particular HCR in the client's repertoire was excessive control of immediate consequences and less control by delayed consequences (Rachlin & Green, 1972) and low frustration tolerance (if the reinforcer did not occur immediately, there was no behavioral variability to achieve it and an emotional explosion occurred). He also believed that the other should guarantee his privileges and didn't accept privations, reinforcer delays, or demands for desired behaviors.

Affective Indifference In the most relevant CRs in Mélvio's HCR, his parents had an SD function to ask for social and physical reinforcements and, to some extent, reflexive establishing operations to require if privileges and admiration were not guaranteed (Guilhardi, 2018). Mélvio did not have to learn to pay attention to feelings ("my father is sad") and behaviors of others ("he doesn't want to give me money") and to analyze the CRs that could have caused the change ("it must be because I didn't go to his birthday"). What the other felt and why he felt wasn't important, as long as "his" reinforcements weren't reduced or curtailed.

Deficit in the Self-knowledge Jesus and Pureza were under control of ensuring reinforcement independent of what the son was doing and they did not ask questions with SD function for Mélvio to pay attention to his own behavior and what controlled it (Skinner, 1953). The client was primarily under the influence of what he felt: the essential thing was to do to feel good, not to understand why he felt good, and to do not to feel bad, without understanding why, for him, that was bad (Guilhardi, 2018).

Throughout the client's history, the procedures used by the parents with Mélvio interacted with new contingencies in the activities outside home. In adolescence, he presented low performance at school, since studying had a high response cost (low frustration tolerance), low magnitude reinforcers (sensoriality) and family did not present differential consequences for desired and unwanted behaviors in the school area. He started to spend time with colleagues who also had educational problems and valued other subjects, such as music and nightlife. Mélvio began to identify himself with the themes proposed by the group, which guaranteed him access to social reinforcements in the form of attention (sensoriality and distorted self-esteem).

The routine with the group went beyond the scope of the school and moved to bars, shows, and nightclubs (entertainment maintained financially by his parents). The environments were functionally similar to the familiar, where the client had social reinforcements (he could be "important"), not being required to do anything. In this underground context, he met PAS, especially alcohol and cocaine. Drug use was initially maintained by the social impact it caused ("he is the craziest of the group!", "he plays guitar even if he is drunk") and the frequency and intensity gradually increased so that he would not be "just like the others" and would continue to stand out.

Upon finishing school, Mélvio entered several colleges without completing any. His low frustration tolerance did not allow him to attend classes every evening, concentrate for up to four hours/class, do assignments, study, etc., at the same time he did not have access to social and pharmacological reinforcements with his friends at night. He gave up the courses because of the difficulty in emitting a high frequency of responses that did not lead to the immediate and intense reinforcers to which he was more susceptible.

His father retired at the end of school and the family changed their financial situation. The maintenance of expenses for Mélvio's was suspended. The client, in the imminence of the deprivation of such reinforcements, sought work in his area of interest (he wouldn't do something he didn't like) and got a job with a friend, working informally. Later he got a position in a company, the moment in which complaints of relationship difficulties arose. The group's demand had changed: it had moved from the *underground* environment (and in the previous work, a tolerant environment for working with a friend) to a professional environment, where he lived with diverse subjects and without focus on a style of music or tours. At this moment, the client developed "two lifes": during the week, he lived with the deprivation of reinforcers (for not having a repertoire to produce them in a different environment), and on the weekend, he had the life he had built since high school (drugs, rock, attention). He kept working exclusively for the money that financed the weekend and, consequently, the social reinforcers.

An addendum. It is interesting to realize that the inability of the father to pay has possibly led to a different outcome than if the father continued working and did *not want to* pay for his son's pleasures. In the second hypothesis, Mélvio could have thought "*they are not giving what is rightfully mine*", "*they are petty*", etc. The story would have been quite different and the problems would probably have concentrated on the relationship with the family (Guilhardi, 2018).

As time went by, Mélvio became more and more deprived, as his interpersonal repertoire at work was not effective and he could not go out as he would like during the week. He also began to get more under control of the pharmacological effects of drugs (not only the social reinforcers), since consumption had a low response cost and produced intense body sensations (sensoriality), increasing the frequency on weekends and causing serious problems (e.g., car accident), but without worrying him (imprudence). Progressively he left aside activities that were not related to use (e.g., sports).

In the places where the client transited, problem behaviors were not only accepted, but susceptible to be admired. Thus, despite the fact that such repertoire presented itself as unwanted by certain groups of the conviviality (which not only deprived him, but also annoyed him), it continued to produce social reinforcers, preventing him from becoming aware of his difficulties: it were certain people who did not understand his "relevance" and "eloquence" for playing, using drugs and talking about "different" subjects and not him, the result of his HCR, who was the slave of the reinforcers who kept him in this fantasy and restrictive role. The cycle did not foster the development of problem-solving skills, the production of feelings and behaviors of responsibility and self-control, and greater behavioral variability to deal with people with other interests.

Once, during a company *happy hour,* deprived of reinforcers, he used the available repertoire to get attention. He drank too much, used cocaine, made bad jokes, and offered drugs to others. The next day he was fired. It was the first time that the environment signaled a behavior as undesirable, and later he was able to experience real deprivation without the salary. The event caused the first anxiety crisis. Mélvio was under control of the consequence (loss of employment), but not under control of previous stimuli to avoid the emission of certain responses in the future, repeating the same path throughout his life: in deprivation, he did not identify the antecedents or undervalued his pre-aversive function, continuing to use drugs and behave in an unwanted way.

The respondent conditioning among PAS and professional losses made the effects of drugs conditioned stimuli that elicited fear and anxiety, referring to the losses of social and financial reinforcers. Let us remember that the lack of money and the hindrance of nightlife were extremely aversive to Mélvio due to his HCR: far from the group he was nobody (low self-esteem) and had no competent repertoire (low self-confidence). Besides, the anxiety bothered a lot (sensoriality) and led to catastrophic conclusions like "*I'm going to have a heart attack*" (low self-knowledge). Thus, with a double life where he was only fully satisfied in periods of the week, with panic attacks and catastrophic thoughts, without knowing why he felt anxiety and without self-criticism of his behavior pattern, Mélvio sought psychotherapy. What about affective relationships? Dating in general was superficial and involved people who valued the "hipster", musical and film repertoire. The phenotype was "*the best boyfriend in the world*" and "*the most f****** couple in the club*", to impress the girlfriend and the group. Unlike his parents, the women with whom he was related deprived him of attention, charged him, demanded, criticized him, which evoked the repertoire of countercontrol with aggressive phenotype. It was as if Mélvio thought "*I want to be loved and important, and I do everything in your direction so that you reinforce my behaviors, but I don't want to behave to really reinforce your behaviors or lose reinforcers for you to be happy*". At the beginning of psychotherapy, self-observation and changing the interpersonal repertoire were not priorities for the client.

Goals

Taking HCR into account and the identification of problem behaviors, the psychotherapeutic goals for Mélvio's case were:

- Making the client able to respond discriminately to occurring CRs (he did not know that he exaggerated with drugs and emitted unwanted interpersonal behaviors due to his HCR and that anxiety was a product of the problems identified).
- Make the client sensitive to the others.
- Propitiate the client to tolerate aversive conditions (frustration tolerance).
- Putting client's behavior under control of delayed consequences.
- Increase the verbal descriptions of feelings and the relationship with occurring CRs (self-knowledge, specifically on anxiety).

Procedures

1. Metaphors (extended tact) as antecedent stimuli to increase the control of analogous conditions over the client's repertoire. The metaphors were used to mitigate the aversive function of the intervention and decrease the chance of countercontrol.

   Example:

T: *You arrive at work and your boss has moved your chair. He knows you liked where the chair was. You go talk to him and he says, "You're fired, get away."*
C: *I get your point.*
T: *She complained about the disappearance. You said you wouldn't live together anymore.*
C: *Out of proportion.*

The psychotherapist handled hypothetical situations where a third party knew the client's preferences, behaviors and feelings, and behaved without taking them into account. Specifically in the example described, the goal was to make the client more sensitive to his girlfriend. Mélvio had been drinking, using drugs, and arriving home late. When Raissa started a conflict, he responded that he "*would no longer live together*". The intervention consisted of making the client aware of his impact on his girlfriend saying "he was leaving" and the inadequacy of his behavior (the behavior of using drugs, arriving late, and being frustrated are worthy of criticism). Accepting he was emitting unwanted behaviors helped to attack the distorted self-esteem ("*I'm not good at what I do, I have behaviors that don't make me everything I thought I was*").

2. Description of the concept of three-term contingency of reinforcement and the anxiety model of Estes and Skinner (1941).

   Example:

T: [therapist explains the components of the triple contingency and the anxiety model of Behavior Analysis].
C: *I'm trying to find the red light of my life.*

The description of the concept of three-term contingency (in several sessions and using client examples) reaches two important issues of Mélvio: the deficit in getting under control and analyze the CRs that affect the behavior of others, and the deficit in analyzing the behavior itself and the variables of which it is a function. The basic unit of Behavior Analysis promotes the knowledge that our behaviors and people are controlled by CRs and are not free choices. Mélvio should learn that the other had reasons to please or annoy him, to do what he wanted or not to do. On the other hand, the client had a certain behavioral pattern because of his HCR and the occurring CRs and not because using drugs, being impulsive, irresponsible, selfish, and arrogant was his decision.

The concept of contingency of three terms facilitated the explanation of the anxiety paradigm, making it easier for Mélvio to understand that "panic attacks" had historical and environmental determinants.

3. Use of timeline with possible SD function to evoke identification responses of the components of the controlling variables.

The psychotherapist separated all the notes on the anxiety reports, as well as the previous sessions in which the client claimed to have used alcohol and cocaine. He then drew a timeline on a paper sheet, marking the dates of each abuse episode and each reported crisis, aiming to increase the establishment of the consumption-anxiety relationship and to install avoidance behaviors of anxiety crises under control of specific events (discriminating that drug use would cause anxiety and avoiding by not using, drinking less, leaving the bar, etc.). Considering Mélvio's impulsive behavior, the original notes were always at the client's disposal for him to compare events and dates (the notes, as verbal stimuli, were present in the environment). It was also expected that, if the intervention was successful, it would increase the chances of generalization and Mélvio would respond under control of other delayed consequences.

4. Description of possible consequences of client response on people.

   Example:

T: *Sounds like a compensation Scheme. I'm good, I deserve to have fun. You didn't find me good-looking, you didn't compliment me, I deserve to make fun. He didn't reply, I deserve to get angry. It's a prize.*
C: [Crying] That'*s it. That's me. How embarrassing! My family will stop loving me.*
T: *Maybe they won't stop loving you, but they might get tired of worrying. Neglect is like disaffection.*

The psychotherapist described the possible responses with aversive phenotype emitted when Mélvio was deprived and frustrated, and the effect of these responses on the client's family, friends and partners. People could feel bad, change their concepts about Mélvio and change the relationship that existed between them.

5. Progressive presentation of consequent stimuli with possible mild aversive function to the self-valorization verbalizations related to drug abuse.

   Example:
   [*Whatsapp* dialog]

C: *That's very crazy! I got cocaine in* [name of the country].
C: *I used it here. I did it. That's pretty crazy.*
T: *Are your activities over?* [changes subject].
C: *No.*
C: *I mean, more or less. There are the guys from* [the work] *who are going to present* [the slides of a project] *and I theoretically just have to watch.*
T: [Pause] *Theoretically?*

C: *Because their work depended on mine and I may have to explain something.*
C: *But look how crazy. I did all this in another country and I wasn't afraid at the time.*
C: *I used coke in* [name of country].
T: *Actually, Mélvio, the place is of little importance. Whether it was in Europe or in a drug den. we have to understand the function of that at the moment. My concern is that this will become another cool story to be told to close friends.*
C: *It won't.*
C: *It can't.*

According to Guilhardi (2010b), before employing any punitive procedure, careful evaluation and failed attempts at positive reinforcement interventions are required. On behalf of the client's HCR, the simple reporting of situations that produced any kind of attention by the verbal community was itself conditioned reinforcement, even if it produced unpleasant bodily sensations. It was important for the client to be under the control of the *CRs that made him or her vulnerable to the effects* of drugs and not just *the effects*. The psychotherapist, throughout the dialogue exemplified above, tried to draw attention away from the exaltation part of the report, taking time to respond or changing the subject, but without success. Since the client continued to select and repeat the part where he boasted about the behavior, the psychotherapist overlooked the verbalization about using drugs in different places ("*a cool story to be told*").

The intervention was also intended to gradually increase Mélvio's frustration tolerance. The psychotherapist, different from the agents that only presented reinforcers or aversive stimuli, turned into an audience that, in part, maintained a pleasant relationship, but did not agree with all of the client's statements. Mélvio should tolerate an interaction in which, although reinforcing, he would not be valued for anything he said.

Results

1. Awareness of occurring CRs and effective escape behaviors in contexts that evoked substance consumption.

   Example:

C: *Crap night.*

In a given situation, upon arriving at a party and identifying that people were using drugs, he reported that it was a "*crap night*" and that it would probably be a precedent to use, which would cause poor performance at the next day's work meeting (delayed punishment). He left the place. In addition, Mélvio began to anticipate social events that would involve drinking alcohol, taking non-alcoholic beer for his own consumption and learning to make soft drinks, despite jokes about his "masculinity" for not drinking alcohol.

Mélvio reported differentiating "friends of the night" and friends more sensitive to his problems. He said he had changed the way he saw them, because what seemed critical before was seen as care and that he began to admire qualities he found "boring" in such people.

2. Decrease in the frequency of behaviors under control of immediate consequences.

   Example:

C: *I finally received* [the payment three weeks late].
T: *What's up?*
C: *I thanked like a gentleman. I didn't even make a scene. It was their mistake, but okay. I don't like not getting paid, but I'm not gonna get misjudged.*

Some impulsive behaviors decreased in frequency and Mélvio reported thinking more before speaking. He mentioned a situation where the salary was delayed due to a human resources error and for two weeks he mentioned in session how much more days had been delayed and the problem had not been solved. In the third week he said that the salary had been paid and that he did not make the "fight" that he would do in other situations.

Mélvio also looked for an accountant to survey his debts and help him with financial planning.

The frequency of substance use has also dropped. According to Mélvio, he still "allowed" himself to use on his birthday (once a year).

3. The client has resumed past activities that produced alternative reinforcers to the substances of abuse.

   Example:

C: *I went to the gym, I liked the place. I thought there would be only professional athletes* [laughs]. *I already signed up.*

Along with the above results, psychotherapist and client began to look for activities that once had considerable reinforcing value for the client. Mélvio returned to the practice of sports and composing music by computer.

4. Emission of behaviors with milder phenotype ("assertive").

   Example:

C: *Don't talk to me like that Raissa, tell me you're worried, plan something with me, otherwise I'll get angry and want to get drugs. I'm not just "someone who uses drugs".*

Mélvio started to emit less aversive behaviors in several contexts. In relation to the family, which he referred to as "*a group of people who put everything 'under the carpet*'" and from whom he replicated models of "inassertive" behaviors in interactions, the client started to pull conversations and talk about himself, including his difficulty in relation to drinking and drugs and about past events that had adverse consequences for him and his family members.

In relation to Raíssa, the client started to behave, especially in situations of conflict, in a more polite way instead of fighting, indicating to the psychotherapist (in the example) a situation where he was going to spend a few days away and that his girlfriend had said "she would be insecure because he was a junkie" and that "the next time he used drugs he would die".

5. Identification that the crises were emotional episodes related to possible aversive consequences of drug use.

   Example:

C: *At least I know I won't die. I already know why I'm like this. I feel bad. I feel that my body is bad, but I can understand that I'm not really going to die. That this is pure anxiety.*
T: *Today you know yourself better.*
C: *Yeah. It's hard, but I know I'm not gonna die.*

Mélvio came under the control of the CRs that produced fear and anxiety, that is, the antecedents that signals that the consumption of SPA would follow the loss of financial, social and pharmacological reinforcers in the future. With this, the catastrophic and spurious interpretations for what I felt diminished. He began to question the relevance of reinforcers in his life.

Final Considerations

TCR is a psychotherapeutic proposal based on BS (Skinner, 1953) and RB (Skinner, 1945) that argues that substance dependence be interpreted as a set of respondent and operant behaviors (e.g., withdrawal syndrome, tolerance, obtaining drug, drug consumption) that should be therapeutically altered by changing the CRs that install and maintain such classes of behavior. Additionally, it requires an analysis and intervention in other more comprehensive behavioral classes (excesses and deficits) that contribute to the installation and maintenance of PAS consumption behaviors, such as low self-esteem, low self-knowledge, low self-confidence, low frustration tolerance, impulsiveness, recklessness, deficits of discipline and healthy activities and excessive dependence on social approval, more easily achieved by bizarre and risky behaviors and excessive sensoriality, as exemplified in the case presented. It also analyzes behaviors that may be unrelated to PAS. The phenotypic similarities of users' behaviors hide that, essentially, each person is different in multiple aspects in their reasons for abusive use and in the multiple repertories that make up their being, which extend far beyond the behavioral classes directly linked to the drug and which need to be changed concomitantly. As such, each individual needs individualized psychotherapeutic treatments, which, guided by general behavioral principles and laws, are presented in interactions with the chemical dependent as individual techniques, adjusted to individual needs (along with submitting to standard procedures, basically those guided by medicine). Two people are not exactly the same; two treatments are not exactly the same. CR presents such a proposal and is prepared to assume it in psychotherapeutic processes conducted with substance dependents.

Acknowledgments To the psychologists Hélio José Guilhardi and Lylian Cristina Pilz Penteado in the construction of this chapter.

References

American Psychiatric Association (APA). (1994). *Diagnostic and statistical manual of mental disorders* (4th ed.). APA.

American Psychiatric Association (APA). (2013). *Diagnostic and statistical manual of mental disorders* (5th ed.). APA. https://doi.org/10.1176/appi.books.9780890425596

Andery, M. A. P. A. (2010). Métodos de pesquisa em análise do comportamento. *Psicologia USP, 21*(2), 313–342. https://doi.org/10.1590/S0103-65642010000200006

Aranha, A. S., & Oshiro, C. K. B. (2017). A identificação de comportamentos clinicamente relevantes em dependentes de substância. In *XXVI Congresso Brasileiro de Psicologia e Medicina Comportamental*. Bauru.

Baer, D. M., Wolf, M. M., & Risley, T. R. (1968). Some current dimensions of applied behavior analysis. *Journal of Applied Behavior Analysis, 1*(1), 91–97. https://doi.org/10.1901/jaba.1968.1-91

Balvedi, C. (2003). Acompanhante terapêutico – a terapia no ambiente do paciente. In M. Z. S. Brandão, F. C. S. Conte, F. S. Brandão, Y. K. Ingberman, C. B. Moura, V. M. Silva, & S. M. Olian (Eds.), *Sobre comportamento e cognição: A história e os avanços, a seleção por consequências em ação* (pp. 294–299). ESETec.

Benvenuti, M. F. (2004). Condicionamento respondente: Algumas implicações para o desenvolvimento de tolerância, síndrome de abstinência e overdose. In C. N. Abreu & H. J. Guilhardi (Eds.), *Terapia comportamental e cognitivo-comportamental: Práticas clínicas* (pp. 186–193). Roca.

Catania, A. C. (1999). *Aprendizagem: Comportamento, linguagem e cognição* (4th ed.). Artmed. (Original work published in 1998).

Diehl, A., Cordeiro, D. C., & Lranjeira, R. (2011). *Dependência química: Prevenção, tratamento e políticas públicas*. Artmed.

Estes, W. K., & Skinner, B. F. (1941). Some quantitative properties of anxiety. *Journal of Experimental Psychology, 29*(5), 390–400. https://doi.org/10.1037/h0062283

Ferster, C. B. (1972). An experimental analysis of clinical phenomena. *The Psychological Record, 22*, 1–16.

Garcia-Mijares, M., & Silva, M. T. A. (2006). Dependência de drogas. *Psicologia USP, 17*(4), 213–240. https://doi.org/10.1590/S0103-65642006000400012

Guilhardi, H. J. (1988). A formação do terapeuta comportamental: Que formação? In H. W. Lettner & B. P. Rangé (Eds.), *Manual de psicoterapia comportamental* (pp. 313–321). São Paulo.

Guilhardi, H. J. (2002). Autoestima, autoconfiança e responsabilidade. In M. Z. S. Brandão, F. C. S. Conte, & S. M. B. Mezzaroba (Eds.), *Tudo (ou quase tudo) que você precisa saber para viver melhor* (pp. 63–98). ESETec.

Guilhardi, H. J. (2003). Tudo se deve às consequências. *Instituto de Terapia por Contingências de Reforçamento*. Recuperado de: http://www.itcrcampinas.com.br/pdf/helio/tudo_consequencias.pdf

Guilhardi, H. J. (2004). Terapia por contingências de reforçamento. In C. N. Abreu & H. J. Guilhardi (Eds.), *Terapia comportamental e cognitivo-comportamental: Práticas clínicas* (pp. 3–40). Roca.

Guilhardi, H. J. (2007). Conceituação de sentimentos. *Instituto de Terapia por Contingências de Reforçamento*. Recuperado de: http://www.itcrcampinas.com.br/pdf/helio/Conceituacao_de_sentimentos2007.pdf

Guilhardi, H. J. (2010a). História de contingências de reforçamento. *Instituto de Terapia por Contingências de Reforçamento*. Recuperado de: http://www.itcrcampinas.com.br/txt/historia.pdf

Guilhardi, H. J. (2010b). Punição não é castigo. *Instituto de Terapia por Contingências de Reforçamento*. Recuperado de: http://www.itcrcampinas.com.br/pdf/helio/Punicao_castigo2010.pdf

Guilhardi, H. J. (2012). Os seis sentidos de "the lady and the unicorn". *Instituto de Terapia por Contingências de Reforçamento*. Recuperado de: http://www.itcrcampinas.com.br/txt/seissentidos.pdf

Guilhardi, H. J. (2013). Alcoolismo: Conceitos da análise do comportamento para superação. *Instituto de Terapia por Contingências de Reforçamento*. (Obra original publicada em 2010). Recuperado de: http://itcrcampinas.com.br/txt/alcoolismo.pdf

Guilhardi, H. J. (2018). Problemas do reforço livre. *Revista Brasileira de Análise do Comportamento, 14*(2), 171–190. https://doi.org/10.18542/rebac.v14i2.7537

Guilhardi, H. J. (2019). Pero, y si no hay amor. Em: I. M. Rodrigues Jr., & J. M. G. Rodríguez (Eds.), *Manual latinoamericano de terapia de pareja volumen 1: temas introductorios*. (pp. 43–68). São Paulo: Instituto Paulista de Sexualidade.

Harris, K. B., & Miller, W. R. (1990). Behavioral self-control training for problem drinkers: Components of efficacy. *Psychology of Addictive Behaviors, 4*(2), 82–90. https://doi.org/10.1037/h0080586

Heyman, G. (1996). Resolving the contradictions of addiction. *Behavioral and Brain Sciences, 19*(4), 561–574. https://doi.org/10.1017/S0140525X00042990

Hunt, G. M., & Azrin, N. H. (1973). A community-reinforcement approach to alcoholism. *Behaviour Research and Therapy, 11*(1), 91–104. https://doi.org/10.1016/0005-7967(73)90072-7

Kanfer, F. H., & Saslow, G. (1976). An outline for behavioral diagnosis. In E. J. Mash & L. G. Terdal (Eds.), *Behavior therapy assessment* (pp. 20–40). Springer Publishing Company.

Leonardi, J. L. (2015). O lugar da terapia analítico-comportamental no cenário internacional das terapias comportamentais: Um panorama histórico. *Perspectivas em análise do comportamento, 6*(2), 119–131. https://doi.org/10.18761/pac.2015.027

Martin, G., & Pear, J. (2009). *Modificação de comportamento: O que é e como fazer* (8ª ed.) (N. C. de Aguirre, Trad.). São Paulo: Roca. (Obra original publicada em 2007).

Miguel, A. D. Q. C., Yamauchi, R., Simões, V., da Silva, C. J., & Laranjeira, R. R. (2015). From theory to treatment: Understanding addiction from an operant behavioral perspective. *Journal of Modern Education Review, 5*(8), 778–787. https://doi.org/10.15341/jmer(2155-7993)/08.05.2015/006

Rachlin, H., & Green, L. (1972). Commitment, choice and self-control. *Journal of the Experimental Analysis of Behavior, 17*(1), 15–22. https://doi.org/10.1901/jeab.1972.17-15

Skinner, B. F. (1945). The operational analysis of psychological terms. *Psychological Review, 52*(5), 270–277. https://doi.org/10.1037/h0062535

Skinner, B. F. (1953). *Science and human behavior*. McMillan.

Skinner, B. F. (1957). *Century psychology series. Verbal behavior*. Appleton-Century-Crofts. https://doi.org/10.1037/11256-000

Skinner, B. F. (1975). The ethics of helping people. *Criminal Law Bulletin, 11*, 623–636.

Skinner, B. F. (1986). What is wrong with daily life in western world? *American Psychologist, 41*(5), 568–574. https://doi.org/10.1037/0003-066X.41.5.568

Skinner, B. F. (1989). *Recent issues in the analysis of behavior*. Merril.

Sobell, M. B., Sobell, L. C., & Sheahan, D. B. (1976). Functional analysis of drinking problems as an aid in developing individual treatment strategies. *Addictive Behaviors, 1*(2), 127–132. https://doi.org/10.1016/0306-4603(76)90005-8

Chapter 13
Motivational Interviewing Under a Behavior Analysis Perspective

César Silva Rodrigues Oliveira and Edson Massayuki Huziwara

Introduction

Motivational interviewing (MI) is a treatment method used in the field of substance use disorders (SUD), developed by William R. Miller from his own clinical experience. MI is largely based on the person-centered approach (Rogers, 1959), as well as on other theories of social psychology and, although its origin is related to the area of substance abuse and dependence, this method has been widely studied and used for several other behavioral domains, such as adherence to the practice of physical exercise, modification of eating habits, and reduction of risky sexual behavior, among others (Lundahl et al., 2010). In addition, it has been shown to be more effective than no treatment and similarly effective than other treatment options, although more cost-effective due to its brief intervention character (Lundahl & Burke, 2009; Smedslund et al., 2011).

The objective of this chapter is to introduce MI to the behavior analysts' community, especially those unfamiliar with methods for treating patients with SUD, as well as to provide an analytical-behavioral understanding of the method and its main strategies.

Motivational Interviewing: Its Origins

According to Miller, in a report presented in the third edition of the book entitled *Motivational Interviewing* (Miller & Rollnick, 2013), in the 1980s, the addiction treatment in the United States was often highly authoritarian,

C. S. R. Oliveira (✉) · E. M. Huziwara
Universidade Federal de Minas Gerais (UFMG), Belo Horizonte, MG, Brazil

S. M. Oliani et al. (eds.), *Behavior Analysis and Substance Dependence*,
https://doi.org/10.1007/978-3-030-75961-2_13

confrontational, humiliating, and relying on a directing style of counseling. People with such problems were characterized as pathological liars, with immature personality defense mechanisms and also with problems to maintain contact with reality. Surprisingly, Miller's first experiences in treating people with alcohol problems revealed that they were often open, interesting, and aware of the problems produced by their behavior. It did not take long for him to realize that the openness or resistance of the patient appeared to be a product of the established therapeutic relationship rather than a personality trait of individuals with such problems.

In a clinical trial of behavioral therapy for alcohol-related problems (Miller et al., 1980), the authors trained nine counselors in self-control techniques and in person-centered approach skills such as accurate empathy. After being trained, the same counselors performed self-control training in outpatients. Three supervisors observed and rated the extent to which each counselor exhibited accurate empathy while conducting the training. The therapist's empathy was able to predict two-thirds of the variance in the patient's alcohol consumption six months after treatment ended. Thus, the results observed suggested the importance of the therapist's emphatic style to engage patients in the proposed treatment.

After these initial findings (Miller et al., 1980), Miller developed the first version of his treatment approach. In a trip to Norway, the author had the opportunity to present and discuss the theoretical and empirical basis of this new approach with a group of psychologists gathered at the Hjellestad Clinic (Miller & Rollnick, 2001). According to Miller and Rose (2009), this environment was important for the clarification of his method, besides it has been an event that helped him in an important way in the writing of his original article, published in 1983 (Miller, 1983). In 1989, on a trip to Australia, Miller met Stephen Rollnick, who reported that MI was very popular in the treatment of SUD in the UK. Rollnick encouraged Miller to write a book,[1] which he co-authored, systematizing and helping to spread knowledge about MI. Since then, much has been produced and modifications have been proposed in relation to the concepts presented in the first edition of the book, such as the inclusion of the notion of the "spirit" of MI in the second edition,[2] in addition to an emphasis on the concept of *change talk* and *sustain talk* gathered in the third edition[3] together with an update of the "spirit" of MI.

[1] Miller, W. R., & Rollnick, S. (1991). *Motivational interviewing: preparing people to change addictive behavior.* New York: The Guilford Press.

[2] Miller, W. R., & Rollnick, S. (2002). *Motivational interviewing: preparing people for change* (2nd ed.). New York: The Guilford Press.

[3] Miller, W. R. & Rollnick, S. (2013). *Motivational Interviewing: helping people change* (3rd ed.). New York: The Guilford Press.

Motivational Interviewing: Definition and Strategies

A basic element of MI refers to the understanding of ambivalence as a common and present behavior in any process of change. That is, having reasons to change and, at the same time, not to change is a normal human experience. According to Miller and Rollnick (2013), when a person presents ambivalence in relation to a subject of interest it is common to alternate the emission of two types of speech during a conversation. One type would be the *change talk*, in which the patient argues for change giving reasons, talking about his or her ability to change or committing to change. Another type would be the *sustain talk,* which corresponds to arguments in favor of maintaining the current behavior. According to the assumptions of MI, the therapist arguing in favor of change is counterproductive, since it causes sustain talk by the patient, which generally reinforces the conception that people with SUD are resistant, opposed, and in constant denial of their problems. In this scenario, one of the main objectives of MI is to modify risk behavior by exploring and solving this ambivalence. Thus, MI is defined as "a client-centered, directive method for enhancing intrinsic motivation to change by exploring and resolving ambivalence" (Miller & Rollnick, 2002, p. 25).

In a more recent definition, the same authors refer to MI as:

> *(…) a collaborative, goal-oriented style of communication with particular attention to the language of change. It is designed to strengthen personal motivation for and commitment to a specific goal by eliciting and exploring the person's own reasons for change within an atmosphere of acceptance and compassion.* (Miller & Rollnick, 2013, p. 40).

At least two notions are important for the characterization of the MI, namely its "spirit" and processes. According to Miller and Rollnick (2013), there is an attitude that must be maintained by the therapist throughout the process, which the authors call "spirit". In the authors' own words, "without this underlying spirit, MI becomes a cynical trick, a way of trying to manipulate people into doing what they don't want to do" (Miller & Rollnick, 2013, p. 23).

There are four elements that make up the "spirit" of MI: partnership, acceptance, evocation, and compassion. Partnership involves establishing a positive interpersonal atmosphere that is conducive to change, but not coercive. The therapist searches for establishing an active collaboration between experts, considering that the patients are undisputed experts on themselves, to value the patient's perspectives, avoiding imposing the therapist's vision on the patient's vision. The deep acceptance derives from four other elements extracted from Carl Rogers' work, namely, absolute worth, accurate empathy, support to autonomy, and affirmation. In short, acceptance would involve recognizing the inherent value and potential of each human being; developing an active interest and effort in understanding the perspective of the other in his/her own way; honoring and respecting the autonomy or the irrevocable right of the person to choose his/her own path; and highlighting the strengths and efforts of the person, rather than what he/she lacks. In turn, evocation refers to the therapist strengthening the motivations for change that are already present rather than focusing on installing that which is absent. Finally, compassion is about promoting the well-being of the other and prioritizing the needs of the other in the relationship.

Besides the "spirit" of the MI, another important notion for its understanding concerns its processes. In the first two editions of the book "Motivational Interviewing", the authors described MI operating in two phases: "building motivation" and "consolidating commitment". This division suggested a linear process of change, which did not correspond with the clinical observations. The process of MI, on the contrary, seems to be a process of phases, in which one overlaps with the other. These processes are thus recursive and, at the same time, sequential. Thus, in the third edition of the book, the authors elaborated four processes, which were expressed in the gerund to better represent its sequence and overlapping: "engaging", "focusing", "evoking", and "planning". "Engaging" consists in the process of building a therapeutic alliance that searches for solutions to the problems encountered. "Focusing" is the process by which a specific direction is developed and maintained in the conversation about change. "Evoking" is about evoking the patient's own motivations for change, i.e., having the patient himself argue for change. Finally, "planning" encompasses both the development of a commitment to change and the formulation of an action plan.

The practice of MI involves the flexible use of communication skills appropriate to the person-centered approach. These skills are present throughout all the processes of MI and are summarized under the acronym OARS,[4] formed from the expressions (1) open questions; (2) affirming; (3) reflections; (4) summarizing. Open questions are invitations to think and elaborate, unlike closed-ended questions, which search for specific information and can be answered by a short answer. In "engaging" and "focusing" processes, they help the therapist to understand the patient's frame of reference, strengthening a collaborative relationship and finding a direction, while in "evoking" and "planning" they help to strengthen motivation and to develop a plan for change. Affirming, on the other hand, is both general and specific, that is, it concerns both the therapist's ability to be attentive to the patient's resources and qualities and also to value his or her abilities, good intentions, or efforts during the sessions. Reflections are very important skills, since they clarify and deepen the meaning of what is said by the patient, as well as keeping him talking and exploring issues related to the desired behavioral change. They can be simple (i.e., literal reproductions of what the patient said) or complex (i.e., reproductions of the sense of his speech). Moreover, in MI, reflections are necessarily selective, which means that the therapist objectively selects what to reflect on, especially in "evoking" and "planning" processes, directing the patient's attention to specific aspects of his speech. Summarizing, in turn, constitutes wider reflections that connect current information with past information, besides being important in moments of transition from one task to another. In "engaging" and "focusing", the abstracts make it clear

[4] Originally, in English, the acronym is OARS, formed by *open questions*, *affirming*, *reflections* and *summarizing*.

to the patient that the therapist was attentive to what was said, valuing the content of the speech. In "evoking" they have the role of bringing together the change talk to continue the process of change, while in "planning" the summaries help to gather specific motivations, intentions, and plans for change.

In addition to the acronym, there is also a fifth skill which is "informing and advising". There are times when it is important to provide the patient with advice or information; however, they do not occur without the patient's consent to receive them and the therapist should make an effort to verify that the information is being well understood, according to the patient's ability to assimilate it. Furthermore, it is important for the therapist to remember that it is his job to allow patients to reach their own conclusions with the information or advice received.

Finally, Miller and Rollnick (2013) suggested that for a therapist to get the full learning from MI, it is important to have mastery of 12 tasks: (1) understand the underlying spirit with which MI is practiced, namely, partnership, acceptance, compassion, and evocation; (2) develop skills and comfort with reflective listening and OARS skills; (3) identify change goals to move toward; (4) exchange information and provide advice within an MI style; (5) be able to recognize change talk and sustain talk; (6) evoke change talk; (7) respond to change talk in a way that strengthens it; (8) respond to sustain talk in a way that does not amplify it; (9) develop hope and confidence; (10) learn the right time to negotiate a change plan; (11) strengthen commitment; and (12) integrate MI flexibly with other clinical skills and practices.

Motivational Interviewing: Mechanisms of Change

For MI, the change in behavior, in addition to a relational component based on its "spirit", which is responsible for reducing patient resistance, also depends on the appropriate use of techniques, which will allow the increase of change talk and decrease of sustain talk (Lundahl et al., 2011; Miller & Rose, 2009). Amrhein, Miller, Yahne, Palmer, and Fulcher (2003) found that a higher number of statements of commitment to change during the session predicted an increase in the proportion of abstinent days in drug abusers. Moyers and Martin (2006) further noted that therapists with speech consistent with the spirit of MI evoked more change talk, while those with inconsistent speech evoked more sustain talk.

Magill et al. (2014) performed a meta-analysis of the causal model established by MI seeking to evaluate the hypothesis that MI strategies produce changes in the discourse of patients and that these changes predict treatment outcomes related to behavior change. The found results confirmed that: (1) therapeutic skills consistent with MI (e.g., open-ended questions, reflections, and affirming) were associated with higher rates of change talk, while therapeutic skills inconsistent with MI (e.g., confrontations, warnings, unsolicited counseling) were associated with fewer change talk and more sustain talk; (2) higher rates of sustain talk were associated with worse treatment outcomes; (3) combined measures of change talk and sustain talk, as well as statements of commitment, were positively related to behavior change, although change talk when taken alone was not associated with change.

Motivational Interviewing and Behavior Analysis: An Approach According to Christopher and Dougher (2009)

Both Behavior Analysis and MI assume the relational nature of motivation for change. For Behavior Analysis, any behavior, including verbal one, is a function of the environmental variables that control its occurrence (Skinner, 1957, 1981). In this sense, a way to reinforce a given verbal behavior would involve the planning of adequate contingencies for the occurrence of such behavior. MI can be understood as a method in which there is a conscious effort by the therapist to come under control of the occurrence of so-called change talk, establishing the occasion for its emission and reinforcing its occurrence. In other words, through the person-centered approach (OARS) communication skills, there is an effort to differentially reinforce the occurrence of change talk within an environment with minimal aversive control (Christopher & Dougher, 2009).

A therapeutic environment with minimum levels of aversive control necessarily requires that the therapist constitutes a non-punitive audience (Skinner, 1953) for the patient. SUD patients usually come to clinical setting brought by family members and have a long history of exposure to coercive strategies to control their behavior which makes a non-punitive posture extremely necessary. Otherwise, an increase in the frequency of speech that topographically resembles change talk (e.g., perceptions of many losses related to the drug use) may be under control of reinforcers other than a real process of change (e.g., avoiding a reprimand by the therapist) (Oliveira, 2007). In other words, the change in the patient's verbal behavior may not be related to a change in the target behavior if coercive strategies are being employed, since such strategies may reinforce the occurrence of responses that reduce the probability of punishment, that is, characteristic responses of countercontrol strategies (Delprato, 2002).

The therapist's attention to the sequential, recursive, and overlapping nature of the four processes proposed by MI (i.e., "engaging," "focusing," "evoking," "planning") probably helps to reduce the occurrence of countercontrol responses. In other words, the differential reinforcement of change talk (i.e., a task proper to the "evoking" process) should not occur without the therapist first establishing a relationship of trust with the patient, establishing himself as a non-punitive audience (i.e., "engaging" task) and differentiating himself from the others who previously punished him. In other words, tasks related to the "engaging" process should occur before tasks related to the "evoking" process. At the same time, a therapist can use strategies of the "engaging" process even when "evoking" process tasks are being performed, which confers the circular character of these processes.

In summary, the therapist is more likely to establish himself as a non-punitive audience behaving in accordance with the "spirit" of MI (i.e., establishing a partnership relationship, not authoritarian, in which he values the knowledge of the patient about himself, not reprimanding or judging his behavior, and strengthening his motivations instead of implanting others), which helps to evoke more precise tact regarding the contingencies that govern his behavior. The more precise the patient is to contact the reinforcers or aversive stimuli associated with his or her risk behavior, the more accurate the patient's functional analysis can be described (Christopher & Dougher, 2009).

For example, an initial statement from an SUD patient may indicate that he would like to know strategies for stopping drug use. Moreover, other statements may also suggest that he does not understand the reasons for maintaining this behavioral pattern or cannot point out positive aspects related to drug use. A more detailed analysis, however, may reveal that tacts regarding the reinforcing consequences of drug use have been punished in the past, which is why the patient would have omitted them at this point.

Additionally, this behavioral pattern at the beginning of a therapeutic relationship possibly also indicates aversive consequences related to being judged by others in daily life. The therapist could even use this situation to explore other behaviors that fulfill the same function (e.g., isolate himself from people who do not use drugs to not be judged) and the distal consequences related to them. In general, faced with a demand as described in the previous example, therapists could focus only on implementing training in self-control strategies, missing the opportunity to expand the patient's contact with the problems related to the use of the substance (e.g., isolation of non-users) as well as to address the reinforcing consequences of this behavior (e.g., drug use euphoria, drug users socialization, escape from the responsibilities of daily life). Such a strategy could be an opportunity to recognize the need to expand contact with other reinforcers or to address alternative behaviors to produce similar reinforcers. In this sense, the use of simple open-ended questions, as proposed by MI (e.g., "what do you like about your cocaine use?" and "and what don't you like?"), can establish the occasion for a more in-depth analysis of the conflicting consequences and contingencies competing with the use of the substance. A more precise tact of the patient on the exemplified situation could be something like this: "I *like the acceleration that cocaine causes me. I talk a lot, I get along easily with the guys, especially after a stressful week that I spend with the care of my son, dedication to work and home. At the same time, I realize that I have become increasingly isolated from my family and friends. I am very embarrassed to face them, especially after nights that I come sniffing around. My son, as he is still very small, does not understand, but he will soon understand*" (sic). That is, by behaving in accordance with the "spirit" of MI and through the use of OARS communication skills (i.e., open-ended questions, affirming, reflections, and summarizing), the therapist indicates the absence of punishment and establishes himself as a discriminative stimulus for the patient to speak freely about their problem, reinforcing tacts from every contingencies related to the target behavior (Christopher & Dougher, 2009).

According to Christopher and Dougher (2009), among OARS communication skills, reflections (i.e., literal reproductions of the patient's speech or meaning) are critical to understand how the method can increase the frequency of change talk. In addition to the fact that the reflections have an autoclitic function,[5] since they increase the effect of the therapist's verbalizations that intend to communicate acceptance, they can function as establishing operations,[6] since they increase the reinforcing properties of the therapist's verbal behavior, thus leading to an increase in the likelihood of the patient emitting previously punished, painful, or sensitive behavior about his problem. In the example mentioned above, a reflection said by the therapist could be something like this: *"you notice that you have become more and more isolated from your family and friends because you feel ashamed. Also, you worry about your child's reaction when he or she can understand what is going on with you"*. In the face of this intervention, it would be likely that the patient would agree with the therapist and continue talking about this relevant clinical issue. Additionally, the patient would be more likely to "react better" to the therapist's future verbalizations. In this way, acceptance, signaled by reflection, can evoke a more precise exploration of the previously avoided contingencies, which can decrease the number of imprecise tacts about the contingencies related to the maintenance of the behavior problem (Christopher & Dougher, 2009).

For a more accurate understanding of how MI increases the change talk, Christopher and Dougher (2009) also sought to functionally define the different types of reflection and their different functions. In general, all of them could be classified as mands, since such reflections are operant behavior maintained by the specific consequence of evoking change talk and diminishing characteristic countercontrol responses, although they can also have an intraverbal function because they are evoked by a verbal discriminative stimulus. Simple reflections, for example, are those in which the therapist merely what repeat some patient's sentences, demonstrating that he understands what the patient said.

Complex reflections are related to a deeper level of demonstration of understanding in which the therapist specifies the contingency that controls the verbalization of the patient. Suppose, for example, that the phrase *"I like the acceleration of cocaine"* is said by the patient after the therapist has encouraged him to abstain from cocaine. In this context, the patient's phrase may be understood as a countercontrol response to avoid the therapist's punishment, who signaled his expectations regarding behavior change. The therapist could respond as follows: *"I understand … it would be difficult for you to stop using"*. In this sense, complex reflection can help reduce countercontrol, while increasing the likelihood that the

[5] The so-called autoclitic operant consists of a verbal unit that occurs together with other basic operants, modifying the effects of these basic operants on the listener (Barros, 2003; Borloti, 2004; Skinner, 1957).

[6] Establishing operations are environmental events that momentarily change the effectiveness of a stimulus as a reinforcer or punisher. This concept, in behavioral terms, is related to what is called motivation in generic terms (Michael, 1993; Miguel, 2000).

patient will talk about the contingencies that control his abilities to change (Christopher & Dougher, 2009). An amplified reflection is a speech in which the therapist usually exaggerates the patient's sustain talk for reducing countercontrol. At the same time, this type of reflection increases the probability that the patient will engage in more exploratory behavior for specifying the contingencies that control the problematic behavior. For example, in the face of a phrase like this: *"using drugs helps me relax,"* the therapist may respond: *"using drugs is the only way you relax"*. In this context, the patient is asked to agree with the speech that restricted the class of relaxing events to cocaine use or to repair it, describing other behaviors that share the same relaxing function. Thus, cocaine use becomes one more among other behaviors of this functional class that can still be distinguished as generating delayed aversive consequences (Christopher & Dougher, 2009).

Another speech by the therapist, named double reflections, relates the change talk with the sustain talk through a connective word such as "*and*", making clear the divergence between the patient's values and his or her current behavior. For instance, the therapist may say a phrase such as: *"you worry about being away from your family and find it difficult to relax without cocaine"*. Christopher and Dougher (2009) point out that in this case, the therapist's reinforcement by the patient having verbally come into contact with these contingencies can, through empathetic reflection, increase the reinforcing value of talking about behavior change, functioning as an establishing operation for the emission of change talk like that: *"maybe I can learn new ways to relax without cocaine"*.

Finally, the summaries, as more extensive reflections, relate the change talk and the sustain talk, trying to describe the full extent of contingencies that compete in controlling behavior. According to the authors, patients would be more inclined to express a commitment to change considering that they have already explored other behaviors that share the same function of the problem behavior without producing aversive consequences and come into contact with the discrepancy between their values and their current behaviors. In these conditions, the therapist reinforces the elaboration of selfmands about the change and helps the patient to elaborate a plan for it.

For the constitution of this plan, MI makes clear the importance of providing the patient with advice or information as long as the therapist has permission or consent to do so. Asking permission to inform or advise is a type of verbalization that performs an autoclitic function over other mands of the therapist, since they alter the aversiveness of the information or advice given, which may increase its effectiveness. To illustrate, a good example could be: *"Would it be ok for you if I told you some strategies that other people use to stop using cocaine?"*

Having explained how empathetic reflections can set the context for reinforcing change talk, Christopher and Dougher (2009) suggest the following functional definition of MI, which is reproduced here:

> *(…)MI evokes change talk by creating a therapeutic relationship of acceptance, collaboration, and client autonomy, which reduces counterpliance and avoidance of contact with painful contingencies related to drinking, while deliberately and differentially reinforcing*

> *change talk by using client-centered counseling skills (OARS) to establish variation in client verbal behavior related to change. The therapist reinforces the client's behavior of accurately tacting the full range of competing contingencies, both historical and current and proximal and distal, that govern drinking behavior. Thus, MI is essentially an environment deliberately arranged for the evocation of change talk and the elaboration of self-mands that are correlated with behavior change.* (Christopher & Dougher, 2009, p. 155).

Christopher and Dougher (2009) therefore highlight the importance of OARS communication skills and the "spirit" of MI in shaping a non-punitive audience environment, which reduces countercontrol responses. The authors also emphasize the importance of differential reinforcement of tacts on the various aversive and reinforcing consequences of risk behavior to collaborate in the elaboration of selfmands related to the desired behavior change. Although several studies highlight the correlations between change talks and behavioral change (Amrhein et al., 2003; Magill et al., 2014), the functional relationships between these two factors have not yet been clearly explored, as the authors highlight. In other words, why does increasing change talk influence post-session behavior? According to these same authors, three processes related to rule-based behavior (Skinner, 1969) would explain such influence. In the first case, the social contingencies present during the session and in the patient's natural environment reinforce the statement of commitment to change, which is a function of the interpersonal contingencies of the session in addition to the description of past and future consequences of the target behavior. This social environment, therefore, begins to monitor and reinforce behaviors congruent with the commitment made. Another process is related to the weakening of the control of certain rules, either when amplifying a class of behaviors that produce relaxation, weakening the rule "*cocaine helps me relax*", or clarifying behaviors necessary to deal with conflicting contingencies, weakening the rule "*my life will be better if I stop using, but I can't*". Finally, the process in which the therapist searches for evoking and understanding the patient's values is highlighted, thus expanding contact with high-magnitude reinforcers, which can help maintain certain behaviors even in the face of the availability of more immediate reinforcers in competing contingencies.

Using a more recent interpretation that presents considerable differences in the interpretation of verbal behavior when compared to Skinner (1957), Christopher and Dougher (2009) still highlight that the literature on function transformation (Hayes et al., 2001) is necessary for the explanation of why the verbal behavior of the patient and the therapist may alter the behavioral patterns emitted in the post-session. As Wilson and Hayes (2000) have pointed out, MI can figure as a potentially effective clinical strategy to alter the stimulus function of the ultimate consequences of a substance use contingency. However, it is beyond the scope of this chapter to present concepts related to RFT (*Relational Frame Theory*), although it is recognized the importance of understanding the effects of verbal contingencies involved in the relational response of substance users.

Final Considerations

According to the presentation, the manipulation of verbal behavior in the therapeutic environment, to some extent, may favor the change of risk behaviors displayed outside the aforementioned *setting*. Despite the differences between the theoretical bases of MI and Behavior Analysis, the propositions made by this method were analyzed in behavior analytic terms by Christopher and Dougher (2009), helping behavior analysts to assimilate effective clinical strategies for the treatment of SUD people.

For both MI theorists and behavior analysts, there is a special interest in understanding how verbal contingencies can participate in behavioral control. Although Christopher and Dougher (2009) have shed light on the likely mechanisms responsible for verbal behavior during MI sessions to change the source of target behavior control, further studies are needed to clarify these issues.

References

Amrhein, P. C., Miller, W. R., Yahne, C. E., Palmer, M., & Fulcher, L. (2003). Client commitment language during motivational interviewing predicts drug use outcomes. *Journal of Consulting and Clinical Psychology, 71*, 862–878. https://doi.org/10.1037/0022-006X.71.5.862

Barros, R. S. (2003). Uma introdução ao comportamento verbal. *Revista Brasileira de Terapia Comportamental e Cognitiva, 5*, 73–82.

Borloti, E. (2004). As relações verbais elementares e o processo autoclítico. *Revista Brasileira de Terapia Comportamental e Cognitiva, 6*, 221–236.

Christopher, P. J., & Dougher, M. J. (2009). A behavior-analytic account of motivational interviewing. *The Behavior Analyst, 32*, 149–161. https://doi.org/10.1007/BF03392180

Delprato, D. J. (2002). Countercontrol in behavior analysis. *The Behavior Analyst, 25*, 191–200. https://doi.org/10.1007/BF03392057

Hayes, S. C., Barnes-Holmes, D., & Roche, B. (Eds.). (2001). *Relational frame theory: A post-Skinnerian account of human language and cognition*. Plenum Press.

Lundahl, B., & Burke, B. (2009). The effectiveness and applicability of motivational interviewing: A practice-friendly review of four meta-analyses. *Journal of Clinical Psychology, 65*, 1232–1245. https://doi.org/10.1002/jclp.20638

Lundahl, B., Kunz, C., Brownell, C., Tollefson, D., & Burke, B. (2010). A meta-analysis of motivational interviewing: Twenty-five years of empirical studies. *Research on Social Work Practice, 20*, 137–160. https://doi.org/10.1177/1049731509347850

Magill, M., Gaume, J., Apodaca, T., Walthers, J., Mastroleo, N., Borsari, B., & Longabaugh, R. (2014). The technical hypothesis of motivational interviewing: A meta-analysis of MI's key causal model. *Journal of Consulting and Clinical Psychology, 82*, 973–983. https://doi.org/10.1037/a0036833

Michael, J. (1993). Establishing operations. *The Behavior Analyst, 16*, 191–206. https://doi.org/10.1007/BF03392623

Miguel, C. F. (2000). O conceito de operação estabelecedora na análise do comportamento. *Psicologia: Teoria e Pesquisa, 16*, 259–267.

Miller, W. R. (1983). Motivational interviewing with problem drinkers. *Behavioural Psychotherapy, 11*, 147–172. https://doi.org/10.1017/S0141347300006583

Miller, W. R., & Rollnick, S. (2001). *Entrevista Motivacional: preparando as pessoas para a mudança de comportamentos adictivos*. Artmed.

Miller, W. R., & Rollnick, S. (2002). *Motivational interviewing: Preparing people for change* (2nd ed.). The Guilford Press.

Miller, W. R., & Rollnick, S. (2013). *Motivational interviewing: Helping people change* (3rd ed.). The Guilford Press.

Miller, W. R., & Rose, G. S. (2009). Toward a theory of motivational interviewing. *American Psychological Association, 64*, 527–537. https://doi.org/10.1037/a0016830

Miller, W. R., Taylor, C. A., & West, J. C. (1980). Focused versus broad spectrum behavior therapy for problem drinkers. *Journal of Consulting and Clinical Psychology, 48*, 590–601. https://doi.org/10.1037/0022-006X.48.5.590

Moyers, T. B., & Martin, T. (2006). Therapist influence on client language during motivational interviewing sessions. *Journal of Substance Abuse Treatment, 30*, 245–251. https://doi.org/10.1016/j.jsat.2005.12.003

Oliveira, M. B. (2007). *Leitura analítico-comportamental da proposta de intervenção terapêutica em Entrevista Motivacional com enfoque na dependência química* (Trabalho de conclusão de curso). Pontifícia Universidade Católica de Minas Gerais - PUCMINAS, Belo Horizonte, MG, Brasil.

Rogers, C. R. (1959). A theory of therapy, personality, and interpersonal relationships as developed in the client-centered framework. In S. Koch (Ed.), *The study of a science* (*Formulations of the person and the social context*) (Vol. 3, pp. 184–256). McGraw Hill.

Skinner, B. F. (1953). *Science and human behaviour*. Macmillan.

Skinner, B. F. (1957). *Verbal Behavior*. B. F. Skinner Foundation.

Skinner, B. F. (1969). *Contingencies of reinforcement: A theoretical analysis*. Prentice-Hall.

Skinner, B. F. (1981). Selection by consequences. *Science, 213*, 501–504.

Smedslund, G., Berg, R. C., Hammerstrøm, K. T., Steiro, A., Leiknes, K. A., Dahl, H. M., & Karlsen, K. (2011). Motivational interviewing for substance abuse. *Cochrane Database of Systematic Reviews*, Issue 5. https://doi.org/10.1002/14651858.CD008063.pub2.

Wilson, K. G., & Hayes, S. C. (2000). Why it is crucial to understand thinking and feeling: An analysis and application to drug abuse. *The Behavior Analyst, 23*, 25–43. https://doi.org/10.1007/BF03391997

Part III
Special Topics

Chapter 14
Interfaces Between Neurosciences and Behavior Analysis on the Use of Psychoactive Substances

Myenne Mieko Ayres Tsutsumi, André Luiz, Carlos Eduardo Costa, and Célio Roberto Estanislau

Introduction

Understanding the variables that influence substance use and abuse behavior is a task of enormous importance. This task becomes even more complex when it is necessary to present possible relationships between two fields of study, in this case Behavior Analysis and the Neurosciences.

First, there is the need to present some concepts from both areas to then outline possible interfaces between them. Before that, it is important to state that the present chapter arose from dialogues between the authors on the subject, which was the best way found to trace relationships between the areas of study, without the bureaucracy of roles playing a control, sometimes unnecessary, in the development of the ideas here present. Thus, the reader is advised not to take the present text as a rule of reasoning to trace relationships between different fields of study. Constructing interfaces is the result of a wide history of conversations which, when translated into written words, seem to occur in a linear manner. It is therefore indispensable to meet people from different areas, discuss, contest, and complement what is written here.

M. M. A. Tsutsumi (✉)
Pontifícia Universidade Católica do Paraná (PUC-PR), Londrina, PR, Brazil

Universidade Estadual de Londrina (UEL), Londrina, PR, Brazil

A. Luiz
Universidade Positivo – Faculdade Londrina, Londrina, PR, Brazil

Universidade Estadual de Londrina (UEL), Londrina, PR, Brazil

Núcleo Evoluir, Londrina, PR, Brazil

C. E. Costa · C. R. Estanislau
Universidade Estadual de Londrina (UEL), Londrina, PR, Brazil

S. M. Oliani et al. (eds.), *Behavior Analysis and Substance Dependence*,
https://doi.org/10.1007/978-3-030-75961-2_14

Behavior Analysis

Behavior Analysis is a science based on the philosophical principles of Radical Behaviorism (Chiesa, 2006). In the preface of the book *Subjectivity and Behavioral Relations* (original tittle: Subjetividade e Relações Comportamentais), written by Tourinho (2009), the psychologist Roberto Banaco defines radical behaviorist philosophy as enchanting and frightening. The enchantment comes from the intensive use of the principle of parsimony, in which one tries to explain natural phenomena in the simplest way possible. Radical Behaviorism would therefore be charmingly simple. The frightening characteristic, in turn, is formed by embracing an explanatory model that is very different from common sense, taking the absolute control of their lives out of the hands of human beings and shedding light on their submission to the Laws of Nature. In other words, it would be frighteningly different from the most common conceptions of freedom.

To say that the human being is under the Laws of Nature should not cause astonishment or strangeness. Organisms are part of the natural world, so are their behaviors. That means, ultimately, that behavior is determined. In this sense, behavior is an event that does not occur at random, but as a result of a set of relationships among other events in the past (Marçal, 2010). Therefore, behavior is the result of a historical process.

"Behavior" does not just refer to what can be directly observed (e.g., kicking a ball). Thoughts, feelings, ideas, emotions, choices, intentions, etc., are also considered behaviors and are therefore the result of a historical process. Here it is possible to perceive the Monistic and Materialistic vision of Radical Behaviorism: there is no distinction between physical and metaphysical in organisms (Chiesa, 2006). Public behaviors (those that can be observed directly) and private behaviors (those that are accessed directly only by the individual himself) occur in the same natural dimension and are subject to the same natural laws (Skinner, 2006).

To refer to private behaviors, Skinner (2006) used the definition "the world under the skin" and said it would be foolish to neglect what occurs in that world because only the person himself is able to establish direct contact with his inner world. Fluent in science, Skinner added that a full description of the "world under the skin" would be provided by anatomy and physiology. It was an idea – probably very well grounded – of what is now called the interface between Behavior Analysis and the Neurosciences.

The "world under the skin" refers to the internal environment of the organism, consisting of visceral, electrical, and neurochemical responses. This is a key point of the Behavior Analysis section, as it is possible to glimpse possible relationships with the Neurosciences. When organisms interact with the world, not only public behaviors are influenced by this interaction, the whole organism is modified (Skinner, 2006). Therefore, when interacting with the world, the visceral, electrical, and neurochemical responses, constituents of the internal environment, are also modified. And, according to Skinner, it is this organism with a modified behavior pattern and internal environment that will behave in the future (Silva et al., 2005).

Since the internal environment is modified by interactions with the world, it is necessary to pay attention to the possible effects of variables that can affect the internal functions and, therefore, affect the way people will then interact with the environment. One of these variables that affect internal functions is the psychoactive substance.

Psychoactive Substance and Behavior

Harmful use and dependence on substances as well as other related problems (e.g., family and marital relationships, financial issues, etc.) are constant concerns in several countries. In the United States, for example, drug addiction is proving to be one of the most serious and costly problems for the health care system (Silverman et al., 2008). In Brazil, a 2017 survey conducted by the Oswaldo Cruz Foundation (FIOCRUZ) on drug use recorded that 4.9 million Brazilians (3.2% of the population) had made use of illicit substances in the 12 months prior to data collection (Bastos et al., 2017).

Medicines and alcohol, two legal types of substances that appear in the survey conducted by FIOCRUZ, deserve special attention. The use of non-prescription drugs or the use of drugs in a different manner than the one prescribed was performed by 0.6% and 0.4% of the Brazilian population, respectively. The authors of the survey described these percentages as alarming. Specifically, the results indicated that about 2.3 million people presented criteria for dependence in the 12 months prior to the survey; more than four million people reported having argued with someone under the influence of alcohol in the same period. Together with the studies of the World Health Organization (WHO), it was observed that alcohol is the substance that was more directly or indirectly associated with health damages that lead to death.

Access to medication and alcohol should be of extreme concern, not only because of the effects on the body and the social problems that can arise from its indiscriminate use, but precisely because they are substances that are easily accessible to a large part of the population and relatively independent of age. "Easy access"can be read, in experimental terms, as "lower cost of response". "Difficult access", on the other hand, can be read as "higher cost of response". Studies on the cost of response show that the lower the cost required to produce a consequence, the higher the response rate presented in that contingency compared to the response rate presented in another contingency with a higher linked cost.[1] The notion of the cost of response then suggests that the indiscriminate use of easily accessible substances (e.g., those considered lawful) may be greater than the use of relatively more difficult to access substances (e.g., those considered illicit). Generally speaking, the greater the

[1] See Soares, Costa, Aló, Luiz e Cunha (2017) for a review on the response cost studies.

indiscriminate use of substances, the more serious the effects will be for both the individual and society.

Knowledge about the cost of the response allows the planning and implementation of public policies that could control more closely – which does not imply the prohibition of any kind of substance – the access of the population to licit substances, rather than the continuation of an indiscriminate fight against what is culturally considered illicit and, in an equivalent way, worse. In addition, the notion of response cost highlights the operant aspects of drug dependency, suggesting that the excessive use of substances is a type of behavior maintained and modified by the interaction between the organism and the environment (Silverman et al., 2008). In line with this notion, research has shown (e.g., Chivers et al., 2008; Roll, 2005) that interventions based on operant principles are effective in increasing the time without substance use, as well as in increasing the adherence and continuity of patients to specific treatments.

Despite the existence of a considerable body of evidence suggesting a great effectiveness of treatments based on the principles of Behavioral Analysis for treating the use/dependence of substances, important questions remain. Silverman et al. (2008) raised at least three issues that need to be evaluated: (1) the need to increase disclosure of the effectiveness of procedures involving contingency management, as well as how they are implemented, so that they are more widely known and, therefore, more widely used (reading volume 41, no. 4 of the *Journal of Applied Behavior Analysis is suggested here)*; (2) the development of more research to assess relapse-related variables (reading research in the areas of resurgence, relapse and renewal is suggested here); (3) despite contingency management interventions are very effective, they do not work with some patients, demonstrating the need for research that refines the applied procedures. For this third point, there is a greater need for knowledge of physiological aspects (e.g., about the nervous system) that may be related to unsatisfactory results. It follows, therefore, to the Neurosciences section.

Neurosciences

The neurosciences gather evidence about the functioning of the nervous system and do so using observation techniques that focus on different units of analysis. With the development of technologies such as electrical recording and neuroimaging, it was possible for the first time to study the nervous system in a non-invasive way, allowing the observation of its functioning in a living organism. In terms of interface between brain and behavioral sciences, this was an important achievement, since it is now possible to observe the activity of the nervous system while the organism behaves (e.g., functional neuroimaging). Before that, these data were separated and their interface only speculative. This development is strongly in line with Skinner's (2006) "prediction" that one day Physiology and Anatomy would provide important data for a more complete explanation of the behavior of organisms.

Before continuing, it is important to highlight just as the Behavior Analysis section was built, this section will start with the definition of some basic concepts in neurosciences. This does not mean, however, that other elements cannot or are not part of the interface between the two areas.

Some Units of Analysis in Brain Sciences

Cells

Ramon y Cajal and Camilo Golgi shared the Nobel Prize in Physiology or Medicine in 1906 for their proposal that the anatomophysiological unit of the nervous system would be the neuron. Golgi's staining technique allowed the observation that the cytoarchitecture of the nervous tissue was composed of numerous cells of unconventional formats that maintained a specialized communication among themselves. Later, this communication was called synapse.

Neurons have an important structural configuration to be described, since only by understanding their structure is it possible to understand the functioning of the next unit of analysis treated in this chapter, the neuronal communication. Neurons are composed by a polarized (i.e., intracellular medium with negative charge and extracellular medium with positive charge) plasmatic membrane, which is lipoproteic and selectively permeable and by structures immersed in the cytoplasm and responsible for its functioning, the organelles (Junqueira & Carneiro, 2008; Schwartz et al., 2014). Despite different morphologies, in general neurons have dendrites (i.e., prolongations that contain proteins called receptors), cell body (i.e., region that contains the cell nucleus and other organelles), axon (i.e., extension wrapped in a layer called myelin sheath, which aids in conducting the electrical signal), and axon terminal which stores vesicles containing neurotransmitters (Junqueira & Carneiro, 2008; Lent, 2002; Machado & Haertel, 2014).

Although neurons are the best known, they are not the only components of nervous tissue. Glial cells take different forms and names, but basically, their function is to protect and nourish neuronal cells. They are more numerous than neurons themselves (Junqueira & Carneiro, 2008; Kolb & Whishaw, 2001b; Lent, 2002). Without the existence of glial cells, the existence of neurons would be compromised.

Neural Communication

The specialized communication that Ramon y Cajal and Golgi (Andres-Barquin, 2001; Ramon y Cajal, 1995) suggested came to be called synapse, which means connection/communication between two neurons (i.e., pre and postsynaptic) or between a neuron and an effector cell (e.g., muscle cells or glands). This connection is made between different structures of neurons: (a) contact between the axon of one neuron and the dendrites of another (i.e., axodendritic synapse), (b) contact between the axon of one and the cell body of another (i.e., axosomatic synapse), and (c) between axons (i.e., axoaxonic) (Kolb & Whishaw, 2002b; Lent, 2002; Siegelbaum & Kandel, 2014). Calling it "communication" usually leads to the interpretation that neurons "exchange information". Next, what neuroscience calls "exchanging information" will be operationalized.

The "information" exchanged in the connection can be (a) ions that pass from the presynaptic neuron to the postsynaptic through the so-called gap junctions, which are channels that form in the physical contact between the two cells, which characterizes the electrical synapses, or (b) chemical compounds that are launched into space between neurons (i.e., synaptic cleft) and which, when attached to receptors in the postsynaptic neuron, have the ability to alter the polarity of the plasma membrane (Kolb & Whishaw, 2002a; Lent, 2002; Siegelbaum & Koestner, 2014). The "message" that the target cell receives can be of inhibitory, excitatory, or modulatory type, which depends on the neurotransmitter-receptor combination.

Neurotransmitters

Different types of neurotransmitters will lead to different responses depending on this neurotransmitter-receptor combination (Schwartz & Javitch, 2014). Among amino acids, for example, glutamate, when binds to the receptors of the target cell, causes depolarization of its plasmatic membrane, characterizing its excitatory effect. The gamma-aminobutyric acid (GABA) is an amino acid that causes hyperpolarization of the membrane of the target cell producing an inhibitory effect. Neuropeptides (e.g., opioids) and amines (e.g., dopamine and serotonin) are neurotransmitters that can have many types of effects depending on the type of receptor they bind and their localization (Kolb & Whishaw, 2002a; Lent, 2002; Schwartz & Javitch, 2014).

Anatomophysiology

The excitatory or inhibitory effect on neuronal activity has different impacts on the functioning of the nervous system depending on the region to which these neurons belong. There are some ways to divide the human nervous system didactically. Using anatomical criteria, the nervous system is divided into central (CNS), composed by the brain and spinal cord, and peripheral (PNS), composed by nerves, ganglia, and nerve endings. Employing functional criteria, it is divided into somatic (SNS), which participates in the interaction between the organism and the external environment, and visceral (VNS), which relates the control of the internal environment of the organism (e.g., viscera, glands, smooth muscle or heart muscle). Both are divided into an afferent and an efferent component. In SNS, the afferent component is the route in which information from peripheral sensory receptors reaches the nerve centers, and the efferent component takes information from the nerve centers to the striated skeletal muscles that participate in voluntary movement. In the VNS, the afferent component is the route in which information coming from the internal structures of the body is forwarded to the CNS and the efferent component takes information in the opposite direction, from the CNS to the internal structures (Machado & Haertel, 2013a, b). This last component of the VNS is called autonomomic nervous system (ANS) and is divided into sympathetic and parasympathetic. More recently, the enteric nervous system (ENS), which characterizes the intrinsic innervation of the ANS by connecting the CNS to the gastrointestinal tract, was included in this division of the ANS (Machado & Haertel, 2013a).

Reward System

The physiological response to events that increase the future probability of a behavior is of vital importance for the normal functioning of any individual in his interaction with the environment and can be altered in several disorders. The set of neuronal circuits activated in these situations is known as the reward system. When, in a given context, a behavior results in a reinforcement, an associative learning is established between that behavior and that reinforcement. Thus, in future opportunities, that context will tend to evoke a similar response. This type of associative learning takes place thanks to the activity within the reward system. A key element for the occurrence of this learning is the release of dopamine through the pathway from the ventral tegmental area (a nucleus with dopaminergic neuron bodies) to the *accumbens nucleus* (one of the base nuclei, which is a set of structures involved in motor, motivational, and emotional aspects of behavior). The integrity of this system is essential for associative learning between context, behavior, and consequence (Kolb and Whishaw, 2002a). Drugs of abuse, by directly or indirectly altering the functioning of this system, produce an important part of their behavioral effects.

Psychoactive Drugs

In pharmacology, the drug is a term used to refer to chemicals that alter the body having a beneficial or adverse effect, which only occur if there is sufficient concentration of this substance in the blood for action in a tissue that has receptors for it (Rang et al., 2016c; Stahl, 2014). It is essential to understand that the relationship between drug and receptor is central to the changes that occur in the body. As mentioned above, receptors are cellular components (i.e., proteins) that interact with substances (e.g., drugs or neurotransmitters) and are the beginning of a series of biochemical events that result in certain effects. Drugs penetrate the CNS in different ways depending on the type of administration (e.g., oral, inhalation, rectal suppositories, skin patches, injectables into the bloodstream, muscles, etc.). The absorption of drugs is also affected by their physical and chemical properties, as well as the age, sex, and body weight of the individual (Rang et al., 2016d; Stahl, 2014).

Drugs influence the chemical exchanges that occur in synapses and, to understand their effects, it is important to look at how they modify the connection between neurons and target cells. Each of the stages of neurotransmission includes a chemical reaction that can be influenced by the increase (i.e., agonists) or decrease (i.e., antagonists) in the efficiency of this neurotransmission (Rang et al., 2016d). For example, drugs that lead to greater release of dopamine into the synaptic cleft, block its reuptake or inactivation are considered dopamine agonists. By remaining in the synaptic cleft, it spends more time stimulating the postsynaptic neuron. Substances that block the production of dopamine or accelerate its inactivation are considered to be its antagonists because they decrease the biochemical effect on synapses (Stahl, 2014). Psychostimulants such as cocaine and methamphetamine are drugs that alter the neural release of dopamine and the number of its receptors (e.g., D2 receptors). This makes this neurotransmitter spend more time stimulating the postsynaptic neuron, something that is part of the explanation of the behavior changes that are seen in users of these substances (e.g., euphoria, suppression of appetite, mood swings). These substances also activate noradrenaline receptors that are related to increased heartbeat, pupil dilation, and body preparation for fighting or escape, functions that are under the responsibility of ANS (Guimarães, 2008; Kolb & Whishaw, 2001a).

Describing and identifying the chemical reactions that occur in synapses is part of one of the levels of explanation of behavior. By saying that there are changes in communication between neurons and that this occurs due to drug influences, the altered behavior is not explained, but only part of it. If the behavior is understood as a response of the organism in interaction with the environment, it makes no sense to assume that one level of analysis is sovereign over the other. This presumption can fall into so-called reductionism, whatever it is. The consumption of psychoactive substances is an example that can be analyzed within each of the different levels and, therefore, different levels of causality can be identified. The correlation between the use of psychoactive drugs and the change in behavior (e.g., mood, thoughts, and emotions) can be explained from the changes that these substances trigger in synapses. There may be an increase or decrease in the release of a certain neurotransmitter, in the reuptake of others, in addition to altering the number of receptors in postsynaptic neurons. This same correlation can be seen from the behavioral point of view when one considers that the behavior emitted, when the biological apparatus is altered by psychoactive substances is selected from the effects it produces in its immediate environment. The levels of analysis are not mutually exclusive, but complementary (Kolb & Whishaw, 2001a; Lent, 2008).

CNS depressants, which can be represented by general analgesics and opioids, hypnosedatives, antihistamines, and anticonvulsants, for example, are drugs that reflect in behaviors such as drowsiness, muscle relaxation, and amnesia in some cases (Rang et al., 2016a). Ethanol (e.g., alcoholic beverages) is a well-known example for most people. It is a lawful substance and, as mentioned at the beginning of the chapter, has a high rate of consumption and development of dependence. Although it is not the only one, one of the targets in the CNS are the receptor regions for the inhibitory neurotransmitter GABA, and the greater its quantity, the more inhibitory effects on neurons in several regions are observed (Rang et al., 2016b). In more caricatured cases of alcohol use, behavioral changes occur such as increased social disinhibition, confused speech, unbridled walking, and loss of accuracy of fine movements. It is possible to relate these behavioral changes to the influences that alcohol has on hypnosedative regions of brain areas, such as pre-frontal cortex and motor cortex (Guimarães, 2008; Machado & Haertel, 2013a).

An important curiosity of the action of alcohol is the development of tolerance, that is, with frequent use the quantity consumed needs to be increasingly greater to obtain the same effect as when used for the first time (Rang et al., 2016a, b). In other words, there is a decrease in the effect over time and with frequent consumption. Still, on CNS depressants, opioid analgesics (e.g., codeine, morphine, and heroin) are another class of drugs that inhibit the functioning of some brain regions, but they act on special μ receptors that are related to pain perception (Guimarães, 2008; Kolb & Whishaw, 2001a).

A Possible Interface

After this compilation of the neuroscientific knowledge about the functioning of the nervous system and the interference of drugs in it, as well as the presentation of some basic concepts of Behavior Analysis, it becomes possible to discuss the possibility of interface between the two areas. Aiming at objectivity and the implementation of a line of reasoning, a classical study will be used to delineate possible relationships between Behavioral Analysis and the Neurosciences. The chosen study was developed by Siegel, Hinson, Krank, and McCully (1982).

These authors proposed to study the tolerance developed along the use of opioids and whether there was environmental interference in the probability of death by overdose. When a psychoactive substance is used, a series of chemical reactions are triggered, as seen in the neuroscience section. These reactions disturb the homeostatic state of the organism that is phylogenetically equipped to recover the lost balance. With the frequent consumption of the drug, anticipatory responses are elicited and prepare the organism to avoid collapse when consuming the substance (Goudie & Emmett-Oglesby, 1989; Siegel et al., 2000). For example, in the case of psychostimulants such as cocaine and methamphetamine, which lead to increased heartbeat, pupil dilation, and preparation of the body for struggle or escape, anticipatory responses of bradycardia, pupil contraction, and muscle relaxation are elicited. It is important to highlight here the Skinnerian notion that the historical relations between the organism and the environment do not only change the observable behavioral pattern, but the organism as a whole (i.e., the internal environment is also altered and starts to function in a differential way).

Extending the analysis, one must not lose sight of the fact that this organism is in constant interaction with the environment around it. This means that the pairing between stimuli occurs and, using the Pavlovian paradigm (classical or respondent conditioning) to discuss tolerance, configurations of the environment in which the drug is consumed are paired with the psychoactive substance, thus acquiring the function of conditional stimulus (Siegel et al., 2000). On subsequent occasions, the environmental configuration in which the drug is consumed may be sufficient to elicit the anticipatory responses. Given genetic variability, organisms may have different amounts of neurotransmitters and receptors. This difference may be related to a greater or lesser ability to present anticipatory responses, increasing or decreasing the probability of organism collapse. The same approach serves to discuss the problems of the effectiveness of contingency management procedures described by Silverman et al. (2008). Differences in the amounts of neurotransmitters and receptors may facilitate or hinder behavioral changes promoted by treatments for substance use and dependence.

To test the application of the Pavlovian paradigm, the researchers investigated the effect of different doses of heroin administered in different environments on the development of tolerance and whether overdose mortality could be a failure in this mechanism. Siegel et al. (1982) exposed groups of rats to increasing doses of heroin (1 mg/kg, 2 mg/kg, 4 mg/kg, 8 mg/kg), and (a) for one experimental group doses were given in the home cage and a potentially lethal dose (15 mg/kg) of heroin in the same environment (ST – similar test), (b) for the other experimental group doses were given in the home cage and the potentially lethal dose in another room (DT – different test), and (c) for the control group doses of saline were given (i.e., sodium chloride solution) in the home cage and the potentially lethal dose of heroin in the same environment. The mortality rate of the rats after the potentially lethal injection of heroin was 32.4% for the ST group, 64.3% for the DT group, and 96.4% for the control group. These results suggest that when the use of the substance is made in the same place, the environmental configuration acquires the ability to elicit anticipatory responses that make the organism prepared to receive the doses, which ends up making increasingly larger doses necessary to obtain the effects as if it were for the first time. The main evidence comes from the second experimental group that, when the location for the administration of the drug was changed, did not have the environmental cues and, therefore, did not present the anticipatory responses, something that made the organism unprepared to receive the potentially lethal dose.

Final Considerations

As initially explained, the interface between two areas is always a difficult task. Writing about the possible relationships between them is something even more difficult. Therefore, there is a need for further discussion between each of the topics mentioned here. It is clear, however, that no matter how independent the sciences of Physiology and Behavior Analysis are (Tourinho et al., 2000; Zilio, 2016), the natural world does not make this distinction and, as described by Silva (1988), an adequate understanding of behavior requires knowledge in these two sciences, especially when it comes to subjects related to the use and dependence of substances.

References

Andres-Barquin, P. J. (2001). Ramón y Cajal: A century after the publication of his masterpiece. *Endeavour, 25*(1), 13–17.

Bastos, F. I. P. M., Vasconcellos, M. T. L., De Boni, R. B., Reis, N. B., & Coutinho, C. F. de S. (2017). *III Levantamento Nacional sobre o uso de drogas pela população brasileira*. FIOCRUZ.

Chiesa, M. (2006). *Behaviorismo radical: a filosofia e a ciência*. Editora Celeiro.

Chivers, L. L., Higgins, S. T., Heil, S. H., Proskin, R. W., & Thomas, C. S. (2008). Effects of initial abstinence and programmed lapses on the relative reinforcing effects of cigarette smoking. *Journal of Applied Behavior Analysis, 41*(4), 481–497. https://doi.org/10.1901/jaba.2008.41-481

Goudie, A. J., & Emmett-Oglesby, M. W. (1989). Psychoactive drugs: Tolerance and sensitization. In A. J. Goudie & M. W. Emmett-Oglesby (Eds.), *The quarterly review of biology* (Vol. 79). Springer.

Guimarães, F. S. (2008). Substâncias Psicoativas. In R. Lent (Ed.), *Neurociência da mente e do comportamento* (pp. 323–348). Guanabara Koogan.

Junqueira, L. C., & Carneiro, J. (2008). Tecido Nervoso. In L. C. Junqueira & J. Carneiro (Eds.), *Histologia Básica* (pp. 153–181). Guanabara Koogan.

Kolb, B., & Whishaw, I. Q. (2001a). Como as drogas e os hormônios influenciam o comportamento? In B. Kolb & I. Q. Whishaw (Eds.), *Neurociência do Comportamento* (pp. 190–233). Manole.

Kolb, B., & Whishaw, I. Q. (2001b). Quais são as unidades do funcionamento cerebral? In B. Kolb & I. Q. Whishaw (Eds.), *Neurociência do Comportamento* (pp. 76–111). Manole.

Kolb, B., & Whishaw, I. Q. (2002a). Como os neurônios se comunicam? In *Neurociência do Comportamento* (pp. 152–189). Manole.

Kolb, B., & Whishaw, I. Q. (2002b). Como os neurônios transmitem as informações? In *Neurociência do Comportamento* (pp. 112–151). Manole.

Lent, R. (2002). *Cem Bilhões de neurônios*. Ed. Atheneu.

Lent, R. (2008). *Neurociência da mente e do comportamento*. Guanabara Koogan.

Machado, A., & Haertel, L. M. (2013a). Anatomia macroscópica do tronco encefálico e do cerebelo. In *Neuroanatomia Funcional* (3rd ed., pp. 43–52). Atheneu.

Machado, A., & Haertel, L. M. (2013b). *Neuroanatomia Funcional* (3rd ed.). Atheneu.

Machado, A., & Haertel, L. M. (2014). Tecido nervoso. In A. Machado & L. M. Haertel (Eds.), *Neuroanatomia Funcional* (3rd ed., pp. 19–35). Atheneu.

Marçal, J. V. S. (2010). Behaviorismo radical e prática clínica. In A. K. C. R. de Farias (Ed.), *Análise Comportamental Clínica: Aspectos teóricos e estudos de caso* (pp. 30–48). Porto Alegre.

Ramon y Cajal, S. (1995). *Histology of the nervous system of man and vertebrates*. Oxford University Press.

Rang, H. P., Dale, M. M., Ritter, J. M., Flower, R. J., & Henderson, G. (2016a). Fármacos ansiolíticos e hipnóticos. In H. P. Rang & M. M. Dale (Eds.), *Farmacologia* (8th ed., pp. 1251–1274). Elsevier.

Rang, H. P., Dale, M. M., Ritter, J. M., Flower, R. J., & Henderson, G. (2016b). Hábito, dependência e uso abusivo de drogas. In H. P. Rang & M. M. Dale (Eds.), *Farmacologia* (8th ed., pp. 1389–1426). Elsevier.

Rang, H. P., Dale, M. M., Ritter, J. M., Flower, R. J., & Henderson, G. (2016c). O que é farmacologia? In H. P. Rang & M. M. Dale (Eds.), *Farmacologia* (8th ed., pp. 28–36). Elsevier.

Rang, H. P., Dale, M. M., Ritter, J. M., Flower, R. J., & Henderson, G. (2016d). Transmissão química e ação de fármacos no sistema nervoso central. In H. P. Rang & M. M. Dale (Eds.), *Farmacologia* (8th ed., pp. 1053–1063). Elsevier.

Roll, J. M. (2005). Assessing the feasibility of using contingency management to modify cigarette smoking by adolescents. *Journal of Applied Behavior Analysis, 38*(4), 463–467. https://doi.org/10.1901/jaba.2005.114-04

Schwartz, J. H., & Javitch, J. A. (2014). Neurotransmissores. In E. Kandel, J. H. Schwartz, T. M. Jessell, S. A. Siegelbaum, & H. J (Eds.), *Princípios de Neurociências* (5th ed., pp. 256–271). Artmed.

Schwartz, J. H., Barres, B. A., & Goldman, J. E. (2014). As células do sistema nervoso. In E. Kandel, J. H. Schwartz, T. M. Jessell, S. A. Siegelbaum, & A. J. Hudspeth (Eds.), *Princípios de Neurociências* (5th ed., pp. 63–88). Artmed.

Siegel, S., Hinson, R. E., & Krank, M. D. (1982). Heroin "overdose" death: Contribution of drug-associated environmental cues. *Science, 216*(April), 436–437.

Siegel, S., Baptista, M. A., Kim, J. A., McDonald, R. V., & Weise-Kelly, L. (2000). Pavlovian psychopharmacology: The associative basis of tolerance. *Experimental and Clinical Psychopharmacology, 8*(3), 276–293. https://doi.org/10.1037//1064-1297.8.3.276

Siegelbaum, S. A., & Kandel, E. R. (2014). Visão geral da transmissão sináptica. In E. Kandel, J. H. Schwartz, T. M. Jessell, S. A. Siegelbaum, & A. J. Hudspeth (Eds.), *Princípios de Neurociências* (5th ed., pp. 157–166). Artmed.

Siegelbaum, S. A., & Koestner, J. (2014). Os canais iônicos. In E. R. Kandel, J. H. Schwartz, T. M. Jessell, S. A. Siegelbaum, & A. J. Hudspeth (Eds.), *Princípios de Neurociências* (5th ed., pp. 89–110). Artmed.

Silva, M. T. A. (1988). Behaviorismo e neurociências. *Biotemas, 1*(2), 41–47. https://doi.org/10.5007/%25x

Silva, M. T. A., Guerra, L. G. G. C., & Alves, C. R. R. (2005). Modelos Comportamentais em Neurociências. *Revista Brasileira de Análise Do Comportamento, 1*(2), 167–185.

Silverman, K., Roll, J. M., & Higgins, S. T. (2008). Introduction to the special issue on the behavior analysis and treatment of drug addiction. *Journal of Applied Behavior Analysis, 41*(4), 471–480. https://doi.org/10.1901/jaba.2008.41-471

Skinner, B. F. (2006). *Sobre o Behaviorismo* (10th ed.). Editora Cultrix.

Soares, P. G., Costa, C. E., Aló, R. M., Luiz, A., & Cunha, T. R. L. (2017). Custo da resposta: Como tem sido definido e estudado? *Perspectivas Em Análise Do Comportamento, 8*(2), 258–268. https://doi.org/10.18761/PAC.2017.020

Stahl, S. M. (2014). In N. Muntner, I. R. Oliveira, & P. L. Voeux (Eds.), *Psicofarmacologia - Bases Neurocientíficas e Aplicações Práticas* (4th ed.). Guanabara Koogan.

Tourinho, E. Z. (2009). *Subjetividade e relações comportamentais*. Paradigma.

Tourinho, E. Z., da Teixeira, E. R., & Maciel, J. M. (2000). Fronteiras entre análise do comportamento e fisiologia: Skinner e a temática dos eventos privados. *Psicologia: Reflexão e Crítica, 13*(3), 425–434.

Zilio, D. (2016). On the autonomy of psychology from neuroscience: A case study of skinner's radical behaviorism and behavior analysis. *Review of General Psychology, 20*(2), 155–170. https://doi.org/10.1037/gpr0000067

Chapter 15
Behavioral Functions of Drug Use in Marital Narratives: From Progression to Treatment of Substance Dependence

Jaqueline Vago Ferrari and Elizeu Borloti

Introduction

This chapter describes behavioral functions in contingencies of the progression of the use of psychoactive substances (PAS), from the beginning up to the treatment of dependence and its outcomes, in the repertoire of substance-dependent individuals in the course of their marital relationships. For that, the functions of the behaviors described by substance-dependent individuals and their wives were inferred, in narrative sequences, using the same methodological model of narrative interviews and narrative analysis, as shown by Germano and Serpa (2008). These authors describe that the sequences built by the narrators during the narrative interview reveal how they model the memories of their past, how they understand the events and their consequences and the general sense of success and failure from them (Germano & Serpa, 2008, p. 15). They use Larivaille's (1974) notion of the narrative sequence as a quinary chronological process, because it consists of five moments or phases, which is useful to the study of behavioral function, since it focuses on behavioral events, antecedents, and consequents in each time. Thus, the analysis of behavioral functions in contingencies of the history of the marital relationship with the presence of drug use has focused on the five phases of the narrative sequence: initial situation, disturbance, transformation, resolution, and final situation.

A behavioral analysis is an analysis of the contingencies responsible for the occurrence of a behavior and/or for changes in it (Matos, 1999). Thus, to functionally analyze a person's behavior is to answer what the function of that behavior is for that person, that is, what is the functional relationship between his behavior and the effects it produces. Considering the five phases of the narrative sequence (Larivaille, (1974) listed above, the behavioral analyses described in this chapter point to functional elements of this sequence in a threefold contingency, a conceptual instrument

J. V. Ferrari (✉) · E. Borloti
Universidade Federal do Espírito Santo (UFES), Vitória, ES, Brazil

S. M. Oliani et al. (eds.), *Behavior Analysis and Substance Dependence*,
https://doi.org/10.1007/978-3-030-75961-2_15

for analyzing relations between organism-environment (Skinner, 1953; Todorov, 1982). Among the elements of the triple contingency analysis scheme, we highlight: (1) the previous context; (2) the response; and (3) the consequent context.

The *antecedent context* can play a relational function with an operant behavior due to differences in responding because this event is present (in this case, as a discriminative stimulus – Sd). It can also exercise a motivational function, increasing the reinforcing value or decreasing the punishing value of the consequence of such operant behavior and, consequently, increasing the probability of its occurrence or the occurrence of another operant behavior related to it (as an establishing operation – EO). Still in a motivational function, it can invert these values, decreasing the probability of the behavior occurring and making its consequences less attractive (like abolishing operation – AO). It can also exercise an eliciting function (as eliciting stimulus – ES) of a respondent which accompanies that operant (as an unconditioned stimulus – US; or as a conditioned stimulus – CS).

The *occurring response* (R) may be evoked (e.g., be an operant behavior) or elicited (e.g., be a respondent behavior) by the presence of elements from that antecedent context. If the element acts as an Sd, an operant behavior will have an opportunity to be emitted, also under the function of some EO; if it acts as an ES, a respondent will have its opportunity to be elicited.

The *consequent context* is called the response reinforcer (or reinforcing stimulus – Sr); it is the product or effect in the environment produced by the occurrence and that increases its frequency. Sr is positive (Sr+) when added to the context and increases the frequency of the behavior that added it; and it is negative (Sr−) when it is removed from the context and increases the frequency of the behavior that removed it.

The response of using any PAS is under the control of all these elements of the contexts that precede and follow it (Borloti et al., 2015). Silva et al. (2001), in his functional analysis of substance dependence, he described these elements associated with vulnerability factors (sensitization) and the phenomenon of tolerance to the use of PAS during the addiction process. The model by Silva et al. emphasizes sensitization and tolerance as relatively permanent changes in the central nervous system, resulting from the recurrent use of PAS. Thus, understanding the function of using PAS from the context of use is essential to interventions in substance dependence. In this context, we have the substance-dependent individual's family members, especially the spouse. However, few studies emphasize interventions in the substance-dependent individual's family or family social support network (Moraes et al., 2009). Thus, considering that elements of the family context, especially those of the marital context, can play a direct or indirect role in modifying or maintaining the use of PAS (Bordin et al., 2004), the relevance of the study that gave rise to this chapter asserts itself.

The objective of this chapter is to present behavioral functions involved in the progression of PAS dependence, from the beginning of the problem regarding the unsafe use to the search for treatment, throughout marital histories of substance-dependent individuals. The behaviors and their contextual functional elements were observed in narrative sequences obtained through the technique of narrative analysis (Schütze, 2011). Behavior analysis was combined with narrative analysis, integrating both methods of analysis.

Narrative Analysis in Substance Dependence: A Brief Review

Research on the love relationship of substance-dependent individuals with their spouses has focused on many topics, highlighting family dynamics (Paz & Colossi, 2013), codependency (Coleman, 1987; Makvand et al., 2009; Van Wormer, 1990), and domestic violence (Subodh et al., 2014; Wekerle & Wall, 2004). What happens in a dependent's love relationship has attracted the attention of researchers because PAS dependence is a complex, multidetermined phenomenon that damages many aspects of the dependent individual's life. In the family and couple's aspect, for example, it can modify the social roles of members, changing their functions in the relationship. Capistrano et al. (2013a, b) highlight conjugal violence as one of the possible effects of these changes.

Therapeutic interventions with drug-dependent individuals consider the family as an essential part of the context of using PAS (Spagnol, 2018). The behavior of family members impacts the improvement or worsening of the consequences of drug use, from recreational use, going through the use of abuse patterns and to the use of dependency patterns. Among these family members, the wife assumes a primary role. She usually plays a role in the stability of the healthy pattern and in her substance-dependent spouse's motivation to face the difficulties of the long course of treatment (Dos Santos et al., 2007). This appears in narratives of the relationship's history, which in turn makes narrative analysis (Schütze, 2011) an important theoretical-methodological proposal for understanding the contingencies present in this story.

Schütze (2011) analysis of narratives is, in fact, a form of verbal report analysis. This is because it is through the verbal report that the narrator recounts situations in his life, describing and arguing about contingencies that give meaning to what he himself produces verbally regarding such situations; and demonstrating how he relates to all of this, in a process that Skinner (1953) would call autoclitic. Narratives, when transcribed, produce texts about personal experiences, in other words, descriptions of contingencies lived by individuals, who tell and interpret them through their own personal, social, and collective histories, in a process of turning themselves to their own. Narrative in an autoclitic manner. From the point of view of their origin theory, however, the histories produced would be inscribed in subjectivity and be implicated "with the space-time dimensions of the individuals when they narrate their experiences, in the domains of education and training" (Souza, 2008, p. 89), showing the influence of the verbal community in its modeling.

In this sense, narrating is, in addition to telling a story, telling a story about whoever narrates it. Therefore, in reports of substance-dependent individuals and their wives about their relationship histories, the paths of each spouse and how they are aligned in making a couple are described. Consequently, the contingencies described in these narratives make it possible to focus on the behavioral functions that materialize the spouse's involvement with the PAS on which he is dependent. The importance of analyzing the contingencies in the analysis of narratives of these couples is emphasized because they allow the observation of relationships between events that define the different stages of the marital relationship, its beginning and its general and specific crises, arising from the progression of the PAS pattern of use, including changes in behavior with the gradual establishment of addiction. Even with this merit, studies of narrative analysis with substance-dependent individuals, single or married, have been uncommon. There are no studies combining functional analysis of behavior and narrative analysis.

Only one study of narrative analysis of substance-dependent individuals was found, the one by Hanninen and Koski-Jannes (1999), which analyzed autobiographical narratives of individuals who stopped using alcohol, multiple drugs, and tobacco, and have managed situations of binge eating, sexual compulsion, and pathological gambling. Its authors are not behavior analysts, however, due to the way they categorized the verbal report (narrative) according to what was described by the narrators, the key contingency for the recovery of dependency is abstracted, in tacts of feelings and emotions and rules on causality, morality, and ethics involving the behavior of using PAS. The verbal report of the dependent participants indicated five self-narratives that followed a chronology in the path of coping with addiction: history of Anonymous Alcoholics; the growth history; the history of codependency; the love history; and the mastery history. As these self-narratives were repeated in the verbal report of all the participants, the authors agreed on a collectivity of factors of the life path in the PAS dependence.

Apart from the study by Hanninen and Koski-Jannes (1999), national investigations of romantic relationships involving substance-dependent individuals do not exist, a methodological fact that endorses the relevance of this study. It is also added that there is a scarcity of studies comparing populations of couples dependent on alcohol and those dependent on multiple substances, among the few that compare individuals. De Moura Kolling et al. (2007), for example, compared individuals dependent on cocaine/crack and alcohol/cocaine/crack, finding a high frequency of Personality Disorder in the latter. They related this to alcohol dependence and indicated the need for further research on emotional and personality changes in both groups for better planning of preventive and therapeutic programs.

Methodology

The behavioral functions inferred from verbal reports of clinical cases presented in this chapter were inferred from data from narrative analysis. In turn, the analysis of narratives, following the theoretical framework proposed by Schütze (2011), was obtained from multiple case studies with couples. Multiple case studies were chosen because they make it possible to detail and systematize circumstantial information about more than one case (Patton, 2002) at a defined time and place (Ventura, 2007). Added to these advantages is the possibility of the case study allowing an increased understanding of the contemporary real phenomenon of marital relationship (Miguel, 2007) by its description (Eisenhardt, 1989; Roesch, 1999). Thus, this chapter tells the story of a current or past event, that is, the marital relationship, through the narrative interview as a data collection procedure (Voss et al., 2002).

In the area of international research involving romantic relationships in the context of drug dependence, the case study was employed by Wetchler and DelVecchio (1996). After observing Systemic Couples Therapy (SCT) sessions in couples with heroin-dependent wives, the authors concluded that SCT produced changes in the wives' behavioral repertoire, both in using the substance and in negotiating or cooperating in marital conflicts. In national surveys, the case study was used to understand the marital dynamics (Santos & Costa, 2004), domestic violence (Torossian et al. 2009), individuality and conjugability (Levandowski et al., 2009) in typical couples and also couples of specific groups, such as riverside couples in the Amazon region (Silva et al., 2011).

The analyses presented in this chapter describe the couple's history by identifying and analyzing the narrative sequences in the verbal reports of both husband and wife, highlighting the descriptions of contingencies evoked in their reports as they are representative parts of the whole history of their relationship. In behavioral terms, the narrative sequences that involve these contingencies are sets of verbal operants involving those who behaved in a time and space from a conflict over the use of the PAS. That said, the model of analysis of narrative sequences, as exposed by Germano and Serpa (2008), was used as the basis in this chapter, using Larivaille's (1974) notion of narrative sequence: initial situation, disturbance, transformation, resolution, and final situation. Thus, what follows next is an analysis of such sequences considering the history of the marital relationship with the progression of drug use, from addiction to its treatment.

Participants were selected in the Health Rehabilitation Program for Substance-Dependent Individuals and Alcoholics (Presta, in Portuguese), at the Military Police Hospital, located in the city of Vitória (ES). Presta offers specialized treatment for substance dependence, focusing on improving self-esteem and rebuilding the life project of patients, military personnel, their families, and community members.

Four couples participated in the study ($N_{TOTAL} = 8$), included according to the following criteria: (a) in a relationship for over 5 years; (b) at least in a civil union; (c) in which one of the spouses has been diagnosed with F10.2[1] (2 couples) or with F19.2[2] (2 couples); (d) and the spouse was undergoing specialized follow-up on an inpatient or post-discharge basis at Presta. Exclusion criteria were: (a) Personality

[1] Mental and Behavioral Disorder due to alcohol use – dependency syndrome.

[2] Mental and Behavioral Disorder due to alcohol use – dependency syndrome.

Disorder (F60);[3] (b) Intellectual Disability (F70), Mild, moderate and severe Cognitive Disorder (F06.7) and Dementia (F0);[4] and (c) Schizophrenia (F20).[5] Some spouses included as participants were in the treatment process; others, in post-discharge. They were all heterosexual. Order of marital union, income, religion, paternity/maternity, and psychological treatment were not exclusion criteria.

The narrative interview was used as the main instrument for data collection for the analysis of narratives and, from it, for the analysis of behavioral functions. The narrative interview aims at reconstructing the verbal repertoire, in general intraverbal, contingencies (events), according to the experience of the interviewees, who are encouraged to retell the story of scenarios of significant moments in their lives. (Bertaux, 2010; Bruner & Weissner, 1995) Schütze (1983), according to Jovchelovitch and Bauer (2002, p. 105), affirms the instrument's trans-theoretical aspect: "it is a technique for generating stories; it is open regarding the analytical procedures that follow the data collection". For this reason, the data collected through these interviews can be subjected to an analysis of contingencies, inferred from the responses to the same "narrative-generating question"[6] which initiates the interviews (Riessmann & Schütze, 1991, p. 353).

Data Analysis Procedures

The analysis process of the narrative interviews was carried out based on the complete proposal by Schütze (2011), which includes the following stages of analysis: (a) Identification of the indexed and non-indexed elements;[7] (b) Analysis of the indexed elements;[8] (c) Analysis of non-indexed elements[9], and (d) Contrasting

---

[3] Because such disorders indicate persistent patterns that cause impairment in social, occupational, or other important areas of an individual's life (American Psychiatric Association, 2014).

[4] Due to the fact that this investigation required responses prepared by the participants in order to achieve the expected objectives.

[5] This diagnosis consists of a set of signs and symptoms associated with impaired professional or social functioning, which could interfere with the objective of the study (American Psychiatric Association, 2014).

[6] *"I would like you to tell about the story of your love relationship, from the day you met, through the establishment of the relationship to the present day"*.

[7] The indexed elements are those that make concrete reference, within the narrative, to the markers of: Who did it? What? When? Where? Why? Non-indexed elements, on the other hand, are those that express values, judgments and a generalized form of "life wisdom". The distinction between indexed and non-indexed elements of each narrative serves to signal that the story told by the interviewee goes beyond the chronological sequence of the narrated events, also expressing itself, by functions, meanings and self-understandings that the narrator makes of his path.

[8] Analysis of the couple's history through the identification and analysis of the narrative sequences, highlighting the events that were evoked by the couple to be described as part of the whole (the history of the relationship).

[9] Analysis of each segment of the narrative in order to identify the descriptive, argumentative and explanatory propositions of the report, which refer to how the narrators report external events

comparison,[10] as presented by Ferrari (2019). However, this chapter presents only part of this analysis: the analysis of indexed elements based on the identification of narrative sequences. After identifying the narrative sequences, behavioral functions were inferred from them in contingencies related both to the progression of the pattern of PAS use of substance-dependent husbands regarding the search for a solution (treatment) and the maintenance of the results of that solution (in this case, abstinence). The following are the procedures for the two analyses conducted together.

Analysis of the Elements Indexed in the Couples' Narratives

The analysis of the elements indexed in the narratives was the decomposition of the couple's history with the dependence on the PAS, through the identification of their narrative sequences, highlighting the events that were evoked in the members' repertoire and described as part of the whole of the history of their love relationship. For this, the model exposed by Germano and Serpa (2008) was used to explain events described in autobiographies (in the authors' study, of young people in conflict with the law).

Analysis of the Functional Elements of the Contingencies of the Progression of the PAS Use Pattern

The analysis of the functional elements of the contingencies of the progression of the PAS use pattern was the decomposition of the behavioral functions narrated in the chronological process of PAS dependence, and their antecedents and consequents, according to the A-B-C model (antecedent-behavior-consequence model). The antecedents As are the Sd's, the EOs, the AOs, and the ESs (which could have functioned as US's or CS's, but which were not distinguished). The Rs, behaviors, or classes of responses observed were described by the responses related to the PAS. These responses are not always made explicit in the narratives, and have sometimes been inferred from the context and effects of use, in antecedent and consequent events. The Cs, consequences, are Sr+ (Positive reinforcement), Sr− (Negative reinforcement), Pn+ (Positive punishment), and Pn− (Negative punishment).

(changes, mourning, labor issues, etc.), their reactions, understanding or interpretation of these events.

[10] Contrasting comparison is a analysis of each segment of the narrative in order to identify the descriptive, argumentative and explanatory propositions of the report, which refer to how the narrators report external events (changes, mourning, labor issues, etc.), their reactions, understanding or interpretation of these events.

Clinical Cases

Table 15.1 shows the main characteristics of the participating couples.

Couples 1 and 2 are made up of husbands with alcohol dependence (ICD F10) and couples 3 and 4 are made up of husbands with addiction to cocaine and multiple drugs (ICD F14 and ICD F19). Wives have no substance dependence.

Couple 1: Jean and Lara. Couple 1's husband, Jean, was addicted to alcohol, was 58 and his wife, Lara, was 53. They had been married for 29 years and were the parents of two children. They were contacted when they were at Presta to participate in post-discharge activities (she, at least once a month; he, every 15 days, since 2008 when he was hospitalized). The couple reports maintenance of abstinence by their husband since 2008, even when they experienced the loss of their youngest child, 5 years ago, in a car accident. This loss strengthened the spouses' bond with Presta, due to the psychological support received, while still remembering the fact, which still touched them very much.[11]

Couple 2: Maurício and Helena. Couple 2 was formed by Maurício, the 53-year-old husband with alcohol dependence, and his wife, Helena, 55. They had been in a relationship for 28 years, with 2 biological children and an adopted daughter. Maurício and Helena were approached on the day they were at Presta to participate in post-discharge activities. Unlike Couple 1, Maurício and Helena participated together at least once a month after discharge, since 2013, when Maurício was hospitalized. According to him, since the end of this hospitalization there had been no (re) occurrence of alcohol use by him; she, in turn, believed that he

Table 15.1 Characteristics of participating couples

Group	Couple	Fictitious names	Age	Relationship duration[a]	Amount of children
Alcohol	Couple 1	Jean and Lara	58 e 53 years	29 years	2 children
	Couple 2	Maurício and Helena	53 e 55 years	28 years	3 children
Multiple substances	Couple 3	Ícaro and Joana	34 e 24 years	9 years	None
	Couple 4	Márcio and Nilda	52 e 45 years	22 years	3 children

[a]From the beginning of dating to the present day

[11] Some of Jean's cognitive and behavioral characteristics influenced the interaction with him in narrative interviews. He repeated words and the evocation of those seemed compromised. He also demonstrated a flight of ideas, as he started answering content evoked by the narrative-generating question and continued or ended with other content, especially in the individual interview. The first author of this chapter had to repeat the question for Jean to verbally issue the narrative related to the objective of the study.

would have used alcohol between 2017 and 2018, during a sergeant course in Vitória.

Couple 3: Ícaro and Joana. Couple 3 was made up of Ícaro, with Cocaine Dependence, 34 years old, and Joana, 24 (they had no children). After 9 years of relationship, they lived together for 5. He was a military policeman; she, a saleswoman. Like Couples 1 and 2, they were also found in post-discharge activities, where they had always been together since 2017, when Ícaro was hospitalized. Ícaro and Joana reported that since the end of hospitalization, in 2017, there was no (re) occurrence of the use of cocaine by Ícaro, nor of tobacco or alcohol, which used to also be consumed before hospitalization.

Couple 4: Márcio and Nilda. Márcio, 52, and his wife, Nilda, 45, made up Couple 4, and he was diagnosed with Cocaine Dependence. They had been in a relationship for 22 years, and in that time they had three children. The couple was contacted when Márcio was hospitalized and both he and she were receptive to the interviews, a fact that perhaps justified the fact that they were thorough in their responses. Added to this were the specific characteristics of the spouses: both were military police officers with higher education (she, in one of the human sciences). Márcio was in the hospital for only 2 weeks when the couple was interviewed, and Márcio's use of alcohol is always present in the history of his relationship with Nilda. Although, through the Presta system, Márcio was diagnosed with Alcohol Dependence, in the interviews he shared that he combined the uses of alcohol and cocaine, given that the couple belonged to the group related to CID F14 and CID F19.

Description and Behavioral Analysis in Narrative Sequences: From Progression to the Treatment of Substance Dependence

The narrative sequences of the stories of marital relationships in clinical cases correspond to descriptions of relationship phases in the progression of substance use: from its beginning (recreational/abusive use) to its end (treatment). Such sequences (Larivaille, 1974) serve behavioral analysis (Fig. 15.1).

Initial Situation: The Beginning of the Love Relationship

Table 15.2 presents the indexed elements of the narrative sequence and the behavioral functions for using the PAS in the beginning of the couples' romantic relationships.

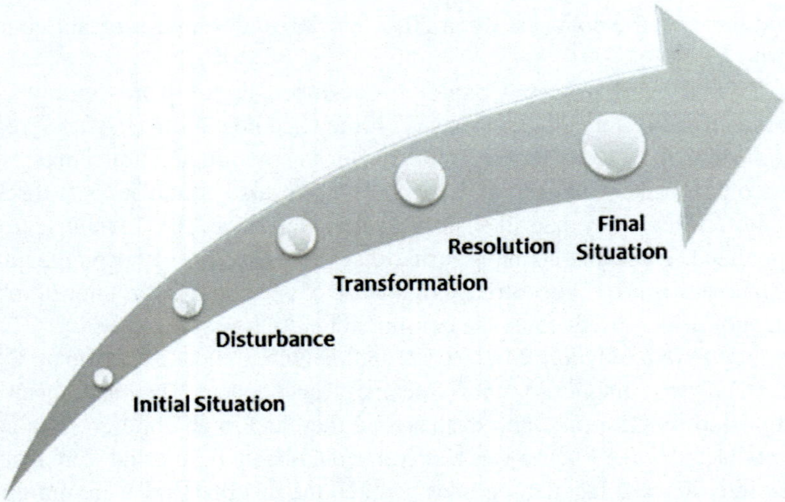

Fig. 15.1 Figure based on the model of Larivaille's model (1974) for analysis of narrative sequences Legend: Initial Situation (beginning of love relationship); Disturbance (relationship between critical points of the PAS use and the love relationship); Transformation (behavior change and its impact on the couple's life); Resolution (substance dependence treatments and other attempts to solve the problem); Final situation (maintenance of the problem solution repertoire)

Disturbance: Relationship Between Critical Points of the PAS Use and the Romantic Relationship

Table 15.3 shows the indexed elements of the narrative sequence of the disorders that the PAS use produced in the love relationship, in its antecedent and consequent behavioral functions.

Transformation

Table 15.4 presents the indexed elements of the narrative sequence of the transformations that the PAS use causes, with its antecedent and consequent events. It is possible to observe how this use changed the marital relationship of the participating couples.

Table 15.2 Initial situation of the marital relationship and use of PAS: Narrative Sequence and Behavioral Functions

Couple	Narrative sequence	Behavioral functions in the initial situation
1	In a city in the countryside of Espírito Santo state, Lara and Jean met when he was having a relationship with her friend. He breaks up with this friend because he started being interested in Lara, who had the condition of only dating him if he was single. After 1 year of dating the couple started organizing the wedding, which took place with a party, preceded by a bridal shower. In 1990 the first child of this "young couple" was born. With no experience, the couple faced financial issues (described by Lara as a problem in Jean's family). As a solution, they had to sell their cars, other goods and live in a city in the metropolitan region of the state. Living in this city, on many occasions, Jean drank "socially" with friends, according to him; according to Lara, he already drank a lot and, also according to both, "without a clue what it was" (alcoholism). For her, this "lack of notion" was due to them being a young couple and still getting to know each other, since it was only afterward that they discovered that it was an addiction.	Deprivation condition due to financial issues and the reduction of living standards (EO) Housing condition in a metropolitan region (EO) The condition of mutual ignorance ("being a young couple") of the dependency (EO) Presence of social occasions for drinking (Sd and ES) "Whenever I have an opportunity, if I drink socially, then there will be no problems" (Jean's rule, also functioning as an EO) Presentation of the affection from his friends (Sr+).
2	The couple met in 1990 at a club. He and she began living together shortly after Helena's employer became aware of the relationship between them, and did not approve it because Maurício was a police officer. After a year living together, Helena got pregnant. They got married. After the wedding, in less than 1 month, the couple's first child was born. Helena only recognized alcohol use as a problem in 2005.	The condition of permissiveness by the wife, for 15 years, of problematic drinking (EO)
3	Joana was introduced to Ícaro in 2013 by his brother. After a few months, they started dating. In 2013, Ícaro already used the PAS, albeit in a smaller quantity, and managed to hide it from Joana, using it where she couldn't see it. Joana was not aware of what cocaine was and only learned that Icarus was using it when the condition of dependence worsened.	The condition of unawareness of the dependency by the wife (EO) The wife's presence (Sd and ES) Snorting less cocaine (R1 of removing aversive stimulation) Snorting cocaine in a location unseen by the wife (R2 of removing aversive stimulation) Reducing the probability of the wife "finding out about the use" and presenting aversive stimulation, such as criticism, or removing reinforcers, such as affection (Sr−)

(continued)

Table 15.2 (continued)

Couple	Narrative sequence	Behavioral functions in the initial situation
4	Nilda and Márcio met during an officer training course. They started going out and afterward dating. In a year of dating, they got engaged and moved in together. At the end of the course, they got married. At the beginning of the relationship, Nilda did not realize Márcio used cocaine, which was consumed by him unnoticed by her, who discovered the use of cocaine at a party at Márcio's parents' house. Since then, they began talking about the use.	The condition of unawareness of the dependency by the wife (EO) The wife's presence (Sd and ES) Snorting cocaine in location unseen by the wife (R of removing aversive stimulation) Reducing the probability of the wife "finding out about the use" and presenting aversive stimulation, such as criticism, or removing reinforcers, such as affection (Sr−). Talk about the use of cocaine (R from both, approaching a solution to the problem)

Note: *Sd* discriminative stimulus, *EO* Establishing Operation, *ES* Eliciting Stimulus, *Sr+* Positive reinforcement, *Sr−* Negative reinforcement, *R* Response

Resolution

Table 15.5 contains the indexed elements of the narrative sequence of possible resolutions for the use of PAS in romantic relationships based on their consequences. It also shows the background to the behaviors involved in these resolutions.

Final Situation

The indexed elements of the narrative sequence of the final situations regarding the impact of the PAS use on love relationships are in Table 15.6. In it, we can find the elements of the antecedent context of the responses related to this outcome.

Discussion

In the narrative sequences, the behavioral functions appeared in common contingencies during the progression of the use of PAS by spouses dependent on alcohol (Couples 1 and 2) and multiple substances (Couples 3 and 4). It stands out, in alcohol-dependents, that this progression, during the marital relationship, was favored by the late perception of the alcohol use as harmful/problematic from the wives and other family members. This late perception marks the narrative sequences of the Initial Situation and the Disturbance. In multiple substance-dependents, their wives'

Table 15.3 Disruption of the marital relationship and the PAS use: Narrative Sequence and Behavioral Functions

Couple	Narrative sequence of disturbance	Behavioral functions in the disturbance
1	Jean and Lara returned to the countryside of the state of Espirito Santo, after receiving a proposal from Jean's uncle for Jean to become a caretaker. As in the metropolitan area, Jean also drank in the countryside and had friends who also drank. Jean quit smoking "overnight", but in relation to drinking, as he had no desire to quit "and so did not try to". Friendships in the countryside made it harder to quit drinking, which became very frequent.	A strong friendship with individuals who drink (EO) The frequent presence of friends who drink (Sd and ES) "When I feel like quitting drinking, if I try to, then I will be able to quit" (rule, also functioning as an EO) The presentation of affection from his friends (Sr+).
2	In 2005, the whole family realized that Mauricio's alcohol use had become daily and of imminent risk. He suffered a heart attack after a party and, at the hospital, it was revealed that the cause was the use of alcohol. Helena took care of him in this and other critical health episodes, also due to the use of alcohol. After these episodes, there was acceptance by the whole family of Maurício's alcoholism as a problem. Maurício was very confident in his wife's protection.	The condition of late knowledge of alcohol dependence by the wife and children (EO of approaching a solution to the problem) The condition of health deterioration (EO of approaching the problem) The condition of acceptance of alcohol dependence by the family (EO of approaching a solution to the problem) Presence of a caregiving wife during critical health episodes (Sd) "When, and whenever I need, if I have health problems, then I will get taken care of by my wife" (rule, also with the function of EO for drinking).
3	The PAS use progressed to the pattern of abuse after Ícaro moved in with Joana, as it was easier to hide it from few people. Nobody was watching him as they did when he lived with his parents. Living with Joana, he needed to hide the use only from her and his mother-in-law. The worsening of substance dependence started to become concerning.	The condition of poor social surveillance (EO for snorting) Snorting cocaine in a place unseen by the wife and mother-in-law (R of removing aversive stimulation) Reducing the probability of the wife and mother-in-law "finding out about the use" and presenting aversive stimulation, such as criticism, or removing reinforcers, such as affection (Sr–) Thinking about the worry pattern "what if it gets worse?" (R of approaching the solution to the problem) "When I feel like snorting, if I do, then the problems will get worse" (rule, also functioning as an AO for the cocaine use)

(continued)

Table 15.3 (continued)

Couple	Narrative sequence of disturbance	Behavioral functions in the disturbance
4	In 2002 the couple's arguments increased. The frequency of the consumption pattern of substances by Márcio increased, following the increased stress in his service. He and Nilda were involved in arguments for several reasons. One of these arguments seems to have been related to the premature birth of the couple's second daughter, because soon after it, Nilda got sick, and the childbirth was anticipated. Márcio was also involved in a conflict with a man in a bar, who he shot with his firearm.	The condition of conflict intensification in the marital relationship (EO for snorting) The condition of intensification of stressors at work (EO for snorting) The presence of reasons for conflict in the relationship (Sd and ES) The presence of reasons for stress at work (Sd and ES) Arguments with the wife (R1 of escaping aversive stimulation) Shooting a man with a gun (R2 of escaping aversive stimulation) Reducing the likelihood of maintaining aversive stimulation (Sr−)

Note: *Sd* discriminative stimulus, *EO* Establishing Operation, *ES* Eliciting Stimulus, *Sr*+ Positive reinforcement, *Sr*− Negative reinforcement, *R* Response

perception of use was also non-existent in the Initial Situation, due to the substance-dependent husbands' strategies to hide their use (Sr−), motivated by their lack of knowledge about what the illicit substance was (EO). From the content of such sequences, one can see that the wives were unaware of the substance dependence, therefore, they did not act to prevent the progression of consumption (Sr). It is then confirmed what Edwards et al. (2005) point out: the perception regarding the harmful use pattern comes up when the family dynamics is compromised by the substance-dependent family member's behavior. Given that the group dynamics involves, among the variables described by communication theorists (Cf., Fulk & Boyd, 1991), the bond (proportion), the reach (amount) and the degree (intensity) of affective bonds, the goal of controlling the consumption and avoiding its negative consequences becomes the daily concern of family members in maintaining group dynamics.

It should be noted that the wives' late perception of their husbands' problematic alcohol consumption may also be associated with the idea presented by Ronzani and Furtado (2010). The authors refer to society's ambiguous way of dealing with the use of alcohol: on the one hand, there is an incentive and glamorization of the use of alcohol by groups, by the media, and by Brazilian culture; on the other hand, when consumption becomes a problem, this use has a negative connotation and is associated with moral weakness, making the alcohol-dependent condemned to exclusion and a series of judgments.

The immediate support of the husband when it comes to excessive alcohol intake, lying to relatives and neighbors about the latter's situation and pretending to be well are common responses in the behavioral functions presented by the wives of alcohol-dependent individuals in the Transformation stage. As they evade aversive

Table 15.4 Transformation of the marital relationship and PAS use: Narrative Sequence and Behavioral Functions

Couple	Narrative sequence of transformation	Behavioral functions of transformation
1	In 2008, living a very difficult relationship with Jean, Lara witnessed her husband's drinking, but pretended that the situation was fine and lied to relatives and neighbors when they asked her about the situation Jean was facing with drinking. It was difficult for Lara to be in the relationship because of his behavior.	The condition of conflict intensification in the marital relationship (EO for drinking) The presence of her drunk husband (Sd and ES, for Lara) Saying "I'm fine" (concealing aversive feeling) (Lara's R1, escaping aversive stimulation) Lying (Lara's R2, escaping aversive stimulation) Presence of questions about how the husband faces the drinking problem (Sd and ES) Reduced likelihood of presenting aversive stimulation (Sr−)
2	The relationship between spouses has become more difficult due to alcohol dependence, with some conflicting situations. Maurício started drinking alcohol excessively. Helena helped her husband when he was ill after these excessive alcohol intakes.	The condition of conflict intensification in the marital relationship (EO for drinking) The presence of conflict in the relationship (Sd and ES). Drinking (excessively) (R from Maurício, escaping aversive stimulation) Providing immediate help to the husband for excessive alcohol intake (R from Helena, escaping aversive stimulation). Reduced likelihood of presenting aversive stimulation (Sr−)
3	Ícaro, having missed days of work, responded to an administrative process. He started distancing himself from Joana, who felt lonely even when he was home. He used to go *clubbing* without his wife and, being there, ended up using drugs. The relationship between them was getting very bad. Situations of disagreement ended in arguments	Aversive condition of punishment at work (EO for snorting cocaine and getting away from people) The presence of an administrative process at work (Sd and ES) The condition of conflict intensification in the marital relationship (EO for snorting cocaine) Being home without her husband's company (ES for Joana, eliciting a feeling of loneliness) Feeling of loneliness at home (R from Joana) Presence of a situation of disagreement with the wife (Sd and ES) Going to clubs without his wife (R from Ícaro, escaping aversive stimulation) Reduced likelihood of presenting aversive stimulation (Sr−)

(continued)

Table 15.4 (continued)

Couple	Narrative sequence of transformation	Behavioral functions of transformation
4	Márcio used to come home later than usual, quiet, and did not talk to his family. He was often transferred to work in other cities, where he used to go to bars and became closer to friends who also used the PAS. The use already affected the relationship and Nilda asked him to undergo the treatment.	The condition of receiving of city transfer request to another city (EO for snorting cocaine) The presence of a transfer document to another city (Sd and ES). The presence of friends who use the PAS (Sd and ES) Going to bars with friends (R1 from Márcio, being closer to the PAS) Returning home late (R2 from Márcio, escaping aversive stimulation) Being silent when arriving home (R3 from Márcio, escaping aversive stimulation) Asking him to undergo treatment of using the PAS (R from Nilda, approaching the solution to the problem)

Note: *Sd* discriminative stimulus, *EO* Establishing Operation, *ES* Eliciting Stimulus, *Sr+* Positive reinforcement, *Sr−* Negative reinforcement, *R* Response

stimulation, such escape-avoidance responses are frequently observed in family members of substance-dependent individuals, and show an insufficiency in the rule-setting repertoires (boundaries) and in the defense of rights and needs, which are usually indicators of the behavioral pattern called codependency (Bortolon et al., 2016). Codependency is an emotionally dependent relationship between a substance-dependent individual and another, who is not substance-dependent. This bond, considered problematic in general, but initially functional to the relationship, causes illness in the codependent individual, resulting in an overload and damages to the mental health of the family caregiver, especially women, as they make up the majority of care providers for substance-dependent family members (Spagnol, 2018).

The presence of a situation involving disagreement with the wife (with the function of Sd and ES) and the condition of conflict intensification in the marital relationship (with the function of EO) are present in all Transformation narrative sequences of couples: in this phase, couples are in stages of the relationship in which they can already describe evident losses caused by the progression of substance use. This improvement in the descriptive capacity is due to the effects of punishment: while difficulties increase the likelihood of use creating conflict followed by negative feelings (Pn+), they also increase the likelihood of use producing an escape from effective communication and opportunities for resolution of conflicts between the couple (Pn−). In different studies of couples with a substance-dependent individual who do not employ the description of phases of the marital relationship, difficult moments are seen, associated with psychological distress and a lower marital satisfaction (Kahler et al., 2003; Kelly et al., 2000; Whisman et al., 2006), which could be equivalent to the moment of Transformation.

In the couples with individuals dependent on multiple substances, the Transformation phase presents behavioral functions related to the work context, such as the condition of receiving a transfer application to work in another city

Table 15.5 Marital relationship resolution and PAS use: Narrative Sequence and Behavioral Functions

Couple	Narrative sequence of the resolution	Behavioral functions in the resolution
1	Jean discovered Presta through contact with a military friend, whom he liked very much. The friend advised him to know the program. Excited, and wanting to prove that he would improve, Jean agreed to be admitted at Presta in 2008. Lara and his friend were very happy with his decision to treat himself.	The condition of friendship and admiration of a military friend (EO of hospitalization) Presence of the admired military friend's advice (Sd and ES) Feelings of excitement/acceptance for the change (R1 from Jean) Thinking "I can, and I will prove that I can improve" (Jean's R2, approaching the solution to the problem) Going to the hospital (Jean's R3, approaching the solution to the problem) Presentation of the satisfaction from his wife and friend (Sr+)
2	Maurício went to Presta in 2013, but without the intention of staying for treatment. He wanted to go home, but his wife "forced" him to try and stay. He stayed for 43 days. He liked it and stayed for treatment, which made Helena very happy.	The aversive condition of treatment imposition (EO for staying hospitalized) Forcing him to stay at Presta for a while (R from Helena, approaching the solution to the problem) "Since I have no intention of being admitted, if I make it clear that I just want to know more about hospitalization, then the others will not insist on it" (Maurício's rule, also with the function of an EO, escaping aversive stimulation) Going to Presta (R1 from Mauritius, to approach the solution to the problem) Mild condition of hospitalization (EO for being hospitalized) The adherence to treatment (R2 from Mauritius, approaching the solution to the problem) The presentation of satisfaction with his hospitalization (Sr+) Presentation of his wife's contentment (Sr+)
3	On Joana and Icaro's brother's initiative, they both got a place at Presta to hospitalize Ícaro. Since it hadn't been Icaro's idea, he thought he would not be in treatment. He went, liked it and stayed; and, together with his wife, he learned more about substance dependence. It was good for improving their marital life.	The aversive condition of having previous knowledge about hospitalization (AO for staying hospitalized) The condition of the initiative of being hospitalized coming from someone else (AO for being hospitalized) Mild condition of hospitalization (EO for being hospitalized) Being in the hospital environment (Sd and ES) Adherence to the treatment (R from Ícaro, to approach the solution to the problem) Presentation of knowledge and learning about substance dependence (Sr+) Presentation of improvement in his marital relationship (Sr+)

(continued)

Table 15.5 (continued)

Couple	Narrative sequence of the resolution	Behavioral functions in the resolution
4	Márcio was admitted at Presta in 2003 and in 2018. Between 2003 and 2018, when he was in his most critical periods of use, he underwent treatment at a CAPS and with independent psychiatrists. In 2003, he was admitted to hospitalization, but the intention was to stay abstinent only during the period of resolution of a lawsuit. In 2018, he went to hospitalization recognizing the need to discontinue the use, adhering to the treatment.	Mild condition of hospitalization (EO for being hospitalized) The adherence to treatment with hospitalization in 2018 (R from Márcio, approaching the solution to the problem) Seeking treatment without hospitalization (R from Márcio, approaching the solution to the problem) The presentation of positive treatment results (Sr+)

Note: *Sd* discriminative stimulus, *AO* Abolishing Operation, *EO* Establishing Operation, *ES* Eliciting Stimulus, *Sr+* Positive Reinforcement, *R* Response

(EO), the presence of an administrative process at work (Sd and ES), the presence of a document transferring the place of work to another city (Sd and ES), and an aversive condition of punishment at work (EO), revealing relations between the work routine and the progression of PAS consumption. It is relevant that the husbands (dependent on multiple substances) of couples 3 and 4 were police officers, a job especially vulnerable to physical and psychological stress. Souza et al. (2013), when investigating military and civil police, mention problems at work (11%) and absence from work (17.1%) as common in this group. They also report that military police officers have a higher percentage of associated consumption of both legal and illegal substances when compared to civilians. Capistrano et al. (2013a, b), when identifying the social impact of drug abuse for substance-dependent individuals, observed that in 21.7% of his sample, job losses were present and, of these, 63.2% have already lost their job as a result of substance dependence.

Going to the hospital (R) and adhering to treatment (R) are responses of approaching a solution to the problem prevalent in the Resolution phase, followed by the presentation of Sr+s for answers on knowledge regarding substance dependence, the perception of positive treatment results, and the contentment of the substance-dependent individual with the hospitalization, as well as for his wife when it comes to the treatment. Learning more about the concepts, phenomena and effects of substance dependence is an important aspect to manage the problems and for effective

Table 15.6 Final situation of the PAS use in the marital relationship: Narrative Sequence and Behavioral Functions

Couple	Narrative sequence of the final situation	Behavioral functions in the final situation
1	Hospitalization in 2008 at Presta. Maintenance of abstinence and the treatment process with the wife's weekly participation at Presta.	Maintaining weekly post-discharge treatment at Presta after hospitalization (R from Jean and Lara, for maintaining abstinence). The presentation of the wife's contentment for maintaining Jean's abstinence (Sr+) The presentation of Jean's contentment for maintaining abstinence since 2008 (Sr+)
2	The husband claims a period of abstinence during the past 5 years. He attends Presta's post-discharge program every 2 weeks. Sometimes with the wife. The wife reports that her husband's aggressive behavior has not changed, that he has just stopped drinking. She believes he used alcohol during the period he was in Vitória, taking the sergeant course, when he experienced stressful situations.	Maintaining the post-discharge treatment every 2 weeks at Presta after hospitalization (R from Maurício, for maintaining abstinence). The presence of the wife's judgment without attempting to solve the problem (Sd). Maurício: Maintenance of aggressive behaviors (Sd) Mauricio: Experiencing stressful situations (Sd)
3	Hospitalization in 2017 at Presta. Maintenance of abstinence for 1 year and 2 months, post-discharge treatment at Presta with his wife. They attend church together and live in harmony.	Maintaining post-discharge treatment at Presta after hospitalization (R from Ícaro and Joana, for maintaining abstinence) Going to Church (Sd and ES) Harmonious marital living (R of maintaining abstinence). The presentation of the wife's contentment by maintaining Ícaro's abstinence (Sr+)
4	Márcio was still hospitalized during the interview, effectively taking part in all activities. The family was also taking part in the treatment.	Adhering to treatment (R from Márcio of approaching the treatment's maintenance and abstinence after discharge) The family's presence during treatment (Sd)

Note: *Sd* discriminative stimulus, *EO* Establishing Operation, *ES* Eliciting Stimulus, *Sr+* Positive reinforcement, *R* Response responses of care and prevention of problems related to substance dependence (Filizola et al., 2006; Rocha, 2011). The lack of knowledge regarding the substance dependence management can lead the relatives of the substance-dependent individual to discourage one from changing, also holding the individual responsible for progressing or relapsing on the use pattern, as well as strengthening the denial of the PAS use evidence. In general, according to Rocha, these behaviors of family members are correlated with ambivalent feelings, such as shame and guilt.

The Maintenance stage is marked by behavioral functions that involve the participation of the substance-dependent individual (both dependent on alcohol and multiple substances) in the continuity of treatment-related activities. In the cases studied in this chapter, these activities are those of the Presta post-discharge follow-up program after hospitalization. The participation of the wife (Sr+), the family's presence in the treatment (Sd), and the harmony between the couple (Sr+) also prevail among couples as a function that favors the maintenance of the treatment and the abstinence in the observed cases. The family's effective participation in the treatment of substance dependence is a protective factor for the substance-dependent individual and a strategy for family members, also affected by the dependency, to be cared for and gain knowledge about what to do and how to contribute to the treatment (Paz & Colossi, 2013).

Final Considerations

The purpose of this chapter was to present behavioral functions involved in the progression of substance dependence and its treatment during the marital relationship. The results highlighted behavioral functions of use progression as contained: in the late perception of alcohol use as harmful/problematic by the wives; the strategies of substance-dependent husbands to hide the use from their wives; their lack of knowledge about what the illegal substance was; pretending to be well (wives), a condition of intensifying conflict in the marital relationship, the presence of a situation of disagreement with the wife, an aversive condition of punishment at work. Among the functions related to solving the problem, the following stand out: going to the hospital; adhering to treatment; learning the concepts, phenomena and effects of substance dependence; participating in the post-discharge follow-up program (substance-dependent individual); participating in the treatment (wife and family) and contributing to the harmony between the couple.

References

American Psychiatric Association (APA). (2014). *DSM-5: Manual diagnóstico e estatístico de transtornos mentais*. Artmed Editora.

Bordin, S., Figlie, N. B., & Laranjeira, R. (2004). *Aconselhamento em Dependência Química*. Roca.

Borloti, E. B., Haydu, V. B., & Machado, A. R. (2015). Crack: Análise comportamental e exemplos das funções da dependência. *Acta Comportamentalia: Revista Latina de Análisis de Comportamiento, 23*(3), 323–338.

Bortolon, C. B., Signor, L., Moreira, T. D. C., Figueiró, L. R., Benchaya, M. C., Machado, C. A., … Barros, H. M. T. (2016). Family functioning and health issues associated with codependency in families of drug users. *Ciência & Saúde Coletiva, 21*, 101–107. https://doi.org/10.1590/1413-81232015211.20662014

Bruner, J., & Weisser, S. (1995). A invenção do ser: a autobiografia e suas formas. Cultura escrita e oralidade. *São Paulo: Ática*, 141–161.

Bertaux, D. (2010). Narrativas de vida: a pesquisa e seus métodos. Natal: Edufrn.

Capistrano, F. C., Ferreira, A. C. Z., Silva, T. L., Kalinke, L. P., & Maftum, M. A. (2013a). Perfil sociodemográfico e clínico de dependentes químicos em tratamento: análise de prontuários. *Escola Anna Nery Revista de Enfermagem, 17*(2), 234–241. https://doi.org/10.1590/S1414-81452013000200005

Capistrano, F. C., Ferreira, A. C. Z., Maftum, M. A., Kalinke, L. P., & de Fátima Mantovani, M. (2013b). Impacto social do uso abusivo de drogas para dependentes químicos registrados em prontuários. *Cogitare Enfermagem, 18*(3), 468–474. https://doi.org/10.5380/ce.v18i3.33556

Coleman, E. (1987). Marital and relationship problems among chemically dependent and codependent relationships. *Journal of Chemical Dependency Treatment, 1*(1), 39–60. https://doi.org/10.1300/J034v01n01_04

dos Santos Lima, R. A., de Almeida Amazonas, M. C. L., & Motta, J. A. G. (2007). Incidência de stress e fontes estressoras em esposas de portadores da síndrome de dependência do álcool. *Estudos de Psicologia, 24*(4), 431–439. https://doi.org/10.1590/S0103-166X2007000400003

Edwards, G., Marshall, E. J., & Cook, C. C. H. (2005). *O tratamento do alcoolismo: um guia para profissionais de saúde*. Porto Alegre: Artmed. (*Original work published in 2003*).

Eisenhardt, K. M. (1989). Building theories from case study research. *Academy of Management Review, 14*(4), 532–550. https://doi.org/10.1177/014920639101700207

Ferrari, J. V. (2019). Contingências de (re)ocorrência do uso de substâncias psicoativas no curso do relacionamento conjugal (Master's thesis, Universidade Federal do Espírito Santo).

Filizola, C. L. A., Perón, C. D. J., Nascimento, M. M. A. D., Pavarini, S. C. I., & Petrilli Filho, J. F. (2006). Compreendendo o alcoolismo na família. *Escola Anna Nery, 10*(4), 660–670.

Fulk, J., & Boyd, B. (1991). Emerging theories of communication in organizations. *Journal of Management, 17*(2), 407–446. https://doi.org/10.1177/014920639101700207

Germano, I. M. P., & Serpa, F. A. D. S. (2008). Narrativas autobiográficas de jovens em conflito com a lei. *Arquivos brasileiros de psicologia, 60*(3) http://www.repositorio.ufc.br/handle/riufc/28091

Hanninen, V., & Koski-Jannes, A. (1999). Narratives of recovery from addictive behaviours. *Addiction, 94*(12), 1837–1848.

Jovchelovitch, S., & Bauer, M. W. (2002). Entrevista narrativa. *Pesquisa qualitativa com texto, imagem e som: um manual prático, 4*, 90–113.

Kahler, C. W., McCrady, B. S., & Epstein, E. E. (2003). Sources of distress among women in treatment with their alcoholic partners. *Journal of Substance Abuse Treatment, 24*(3), 257–265. https://doi.org/10.1016/S0740-5472(03)00033-3

Larivaille, P. (1974). L'analyse (morpho) logique du récit. Poétique, 19, 368–388.

Levandowski, D. C., Piccinini, C. A., & Lopes, R. D. C. S. (2009). O Processo de separação-individuação em adolescentes do sexo masculino na transição para a paternidade. *Psicologia: Reflexão e Crítica, 22*(3), 353–361.

Kelly, A. B., Halford, W. K., & Young, R. M. (2000). Maritally distressed women with alcohol problems: The impact of a short-term alcohol-focused intervention on drinking behaviour and marital satisfaction. *Addiction, 95*(10), 1537–1549. https://doi.org/10.1046/j.1360-0443.2000.951015378.x

Moura Kolling, N., da Silva, C. R., Carvalho, J. C. N., da Cunha, S. M., & Kristensen, C. H. (2007). Avaliação neuropsicológica em alcoolistas e dependentes de cocaína. *Avaliaçao Psicologica: Interamerican Journal of Psychological Assessment, 6*(2), 127–137.

Makvand, H. S., Bigdeli, I., & Agha, B. A. (2009). *Codependency and mental health in wives of opioid drug abusers*. https://doi.org/10.1590/1413-81232015211.20662014

Matos, M. A. (1999). Análise funcional do comportamento. *Estudos de Psicologia, 16*(3), 8–18. https://doi.org/10.1590/S0103-166X1999000300002

Miguel, P. A. C. (2007). Estudo de caso na engenharia de produção: estruturação e recomendações para sua condução. *Production, 17*(1), 216–229. https://doi.org/10.1590/S0103-65132007000100015

Moraes, L. M. P., Braga, V. A. B., Souza, A. M. A., & Oriá, M. O. B. (2009). Expressão da codependência em familiares de dependentes químicos. *REME Revista Mineira de Enfermagem, 13*(1), 34–42.

Patton, M. Q. (2002). Two decades of developments in qualitative inquiry: A personal, experiential perspective. *Qualitative social work, 1*(3), 261–283.

Paz, F. M., & Colossi, P. M. (2013). Aspectos da dinâmica da família com dependência química. *Estudos de Psicologia, 18*(4), 551–558.

Riemann, G., & Schütze, F. (1991). Trajectory as a basic theoretical concept for analyzing suffering and disorderly socialprocesses. In D. R. Maines (Ed.), *Social organization and social process: Essays in honor of Anselm Strauss* (pp. 333–357). De Gruyter.

Rocha, A. P. (2011). *As problemáticas enfrentadas pelas famílias co-dependente no tratamento da dependência química no âmbito do programa amor-exigente no município de Ponta Grossa-PR*. Undergraduate thesis, Universidade Estadual de Ponta Grossa, Paraná.

Roesch, S. M. A. (1999). *Projetos de estágio e de pesquisa em administração* (p. 2). Atlas.

Ronzani, T. M., & Furtado, E. F. (2010). Estigma social sobre o uso de álcool. *Jornal brasileiro de psiquiatria, 59*(4), 326–332.

Santos, L. V. D., & Costa, L. F. (2004). Avaliação da dinâmica conjugal violenta e suas repercussões sobre os filhos. *Psicologia: teoria e prática, 6*(1), 59–72.

Schütze, F. (1983). Biographieforschung und narratives interview. *Neue praxis, 13*(3), 283–293.

Schütze, F. (2011). Pesquisa biográfica e entrevista narrativa. In W. Weller & N. Pfaff (Eds.), *Metodologias da pesquisa qualitativa em educação: teoria e prática* (pp. 210–222). Vozes.

Silva, M. T. A., Guerra, L. G. G. C., Gonçalves, F. L., & Garcia-Mijares, M. (2001). Análise funcional da dependência de drogas. In H. J. Ghilardi, M. B. B. P. Madi, P. P. Queiroz, & M. C. Scoz (Eds.), *Sobre comportamento e cognição* (pp. 422–442). ESEtec.

Silva, S. S. D. C., Lima, L. C., Pontes, F. A. R., Bucher-Maluschke, J. S. N. F., & Santos, T. M. D. (2011). Qualidade conjugal: estudo de caso de ribeirinhos na Amazônia. *Gerais: Revista Interinstitucional de Psicologia, 4*(1), 50–59.

Skinner, B. F. (1953). *Science and human behavior*. Simon and Schuster.

Souza, E. C. (2008). Modos de narração e discursos da memória: biografização, experiências e formação. *(Auto) biografia: formação, territórios e saberes. Natal: EDUFRN*, 85–101. https://doi.org/10.1590/0103-7307201507611.

Souza, E. R. D., Schenker, M., Constantino, P., & Correia, B. S. C. (2013). Consumo de substâncias lícitas e ilícitas por policiais da cidade do Rio de Janeiro. *Ciência & Saúde Coletiva, 18*, 667–676. https://doi.org/10.1590/S1413-81232013000300012

Spagnol, S. C. B. (2018). *Familiares de dependentes químicos na rede de atenção psicossocial: panorama atual e perfil do grupo*. Master's thesis, Universidade Federal do Espírito Santo.

Subodh, N. B., Grover, S., Grewal, M., Grewal, S., Basu, D., & Mattoo, S. K. (2014). Interpersonal violence against wives by substance dependent men. *Drug and Alcohol Dependence, 138*, 124–129. https://doi.org/10.1016/j.drugalcdep.2014.02.017

Todorov, J. C. (1982). Behaviorismo e análise experimental do comportamento. *Cadernos de Análise do Comportamento, 3*, 10–23.

Torossian, M. S., Heleno, M. G. V., & Vizzotto, M. M. (2009). Relacionamento conjugal e o fenômeno da violência doméstica: Um estudo de caso. *Mudanças-Psicologia da Saúde, 17*(1), 12–16. https://doi.org/10.15603/2176-1019/mud.v17n1p12-16

Van Wormer, K. (1990). Co-dependency: Implications for women and therapy. *Women & Therapy, 8*(4), 51–63. https://doi.org/10.1300/J015v08n04_04

Ventura, M. M. (2007). O estudo de caso como modalidade de pesquisa. *Revista SoCERJ, 20*(5), 383–386.

Voss, C., Tsikriktsis, N., & Frohlich, M. (2002). Case research in operations management. *International Journal of Operations & Production Management, 22*(2), 195–219. https://doi.org/10.1108/01443570210414329

Wekerle, C., & Wall, A. M. (Eds.). (2004). The violence and addiction equation: Theoretical and clinical issues in substance abuse and relationship violence. Routledge.

Wetchler, J. L., & DelVecchio, D. L. (1996). Systemic couples therapy for a female heroin addict. *Journal of Family Psychotherapy, 6*(4), 1–13.

Whisman, M. A., Uebelacker, L. A., & Bruce, M. L. (2006). Longitudinal association between marital dissatisfaction and alcohol use disorders in a community sample. *Journal of Family Psychology, 20*(1), 164. https://doi.org/10.1300/j085V06N04_01

Chapter 16
Drugs Use in Romantic Relationship and Violence Against Women

Vânia Lúcia Pestana Sant'Ana and Débora Barbosa de Deus

Introduction

Violence against women is a subject that must be discussed from the perspective of developing prevention and intervention strategies that aim to curb its occurrence, mainly due to the frequency and severity of the cases. According to the World Health Organization (WHO), violence is understood as the "use of physical force or power, real or threat, against yourself, against other person, or against a group or community, that results or is likely to result in injury, death, psychological damage, developmental disability, and deprivation" (WHO, 1996, p. 5). Although this definition covers almost all classes of aggressive behavior against women it is necessary to recognize that this pattern is not recent nor determined by a single factor. It is important to know historical aspects of women's role in society and the evolution of their representation as female gender.

In the human evolutionary process, men begin to exercise control over women when they discover their role in conceiving children. This discovery meant that men only accepted to create those who were his descendants of blood and who would inherit their properties. For this, it was necessary that women had sexual relationship exclusively with just one man, and to ensure that it should be delimited the possibilities of encounters between women and men, ensuring that these meetings took place only with the one with whom the woman would join to form a family.

V. L. P. Sant'Ana (✉)
Universidade Estadual de Maringá (UEM), Maringá, PR, Brazil

Instituto Maringaense de Psicologia Analítico Comportamental (IMPAC), Maringá, PR, Brazil

D. B. de Deus
Pontifícia Universidade Católica do Paraná (PUC-PR), Maringá, PR, Brazil

Centro Universitário Cidade Verde (UniFCV), Maringá, PR, Brazil

S. M. Oliani et al. (eds.), *Behavior Analysis and Substance Dependence*,
https://doi.org/10.1007/978-3-030-75961-2_16

From now on, women become first father's property and then husband's property, the rules about gender roles are expanding and becoming "natural and/or biological" social norms (Ariès, 1986), whose aim was to limit as much as possible the social mobility of women, making their operating spaces always controlled by a man and restricted to home limits.

It is presumed that, in general, rules formulated in relation to women started from the assumption that the primary duty and mission of their existence was to procreate and care for their offspring, the man, and the house, while the man's role would be to provide financial support for the family and to dictate the rules that everyone should follow. Such family and social organization began to be openly questioned only after the second half of the twentieth century and several actions and movements took place to make some changes in the female role.

Among the factors that decisively contributed to female emancipation, it can be mentioned industrialization, the departure of men to war, the counterculture movement of the 1960s, the discovery and commercialization of the contraceptive pill (Sant'Ana, 1995). Such factors led to a major change in the customs and morality of that period.

Although the 1960s was a period of liberalization of customs and changes in women's social and moral behavior, there was still a strong social component to impel women to return or remain in maternal and domestic functions: the attribution of a disorganization and the dismantling of the family with the departure of women from domestic boundaries. Feminist movements had to act since long before counterculture movements for these changes to solidify and generate changes in the rules that prescribed which behaviors should be emitted by women, with the initial milestone being women's struggle for the right to vote.

This struggle, called the suffragist movement, began timidly in the USA at the turn of the seventeenth century to the eighteenth century and exploded as an organized movement in the nineteenth century, culminating in August 1920, with the approval of an amendment to the Constitution that granted everyone the right to vote, regardless of race or sex.

In Europe, two events brought about profound changes in the structure of society. The French Revolution (1789) and the Industrial Revolution (1848) triggered a period of great material, intellectual, and social growth for the entire world population (Hosbawm, 2009). In the light of these revolutions, especially the French Revolution, the feminist movement in Europe was born. Initially, the main demands of the feminist movement were based on universal suffrage, divorce, education, and work. In a microstructural sense, the feminist movement gave visibility to the phenomenon of violence based on articulated actions with women in situations of violence (Teles, 2007).

Feminist ideas and women's rights movements reached Brazilian women. The struggle for women's rights in Brazil can be divided into two major phases: the suffragist movement and the inclusion of women in the labor market as a result of the second world war (Alves, 1980). In addition to these, many minor movements occurred both daily and in the political and social scenarios, which enabled the struggle for the right to vote (Karawejczyk, 2013), which culminated, in 1927, in

Rio Grande do Norte state, in the institution of the female vote and, finally, in 1932, this right was extended to all women in Brazil. Regarding the inclusion of women in the labor market, it is important to highlight, in Brazil, in addition to the post-war scenario, the Constitution of the 1930s in which labor rights were instituted for Brazilian women (Guiraldelli, 2007).

The institution of women's right to vote, as well as their insertion at the labor market can be seen as historical and political conquests, however, the acquisition of some rights and the exercise of female citizenship cannot be considered to have been accompanied by behavioral changes in the male population about how to treat and perceive women. There was a strong division between what it was like to be a woman "to get married" and to be a woman "to have fun", the latter should not be considered worthy of respect, which meant, ultimately, that she would not be "honored" with a husband's last name. The cultural practice of men as provider and head of the family was also maintained so that division between these types of women remained active.

The woman legally needed her husband's permission to perform various civil acts and even to decide on a sterilization to avoid further children. Furthermore, the man was allowed a much freer life and without those many restrictions, as long as he fulfilled his role as provider and had the authority to give the final say in all relevant decisions of his family. In order to have authority, he was allowed to physically punish both his children and wife. The intensity of punishment would be related to the man's assessment of the seriousness of transgression committed, ranging from the imprisonment of woman in a convent, physical aggression, torture, and even death. This structure allowed violence against children and women to be seen as normal and even desirable in order to maintain family hierarchy and obedience. It can be assumed that the way in which we perceive and evaluate women has formed a cultural bias in which assaulting, raping, killing a woman or a girl has become common and tolerated throughout history in almost all so-called civilized countries within the most different economic and political regimes.

As an example of such a culture, in Brazil, under the pretext of adultery, the murder of women was legitimate before the republic. Koerner (2002) shows that woman's sexual relationship outside of marriage was considered adultery, which allowed her husband to kill them both. For man, there was no adultery, but concubinage. Subsequently, the Civil Code of 1916 changed these provisions considering the adultery of both spouses as the reason for divorce, the only form of legal marital separation before 1977 when the divorce began to exist in the country. However, changing the law did not change the century-old custom of killing a woman, whether she was a wife, lover, partner, girlfriend, concubine, or daughter. At the beginning of the twentieth century, the Brazilian population began to have a closer contact with behavior and values of other countries, which began to be confronted with local patriarchal traditions still in force, although more weakened.

In the 1920s and 1930s, there was an intense movement of women and some sectors of society that denounced the problem of women's murder. This movement progressed almost silently and emerged in the 1970s with the murder of Minas Gerais columnist Ângela Diniz, the victim of her boyfriend who did not accept separation. News reports at the time describe the murderer's defense attorney's surprise at the social outcry for him to be convicted.

The demonstrations, in 1970, for the defendant to be convicted had the slogan "Who loves does not kill". In that decade, continuing a counterculture movement in the 1960s, several groups, such as militants against the military dictatorship (instituted in Brazil after 1964), intellectuals, union members, and workers from different sectors joined feminists in a daily struggle for rights and better living conditions and for equality between men and women. Unlike the early decades of the twentieth century, reports of crimes that were previously hidden and perpetrated against women became public.

Violence against women was an expression coined by feminist movements a few decades ago and refers to situations as diverse as physical, financial, moral, sexual, psychological violence; harassment at work; traffic of women and girls; sex tourism; ethnic and racial violence; violence committed by State (through action or inaction); the mutilation of female genitals; dowry-related violence and murders; mass rape in wars and armed conflicts (Brasil, 1995; Grossi, 1995).

In the understanding of violence against women, it is emphasized that this is a feature of a patriarchal society, marked by sexism, which imposes a role of submission and social neutrality on women, both in the family context and in the community in which they are inserted. These characteristics are currently present both in the rules that determine women's socialization as being more linked to the care of others and in the application of laws that are mostly ignored when referring to women's rights. This condition can be understood by the lack of access of women, for a long time, to a quality formal education directed to scientific thinking and not to the care of the home and children. By limiting such access, the scope of action of women in the professional field, which is made up of people who legislate or enforce laws, becomes limited, forming a barrier that is difficult to overcome. The first reports of violence against women were initiatives of articulated actions, providing strategic formulations to face the issue that today is called gender violence. From this context, violence against women came to be considered a violation of women's human rights, moving from the private to the public sphere (Teles, 2007). Thus, we can mention the Lei Maria da Penha (11.390/06), which was enacted with the objective of "restraining and preventing gender violence in the domestic, family or in an intimate relationship of affection" (Brasil, 2006 , p. 11), and which encourages the creation of public policies for possibilities of confronting violence against women.

Understand what keeps the high frequency of occurrence of aggressions, the continuity of romantic relationships in this condition, the silence of the victims, as well as a possible connection between these aggressions with the use of legal and illegal substances could lead to the elaboration of public policies aimed at both the general health of population and the mental health of those involved in behavioral patterns that are harmful to themselves and others. Harmful behaviors are those that, in a direct or indirect way, prevent or hinder the full development of individual potentialities and the full exercise of human rights universally defined as inherent to each person.

Drug Use in Romantic Relationships and Violence Against Women

Violent or abusive relationship between man and woman goes against the ideal scenario for romantic relationships that, a long time ago, started to be discussed and sought by many people as the formula for obtaining happiness. Although marriage based on romantic love is relatively recent in Western cultures, relationships built on this concept – love – have become the object of fantasy for the vast majority of people who dream of finding someone to complete them. Such an encounter would generate, in this fantasy, an internal state of deep peace and joy, in other words, it would produce happiness in all moments of life.

Considered a traditional practice, especially in romantic relationships, violence committed by intimate persons is deeply rooted in social life, being perceived, in most cases, as a normal or natural condition. The victim goes into a cycle of violence in which her self-esteem and self-confidence are being undermined daily, leaving her immobilized or unable to react and resort to legal measures that punishes the aggressor and protects the victim. It can be considered that one of the factors that contribute to the maintenance of the cycle of violence and non-denunciation of the aggressor is the woman's perception of the ineffectiveness of legal measures in bringing the necessary security to prevent future aggressions.

Although the victim's affection is mixed with the anger of being beaten, there is love or what the victim has learned to call it by this concept. Due to the phenomenon of habituation (Aló & Costa, 2019), even though it is an aversive situation, violence becomes a necessary element for maintaining the relationship and, however paradoxical it may seem to other people, violence sustains a significant number of romantic relationships. Here it is worth remembering that in the face of a situation that is poor in positive reinforcement stimulation, some stimuli classified as aversive by most people can assume the role of positive reinforcers and maintain behaviors that produced them in the past. In addition, the cycle of violence, characterized by a phase of tension, followed by aggression and, finally, regret and requests for forgiveness with promises regarding the non-repetition of aggression (honeymoon[1]) promotes a mixture of aversive and positive stimuli that, under an intermittent reinforcement scheme, can indefinitely maintain the woman's behavior of remaining in an abusive or violent relationship.

In addition, it can be assumed that aggressive behavior is reinforced by an escape/avoidance pattern from the victim that tries, in many ways, to prevent the occurrence of a new aggression, either by submitting, or by agreeing with all the aggressor's requirements. The escape/avoidance responses of the abused woman would act as positive reinforcers for the aggressor who has his demands promptly met. When attempting to modify this scenario, with occasional refusals and disagreements, the victim selects responses in the aggressor with increasingly intense topographies or

[1] Honeymoon is an expression used for the interval period in which there is no aggression in the relationship, which occurs in cycles of violence against women.

magnitudes, which may reach those that lead to her death. The cultural determinants that also act strongly in female education make women, since childhood, directed to roles related to caring for others, to be patient, tolerant, submissive, and non-assertive. And boys are educated to behave in the opposite way, which can make aggressive behavior an acceptable form of conflict resolution.

Among the risk factors that make up the scenario for violence against women, unemployment, low education, and the use of legal or illegal drugs are also considered as relevant variables. It is hypothesized that the use of drugs, loving union between two people, and the permanence in an abusive or violent relationship adheres to the same rule: the fantasy of finding happiness or well-being outside the individual (or his behavior), in other words, the fantasy of something or someone that supplies all needs and desires of the other (the lack of self-reinforced behavior in the affective situation).

With the appreciation (of social character) of the contingency of lasting happiness and well-being dependent on a loving relationship, it is observed that this is a cultural practice that makes up the scenario for the constitution of the subjectivity of individuals, which can be more significant depending on each person's life history, including the development of autonomy and self-control (Tourinho, 2009). According to Skinner (2003), autonomy and self-control are behaviors developed fundamentally by social interactions, in which certain choices (changes in environmental variables made by individual who behaves) outline the responses that will be emitted, of autonomy and/or self-control, such as, for example, in staying (or not) in a loving relationship.

Given that autonomy and self-control are related to cultural practices (Tourinho, 2009) of romantic relationships, another explanation, also of a social character, would be a correlation between drug use and cases of violence. Regarding the use of licit or illicit drugs, in addition to being a risk factor, there is in the common sense, the perception that their use would lead or trigger male aggression against women. The understanding of behaviors that have guiding rules happens from a verbal community in which a speaker and a listener are interacting, in other words, a person or group that issues a rule and another that follows (or not) this rule (Matos, 1969). It is observed that in Brazilian culture, until recently, the use of legal drugs was an attenuator to reduce social and legal responsibility of behaviors practiced under its effect.

Therefore, within the social context in which there are rules that determine when the use of drugs would be responsible for aggressive action, the individual under its effect would tend to commit violent acts more frequently than in the absence of these substances since he would not be responsible for the violent behavior, but the drug. It would seem, therefore, that aggression would be more under the rule of how he could behave under influence of drugs than the actual effects of the drug used.

The use of substances that modify the functioning of the psyche seems to have been present in the most varied periods of human evolution, both with regard to a religious character and to an escape pattern from the daily difficulties encountered by people from most diverse social classes, educational level, and cultural model. It can be seen that for each type of use there are specific rules dictating how they would work in that context. The use of drugs, in this case, supports the possibility of justification for violence, which also corroborates that the victim remains in the relationship, since the partner is under the effect of substances and not in his "normal" state, in a movement that individualizes the problem, disregarding cultural characteristics, such as the establishment of rules that make up its context.

Several studies search for a causal relationship between the use of legal and illegal drugs and the increase in violence in general and, specifically, domestic violence (Amaral, Vasconcelos, Sá, Silva, & Macena, 2016; Barros et al., 2016; Fonseca et al., 2009; Leite et al., 2017; Minayo & Deslandes, 1998; Rabello & Junior, 2007; Vieira et al., 2008; Vieira et al., 2014). According to Minayo and Delandes (1998), the complexity in understanding the relationship between violence and drugs lies in the difficulty of measuring and/or verifying behaviors or effects from the use of legal/illegal substances. Still, according to these authors, the correlation of frequency between violence and drugs varies depending on the measurement between serious events or events that become worse on these occasions.

Abuse of drugs by the partner seems to make women even more vulnerable in situations of violence in marital and family relationships by the justification established by the woman that the aggressor is not a violent person but is behaving under the effect of something stronger than him, the drug. Although alcohol abuse and violence are approached as a causal relation, it is noteworthy that such a relation is not confirmed since drugs can be one of the factors that contribute to violence, but not exclusively, as already stated when discussing the control of rules on violent behavior presented after drug use. It is also observed that social consequences, even if delayed, are relevant to the maintenance of certain cultural practices and some social contingencies occur so that the individual can deal with the world based on relational networks (Das Neves, 2017).

Drug abuse and violent behavior is a complex relation involving several aspects, such as types of positive reinforcers involved in the relation, magnitude of these reinforcers, reinforcement scheme under which violence was initiated and maintained, and the escape/avoidance behavior of those involved in the violent episode, among other aspects. When we understand that the use of alcohol, as well as other drugs, and episodes of violent behavior do not have a clearly defined interaction, we do not know the direct and/or indirect influences of environment; the individual characteristics of users of alcohol and other drugs; the prevalence and the precise correlations between such influences (Amaral et al., 2016; Barros et al., 2016; Fonseca, et al., 2009; Rabello & Junior, 2007), it is important to research and discuss results that assess the complexity of the context, the social dynamics, the cultural norms historically constructed (such as gender issue), factors of development and individuality, and from that, to institute public policies that meet the needs of those involved.

It is considered that behaviors and roles culturally delegated to men and women prevent those from learning to demonstrate their weaknesses, insecurities, and feelings, while girls learn, from an early age, to behave in terms of submission and agreement. In Western society, during the initial periods of schooling, boys are expected to be more object-oriented, more competent for physical activities, more aggressive, to be achievement-oriented, independent, and dominant in relation to girls for whom the expectations are contrary to those of boys (Sant'Ana, 1995). One of the effects of this socializing process would be that many men have problems in relating to their partner, their children, and the community they belong to. The socialization of boys also points to the use of alcohol as a pattern rooted in social and cultural contexts considered acceptable for relating such use to disinhibition and improvement of mood and also as a symbol of virility and physical resistance in men. In addition, it can increase the concentration on immediate events by reducing awareness of future events or those that are distant in time, producing effects that reduce social stress in men. As a mood enhancer, this substance can also increase existing feelings of anger and frustration, changing men's perceptions of women, making these an immediate and vulnerable target.

In a context in which the aggression response occurs, while the individual is under influence of drugs, this response can be maintained, for example, by the victim's self-silencing (non-denunciation), which brings evidence of the power that this man has over this woman, as it is culturally perpetuated as the hegemonic pattern. Some of these situations of violence happen at home with the couple's children present, or even children of other relationships (Souza & Da Ros, 2006). The repetition of similar situations produces, in the long term, behaviors called low self-confidence and low self-esteem, which would provide a favorable condition for violence to be repeated without making complaints, which would be the first step toward subsequent legal protective measures. The absence of denunciation or non-provocation of marital separation by women is, in most cases, due to financial dependence, especially thinking about the care of children, the fear of the partner suffering some type of punishment, the hope that the partner will change, the living with fear – something even worse can happen with the denunciation or separation – as well as the time of life together and the annulment of women in this relationship (Souza & Da Ros, 2006). Such facts help us to understand woman's difficulty in breaking the violent relationship.

It is also worth reflecting on the degree of aversiveness of certain stimuli, because the functionality of this stimulus is initially expressed by weakening a response (Skinner, 2003); however, it is possible to discuss a binary relationship (Hunziker, 2017) in which certain situations at the same time that they are aversive also contain reinforcing aspects. The woman's behavior of maintaining a relationship in which she suffers violence can be understood by the fact that aggression has aversive characteristics – which would weaken probabilities of the relationship continuing – while there are positively reinforcing aspects, such as having a partner (on whom the woman depends financially, has minor children, religious rules or avoidance of social judgments, etc.) which increases the probability of emitting behaviors that maintain a violent or abusive relationship.

The analyses presented so far help us to understand situations of violence, both from the perspective of woman's permanence in this relationship, as well as from the maintenance of aggressive acts by the man, which leads us to reflect on the importance of public policy projects that favor the possibility of specialized assistance to female public, also considering the importance of projects that involve these men for effective changes.

To recognize the social and assistance needs of women in situations of violence, it is essential to understand the relationships they establish with partners, children, family members and the care demands arising from these relationships, such as protection of children and actions to combat abusive use of alcohol and other drugs by partners.

The woman's desire to break the cycle of violence after the denunciation was made or to abandon her life to end the suffering can be attributed to the intensity and perception of the violence suffered, which leads to a lowered self-esteem, the destruction of self-confidence, and an intense psychic suffering.

Changes in the population's health needs, as well as the history of use of alcohol and other drugs, are considered to require implementation of new services and professional performance strategies, in addition to a strictly biological approach, emphasizing also social aspects. It is necessary to incorporate the perspective that the mental health of women and their partners is determined by issues of gender, socioeconomic and cultural conditions, and general health practices and habits.

Clinical Case Report

This work, carried out through an extension project, was developed at the Clinical School of Psychology of the State University of Maringá (UEM) and had 200 participants/year, including men, women, and children involved in violent relationships or legally denounced for conjugal aggression. The consultations took place in individual and group service rooms, which are equipped with chairs, table, stereo, multimedia device, and laptop. For the development of this work, a partnership was established with SETI-PR (General Superintendence of Science, Technology and Higher Education), fifth Court of Women, Childhood and Youth and the Municipal Secretary of Women and aimed to offer women some instruments that would enable them to fight for the consolidation of their rights, including gender as a guiding category for local public policies; to aggressors, the service aimed to enable them to acquire behavioral patterns to resolve conflicts that were incompatible with the aggression. The service was extended to all members participating in family life[2] exposed to the situation of domestic violence.

In order to achieve the objective, the profile of both aggressors and victims of violence was outlined (data from 2018) and then psychological assistance was offered to women in situations of violence, in order to change some factors that make them more vulnerable to aggression, such as staying physically close to the aggressor, not reporting the aggression suffered, having a pattern of submissive behavior, among others, and assisting male aggressors in order to remodel violent

[2]This text does not address the work done with other family members exposed to violence.

behavior patterns. An important factor in the aggressors' permanence in psychological care was the exchange of alternative sentences of community services for the frequency of those sentenced to weekly sessions. Although it is a coercive measure, it was seen, by aggressors, as an advantageous exchange and, if it did not guarantee unconditional adherence to the proposed activities, it enabled the knowledge and recognition of aggression as illegal and subject to legal sanctions, since in first sessions their assaults were assessed by them as a right over women and not as a crime.

Among the data obtained on the behavior of the aggressors, it is found that, of the 21 participating men, the majority (82.1%) uses alcohol or other drugs during the week and, of these, the majority (76%) is more violent when they are under influence of alcohol or other drugs (according to the victims' reports). A small portion (10.9%) would be willing to undergo treatment for alcohol and other drug addiction. This result seems to confirm the rule that emission of aggressive behavior is influenced by alcohol. We cannot state, however, whether the emission of the aggressive behavior is due to the lowering of the assessment of current and future contingencies or to other variables such as the perception of women as vulnerable and submissive.

Of the 21 women in situations of violence who were attended, the majority sought the women's police station within 48 hours after the fact (77.2%); previously separated from the perpetrator of violence (74.3%); previously registered police occurrences (50.7%); they feel they are an isolated person (45.6%) and attribute this feeling to the violence suffered (48.1%); already had psychological or psychiatric treatment prior to that provided by the project (29.8%).

The service with men occurred in a standardized way, constituting a service protocol. In total, twelve weekly sessions of fifty minutes each were conducted for a period of three months. The service was divided into two phases: the first phase consisting of four individual sessions, and the second phase, with eight sessions in groups composed of up to 10 participants. The sessions were conducted by a psychologist and a student, both members of the extension project and guided by the first author of this chapter.

In the first phase, we sought to create a therapeutic bond and collect the client's life and love relationship histories. In the second phase, eight group sessions lasting 1 h and 30 min each were held, coordinated by one of the project professionals with experience in assisting men who committed domestic or intrafamily violence and an intern, and aimed to create conditions for the occurrence and functional analysis of behaviors that are configured as requirements for an adequate and non-violent social performance (Del Prette & Del Prette, 2003; Villa & Del Prette, 2012), these behaviors being: (a) self-knowledge (emotional expressiveness), (b) self-control, (c) empathy, and (d) assertiveness. Each of the skills-themes was approached in two meetings with a theoretical discussion about the target concept or skill and practical activities: identification training or contextual proposition for emission of the behavior or skill.

Women were attended in at least 12 individual sessions and the topics covered were about types of violence suffered, feelings that emerged before, during, and after the episodes of violence, behaviors presented in each episode of violence and in the intervals between each episode, and the way of perceiving both the aggressions, and the social consequences they received, in other words, we seek a functional analysis of women's behavior and the search for viable alternatives to interrupt the cycle of violence suffered by them. Therapists also discussed any topics that these women considered relevant whether or not they were linked to situations of domestic violence.

In the context of Pro-Mulher, it was possible to verify that the majority of abusive men consumed alcohol and/or other drugs and this, as previous studies already describe, seems to have some relation with violent act, although this fact cannot be considered as the variable more relevant or even the one that would trigger the aggression. Considering that this data may show a relationship between drug use and violence in a love relationship, it is necessary to expand studies to understand and analyze culture and cultural practices as a determining part of situations of violence.

With the conclusion of the proposed work, it was possible to verify that the women attended had a higher frequency of assertive verbalizations about their rights and a greater ability to not expose themselves to risk situations by emitting behaviors different from those of submission and agreement initially presented and that culminated in aggression by their partners. Men demonstrated a greater ability to discriminate and report feelings and emotions, presented a greater number of verbalizations about being able to control themselves by emitting behaviors incompatible with those of aggression and demonstrating verbalizations of understanding and empathy with their women. It was not possible to discriminate if the report of self-control was due to the development of empathy with victims or a greater sensitivity to contingencies, in other words, an avoidance of legal punishments.

Final Considerations

The central discussion in this chapter was about violence against women in a romantic relationship, as well as a possible correlation between violence and the use of legal and illegal drugs. Violence against women has a multi-determined explanation, the cultural context, in its cultural practices, directly interferes with the maintenance of these relationships, silencing women in abusive or violent romantic relationships. From these cultural practices, we can point out possible rules that relate drug use and violence. Although there is an understanding that drug use is a risk factor for cases of domestic violence, it is not possible to establish such a correlation as a constant.

The woman's desire to break the cycle of violence (from denunciation and/or separation) seems to be related to the intensity and perception of the violence suffered, which would generate a pattern of behaviors called lowered self-esteem and self-confidence. This pattern would be acquired during the constitution of subjectivity of each woman in particular and would provide the prerequisites for emission of escape and avoidance behaviors effective to eliminate or minimize the possibility of being assaulted.

Data obtained from the population that participated in the Pro-Mulher program indicate that aggression of men against women can be explained by culturally transmitted behavioral patterns, among which are the incentive to drug use, especially licit ones like alcohol, that would generate, for both, women and men, the construction of an image about aggression, as if this would only have occurred because the aggressor was under influence of drug, in other words, it would not be a constant behavioral pattern, but an exception for being "out of mind" or "high". Thus, there was a devaluation of aggression as a learned and maintained behavior due to its consequences in conflict resolution. During the sessions with the aggressor men, it was possible to perceive verbalizations that denoted possession of man over the woman (for example, "it is a lie that I beat women ... I beat only mine"), and that she must be punished when she violates rules imposed by man ("and I hit because she disrespected me"). The work developed proved to be effective in reducing submissive and risky behaviors among women victims of aggression and in increasing defense and assertive exercise of their rights. For men, the behaviors of aggression and non-compliance with protective measures had their frequencies reduced when compared to events described by them in the initial sessions, and verbalizations with negative content about women assaulted by them had a decrease in intensity and frequency when compared with those of initial sessions.

References

Aló, R. M., & Costa, C. E. (2019). Força da resposta e resistência do comportamento à mudança: por que insistimos tanto? In P. S. Guerra, J. H. Almeida, & C. R. X. Cançado (Eds.), *Experimentos clássicos em análise do comportamento*. Instituto Walden4.

Alves, B. M. (1980). *Ideologia e feminismo: a luta pelo voto no Brasil*. Vozes.

Amaral, L., Vasconcelos, T., Sá, F., Silva, A., & Macena, R. (2016). Violência doméstica e a Lei Maria da Penha: perfil das agressões sofridas por mulheres abrigadas em unidade social de proteção. *Revista Estudos Feministas, 24*(2), 521–540. https://doi.org/10.1590/1805-9584-2016v24n2p521

Ariès, P. (1986). *Sexualidade Ocidental*. Brasiliense.

Barros, É., Silva, M., Falbo Neto, G., Lucena, S., Ponzo, L., & Pimentel, A. (2016). Prevalência e fatores associados à violência por parceiro íntimo em mulheres de uma comunidade em Recife/Pernambuco, Brasil. *Ciência & Saúde Coletiva, 21*(2), 591–598. https://doi.org/10.1590/1413-81232015212.10672015

Brasil. (1995). *Convenção Interamericana para Prevenir, Punir e Erradicar a Violência Contra a Mulher*. Retrieved from http://bvsms.saude.gov.br/bvs/publicacoes/convencaobelem1994.pdf

Brasil. (2006). Lei n. 11.340, de 07 de agosto de 2006. *Lei Maria da Penha*. Retrieved from https://www2.senado.leg.br/bdsf/bitstream/handle/id/496319/000925795.pdf.

Das Neves, A. (2017). Uma interpretação analítico-comportamental de aspectos culturais e simbólicos da fogueira de São João. *Perspectivas Em Análise Do Comportamento, 8*(1), 79–96. https://doi.org/10.18761/pac.2016.035

Del Prette, A., & Del Prette, Z. A. P. (2003). *Habilidades sociais, desenvolvimento e aprendizagem: questões conceituais, avaliação e intervenção*. Alínea.

Fonseca, A. M., Galduroz, J. C. F., Tondowski, C. S., & Noto, A. R. (2009). Padrões de violência domiciliar associada ao uso de álcool no Brasil. *Revista de Saúde Pública, 43*(5), 743–749. https://doi.org/10.1590/S0034-89102009005000049

Grossi, M. P. (1995). O Significado da violência nas relações de gênero no Brasil. *Sexualidade, gênero e sociedade, 2*(4).

Guiraldelli, R. (2007). Presença feminina no Mundo do Trabalho: História e Atualidade. *Revista da RET – Rede de Estudos do Trabalho, 1*(1).

Hosbawm, E. J. (2009). *A Era das Revoluções – 1789 – 1948*. Paz & Terra.

Hunziker, M. H. L. (2017). Dogma sobre o controle aversivo. *Acta Comportamentalia: Revista Latina de Análisis Del Comportamiento, 25*(1), 85–100.

Karawejczyk, M. (2013). *As filhas de Eva querem votar: Dos primórdios da questão à conquista do sufrágio feminino no Brasil (c.1850–1932)* (Doctoral dissertation, Universidade Federal do Rio Grande do Sul). Retrieved from https://lume.ufrgs.br/handle/10183/72742

Koerner, A. (2002). Posições doutrinárias sobre direito de família no pós-1988. Uma análise política. In L. Fukui (Ed.), *Segredos de Família*. São Paulo.

Leite, F., Amorim, M., Wehrmeister, F., & Gigante, D. (2017). Violence against women, Espírito Santo, Brazil. *Revista de Saúde Pública, 51*(0). https://doi.org/10.1590/S1518-8787.2017051006815

Matos, M. (1969). Comportamento governado por regras. *Revista Brasileira De Terapia Comportamental E Cognitiva, 3*(2). https://doi.org/10.31505/rbtcc.v3i2.135

Minayo, M., & Deslandes, S. (1998). A complexidade das relações entre drogas, álcool e violência. *Cadernos de Saúde Pública, 14*(1), 35–42. https://doi.org/10.1590/S0102-311X1998000100011

Rabello, P., & Caldas Júnior, A. (2007). Violência contra a mulher, coesão familiar e drogas. *Revista de Saúde Pública, 41*(6), 970–978. https://doi.org/10.1590/S0034-89102007000600012

Sant'Ana, V. L. P. (1995). *Características Comportamentais em Populações Masculinas com Diferentes Orientações Sexuais* (Doctoral dissertation, Universidade de São Paulo).

Skinner, B. F. (2003). *Ciência e comportamento humano*. Martins Fontes.

Souza, P. A., & da Ros, M. A. (2006) Os motivos que mantêm as mulheres vítimas de.

Teles, M. A. A. (2007). *O que são os direitos humanos das mulheres*. Brasiliense.

Tourinho, E. Z. (2009). *Subjetividade e relações comportamentais*. Paradigma.

Vieira, L., Pordeus, A., Ferreira, R., Moreira, D., Maia, P., & Saviolli, K. (2008). Fatores de risco para violência contra a mulher no contexto doméstico e coletivo. *Saúde E Sociedade, 17*(3), 113–125. https://doi.org/10.1590/S0104-12902008000300012

Vieira, L., Cortes, L., Padoin, S., Souza, I., Paula, C., & Terra, M. (2014). Abuse of alcohol and drugs and violence against women: Experience reports. *Revista Brasileira de Enfermagem, 67*(3). https://doi.org/10.5935/0034-7167.20140048

Villa, M. B., & Del Prette, Z. A. P. (2012). *Inventário de Habilidades Sociais Conjugais (IHSC)*. Pearson Clinical Brasil.

violência no relacionamento violento. Revista de Ciências Humanas, 40.

World Health Organization (WHO). (1996). *Global consultation on violence and health*. WHO.

Chapter 17
Challenges of Clinical Behavior Analysis in Legal Substance Use: Alcohol and Tobacco

Fernanda Calixto

Introduction

According to the World Health Organization (2018), five million people die due to smoking-related factors worldwide. Approximately 50 diseases – including cancer, high blood pressure, emphysema, and stroke – relate to the consumption of cigarettes, cigars, and pipes (i.e., tobacco products). Such data place smoking as the world's leading preventable cause of death. WHO data on alcohol consumption are also alarming. As of January 2019, the organization reported that harmful use of alcohol is one of the risk factors with the greatest impact on morbidity and mortality worldwide, associated with 3 million deaths in 2016. Of alcohol-related deaths: 28% are related to those caused by traffic accidents, self-harm, and interpersonal violence; 21% are due to digestive disorders; 19% to cardiovascular diseases; and the remainder are due to infectious diseases, cancer, mental disorders, and other health conditions.

In a national context, according to an estimate by the Brazilian Ministry of Health, 200.000 people die annually because of smoking and this number is likely to remain steady if the prevalence of smokers does not decrease (Ministry of Health/ National Cancer Institute – INCA, 2019a, b). Regarding alcohol consumption in Brazil, the Ministry of Health announced in 2018 through the Global Report on Alcohol and Health[1] that approximately 2.3 million people met the criteria for alcohol dependence within the 12 months preceding data collection. The survey – which

[1] Relatório Global sobre Álcool e Saúde: https://cisa.org.br/index.php/pesquisa/dados-oficiais/artigo/item/71-relatorio-global-sobre-alcool-e-saude-2018

F. Calixto (✉)
Universidade Federal de São Carlos (UFSCAR), São Carlos, SP, Brazil

Centro Paradigma de Ciências e Tecnologia do Comportamento, São Paulo, SP, Brazil

S. M. Oliani et al. (eds.), *Behavior Analysis and Substance Dependence*,
https://doi.org/10.1007/978-3-030-75961-2_17

heard about 17,000 people aged between 12 and 65 across Brazil between May and October 2015 – is considered one of the most thorough for its scope.

Due to their deleterious effects on health, tobacco and alcohol consumption have become a target of public policies and interventions offered by Brazil's healthcare network. The National Tobacco Control Program,[2] for example, has been offered by the country's Unified Health System[3] since the 1980s. Also, in 2007, a decree approved the National Policy on Alcohol[4] that provides measures to reduce its misuse. Anti-smoking laws (Law No. 9294) were also adopted in Brazil aiming to restrict the use and advertising of tobacco products in public places and the media. In addition, Brazilian legislative institutions have enacted laws that restrict the use of alcohol before driving and the publications of advertisements for alcoholic beverages (Brasil, 1996; Article 306 of Law No. 9.503 and Law No. 9.294). These measures show that regulating legal psychoactive substances has been a common governmental measure to control their excessive consumption.

Although these laws and measures aim to regulate alcohol and tobacco (by not allowing smoking in closed public spaces or driving under the influence of alcohol, for instance), the consumption of such substances is considered legal both in national and international contexts. Cigarettes have not been advertised on Brazilian television since 2000, although beer and other alcoholic products are still commonly advertised in the mainstream media.

Alcohol and tobacco are psychoactive substances that have been present in different societies for decades. Elevated consumption rates are related to their addictive effects as well as cultural practices. In general, the power of psychoactive substances resides in their activation of the brain's reward system – i.e., their use causes immediate pleasure – commonly resulting in physical and psychological dependence. Physical dependence can be observed through body changes in the absence of the substance. As an example, we can cite withdrawal crises in which several extremely unpleasant symptoms may be present depending on the drug used. In tobacco withdrawal, the individual commonly experiences nausea, anxiety, and headaches whereas in alcohol, they experience tachycardia, sweating, and tremors, among others. Psychological dependence is observed in cases in which the individual starts presenting habits to ensure the consumption of the substance. In cases of addiction, users commonly direct all their money to using the substance. Their social circles also become predominantly formed by both friends and acquaintances who are users and people who are part of substance-use-related environments.

For causing great direct harm to an individual's health, addiction to psychoactive substances (legal and illegal) is the target of analysis and intervention in clinical behavior analysis. According to behavioral-analytic principles, the pattern understood as "chemical dependence" is learned and governed by the same principles and

[2] Programa Nacional de Controle do Tabagismo.

[3] Sistema Único de Saúde (SUS).

[4] Política Nacional sobre o Álcool.

laws of any behavior (Higgins et al., 1991). Behavioral-analytic therapists thus hold the challenge of identifying from the client's history how such a complex consumption pattern emerged and what variables account for its maintenance.

From the same perspective, smoking and alcohol cessation is unlikely to occur in cases of addiction as consumption is maintained by powerful immediate reinforcers (Rachlin, 2000). We say that a consequence is reinforcing when it increases the probability of evoking a certain class of responses. Regarding the consumption of psychoactive substances, an immediate effect is the physiological changes that the substance causes in the body with the activation of the reward mechanism and dopamine release (Robbins & Everitt, 1996). Such change may suffice to increase the probability of evoking a whole chain of responses that result in access to the substance. In addition, other consequences may control the same responses. Social reinforcers – such as attention and companionship during consumption – can be functionally related to both drinking and smoking. Also, negative reinforcers generally relate functionally to consumption since smoking can eliminate or delay contact with aversive events. For example, users commonly report that drinking reduces anxiety and stress, and increased consumption generally occurs in situations known to be difficult such as family or work-related problems.

We consider addiction a state in which consumption occurs to avoid negative organic effects in the absence of the substance (McLellan et al., 2000). In these cases, physical discomfort such as nausea, body aches, shaking, among others are regarded as craving states when individuals are abstinent. In sum, for every user of psychoactive substances, either a specific or a group of consequences may be maintaining the consumption chain.

A special aspect of alcohol and tobacco – in comparison to other substances such as marijuana and cocaine – is the fact that they are considered legal in Brazil, which influences consumption patterns as well as the possibilities of intervention. This chapter addresses specific challenges observed in clinical behavior analysis interventions regarding the use of legal substances. Due to their overwhelming effects on users' health, alcohol and tobacco constitute the focus of analysis. The following topics will be discussed: (1) Social acceptance; (2) Response Cost in Obtaining and Consuming; and (3) Diverse Pairings and Functions. Lastly, as examples of effective behavioral-analytic interventions, I present one study focused on tobacco and one on alcohol reduction.

Public Opinion – Social Acceptance

In 2017, Venture conducted a survey on the public opinion and morale of legal and illegal drug use in Brazil. Results showed an adverse public opinion in relation to consumption and consumers (41% in feelings of *disgust or hatred* plus *dislike*) and the vast majority were favorable to maintaining the prohibition of commercialization and consumption of crack (94%), cocaine (94%), and marijuana (80%). Despite not directly comparing public opinion between licit and illicit drugs, Venture's

(2017) findings reveal that the consumption of the latter is potentially followed by social punishment since the theme is vastly judged using negative adjectives.

Considering that a group feels repulsion, hatred, or animosity toward a habit (in this case, using illicit drugs) we can say that such consumption is likely to be followed by aversive social contingencies. For example, a mother may threaten to remove reinforcers after discovering or suspecting that her daughter is using marijuana, or even curtailing her freedom by demanding her hospitalization. Regarding the consumption of legal substances, although there are indications of a negative public opinion, results do not show manifestations in favor of its prohibition. This may show that social punishment for the consumption of legal substances, when present, occurs in smaller magnitude compared to illegal ones. For example, despite the enormous harm caused by tobacco to the health of smokers, no institution specializes in hospitalization for compulsive use of cigarettes; whereas, in Brazil, there are legally supported clinics that perform involuntary hospitalization for marijuana addicts.

Opinions can be understood as verbal descriptions of an event. When they point to causal functional relations such as "cocaine should be prohibited", "whoever uses it must be hospitalized or arrested" we are referring to a verbal description of a contingency, aka a rule (Skinner, 1953). In this case, Venture's (2017) findings show that verbal descriptions (i.e., rules) regarding the consumption of illicit substances in Brazil often specify aversive consequences. Considering that rules control both verbal and non-verbal behavior (Matos, 2001), comparatively, the use of licit substances such as alcohol and tobacco is likely to be accompanied by verbal descriptions that specify less aversive consequences.

We must note that the aversiveness of an event is defined by both its historical and present consequences, as well as specific and individual ones (Sidman, 1995). Verbal descriptions – such as "cocaine users must be arrested" –are likely to be ineffective in differentially affecting users' behaviors while having opposite effects in others. On the other hand, Venture's (2017) findings help us differentially understand social judgment toward users of both licit and illicit drugs.

The social acceptance of substances such as alcohol and tobacco consists of a challenge to interventions focused on the reduction of excessive consumption since many cases result in powerful social reinforcers. Reports such as "I knew I would feel miserable the next day, but I didn't want to be the only one not drinking", "I tried to pace myself, but everybody started talking about the cocktails in the menu", "they offered me beer about six times, I declined five of them…", "I want to stop, but everybody in the office smokes after lunch and gossip about the people in the division" are common in the clinical setting and reveal that inadequate behaviors – for being either excessive or harmful – can be acceptable and even encouraged depending on the social context.

Response Effort in Obtaining and Consuming

What is common about the consumption of alcohol and tobacco is how easily they can be accessed and purchased. In Brazil, tobacco products are found in tobacco shops, service stations, bakeries, and grocery stores. Given that cigarettes are consumed in social contexts, another facilitator is the possibility of asking a smoker for a cigarette. Alcohol can be accessed just as (if not more) easily. Alcoholic beverages are sold in bars, restaurants, stores, and service stations, among other establishments, in addition to being present in various social gatherings such as birthdays and celebrations. Illicit substances, however, tend to be sold with more discretion (the dealer quietly stands at a specific place in the club) and in illegal places ("*bocas de fumo*", for instance, which are earmarked places for drug dealing and use in Brazil).

Easy access to licit substances favors a lower response effort, that is, I can get whatever substance I want without major physical or financial efforts. Response cost is usually referred to as the physical, financial, and temporal requirements of a response to enable access to its reinforcers (Alling & Poling, 1995). Having the substance available for purchase in the local market around the corner configures a smaller response cost when compared to having to go to a remote *boca de fumo*, for instance.

According to Weiner (1962), the response effort affects the likelihood of a behavior, so it must be understood as a variable of its function. Experimental behavior analysis studies with humans and non-humans (Alling & Poling, 1995; Luce et al., 1981; Pietras & Hackenberg, 2005) showed that, depending on the response cost, the probability of occurrence of behaviors changes.

Easy access to legal substances is a recurring theme in the definition of policies and, despite maintaining alcohol and tobacco as legal substances, many decisions aim to make the access more difficult, either by restricting authorized retail places, or by increasing taxes and, by extension, the end price of the product. Countries such as Brazil, the United States, and England pose restrictions on authorized locations of tobacco consumption. In California, for example, smoking is prohibited even in several beaches and parks. Regarding costs, a survey carried out in 2018 by Forbes reported that, while a pack costs an average of 2.22 USD in Brazil, it can cost up to 20,14 USD in Australia – country that used taxation as a restriction measure. Recent data indicate that, although price increase may lower the number of smokers (Forbes, 2018), the measure is controversial. Additional data show that, as taxes rise, the purchase of taxed products decreases while black market products become more popular (Exame, 2019). For this reason, Brazil's Ministry of Justice announced in 2019 the possibility of reducing cigarette-related taxes to contain smuggling (O Globo, 2019).

Increasing taxes and restricting consumption places of alcohol, however, has been discussed and adopted very scarcely – mainly occurring for religious reasons. India and the United Arab Emirates, for example, have laws to prevent the commerce and consumption of alcoholic drinks, which raises the price of products and narrows their consumption to touristic contexts only. It is important to mention that the response cost involved in consuming a psychoactive substance is directly related to its social acceptance. Substances with lesser social acceptance – for religious reasons, for example – tend to be related to a higher response cost of obtention.

Such response cost thus configures a challenge to interventions focused on reducing excessive consumption of alcohol and tobacco, as these products can be accessed with little to no effort. Reports such as "it's hard to avoid, because I can buy it right next to the office", "I didn't even have cigarettes on me, but I ended up asking for one in the club", "I felt more like drinking after I saw everyone else doing so" are extremely common in session. Low response cost implies that consumption can easily happen in multiple contexts. Social acceptance also increases the likelihood of drinking in multiple places, in the presence of various people. Given that substance consumption involves respondent and operant processes, an additional challenge – addressed in the next topic – refers to the multiple functions it can have in the life of an individual.

Multiple Pairing and Functions

By asking the client to self-monitor cigarette consumption to understand its controlling variables, we commonly hear reports such as "I smoke when I arrive at work, I smoke another cigarette at break, one before lunch, another one with coffee after I eat … I smoke when I get home after work and at college before class…". In these cases, smoking is clearly related to multiple contexts. Therefore, different events – constantly present in the client's life – are likely to evoke smoking. When analyzing the consequences of smoking, it is not uncommon to find that this behavior has multiple functions.

Control by social reinforcement can be illustrated by the following reports "I asked the guy I found cute for a cigarette at the party yesterday", "I always smoke at break between classes with my classmates", "if you want to know what's going on at the company, just join the people smoking outside". Regarding control of tasks by negative reinforcement we find the following reports: "I need a smoke before I start", "when I finish a document, I have a smoke to gather the courage to continue working on the spreadsheets". Also, behaviors can be controlled by avoidance or escape of covert events, which can be identified in reports such as "I was too nervous, so I had a smoke and I managed to take a breath and relax" and "I already had a headache for staying 5 hours without smoking". Regarding alcohol consumption, drinking is also extremely common in multiple contexts (e.g., at friends' houses, bars, restaurants, celebrations, among others) with multiple functions (e.g., social reinforcement of friends, escape, and avoidance of aversive events).

All reports mentioned previously refer to a single clinical case and they show that this client (a 28-year-old male) habitually smoked at work, college, and home, either alone or in the presence of friends. Regarding the consequences that control smoking, we have both social as well as negative reinforcement (avoidance of tasks, covert states, and nicotine craving). In clinical practice, cases such as the previous one are recurring and they show that therapists must thoroughly analyze variables that may have a function on that client's smoking and drinking habits.

Comparatively, when we analyze environmental variables involved in consuming illegal substances (e.g., cocaine), due to an increased chance of punishment and high response costs, such consumption is likely to be related to specific contexts (e.g., the client reports having a single cocaine dealer and generally uses it when alone or in the presence of other user friends). However, the controlling variables of any behavior are different depending on the learning history. Therefore, users may do cocaine in multiple contexts, with various functions, just as alcohol users may have single, specific controlling variables. However, due to social acceptance and large availability, licit substances are more likely to be consumed with various functions – which consists of an additional challenge while defining effective intervention plans.

Examples of Clinical Behavior Analysis Interventions

In relation to tobacco, the study by Cole and Bonem (2000) demonstrates a procedure based on a functional analysis of smoking. They propose a procedure of gradual nicotine decrease that aims at reducing the aversiveness of substance withdrawal. Two college students participated in the study: Sue (18 years old) and Tom (21), both smokers. The study was held in four 45-minute group therapy sessions and used a multiple component experimental design. In Phase 1 (baseline), participants provided carbon-monoxide (CO) measures and self-monitored smoking rates – which continued to be measured across the study. In Phase 2, participants received tools to register events related to smoking aiming at analyzing it functionally. In Phase 3, the interval between two smoking events progressively increased. In Phase 4, participants were instructed to implement self-management strategies according to the functional analysis in Phase 2, which involved changing antecedent situations functionally related to smoking, as well as the promotion of either alternative or concurrent skills. At the end of Phase 4, participants were re-exposed to baseline conditions. Follow-up measures were collected 14 days and 6 months after the conclusion of the study.

Sue presented a baseline of 6.5 cigarettes a day. She was able to lower daily cigarette consumption to 3.5 during Phases 2 and 3 and maintain it in Phase 4 and baseline regression. CO measures remained close to behavioral ones, except in Phase 3 in which CO measures were higher. Tom smoked 13 cigarettes a day during baseline, progressively lowered to 2 during Phases 2, 3, and 4, maintained Phase 3 performance on baseline regression, but returned to Phase 1 rates during follow-up. Tom's CO measures remained close to behavioral ones across the study. Results showed that the intervention can be considered effective for Sue in lowering by 70% and maintaining low smoking rates at follow up whereas Tom's smoking rates lowered by 60% during the study and failed to remain low during baseline regression.

Results show the importance of understanding the function of smoking and gradually lowering nicotine consumption to decrease the likelihood of aversive states related to withdrawal.

The second study refers to an intervention on Acceptance and Commitment Therapy (ACT) which consists of a contextual functional approach based on the Relational Frame, known as a third-wave therapy. The study was conducted by Thekiso et al. (2015) and aimed to compare the effectiveness of ACT with a standard treatment in reducing both alcohol dependence and anxiety-depression states. Participants were 26 patients with alcohol dependence and minimum age of 18 sorted into two groups. The first one consisted of a five-week protocol with core ACT interventions: Acceptance, Cognitive Diffusion, Being Present, Self as Context, Values, and Commitment Actions (for details, see Hayes et al., 2008). The second one received standard treatment which consisted of psychoeducation about epidemiology, medical complications of alcohol dependence and affective disorders, the interaction between mood and substances, psychotherapy, and pharmacotherapy. Dependent variables were scores on the Beck Depression Inventory (BDI), Beck Anxiety Inventory (BAI), and Obsessive-Compulsive Drinking Scale (OCDS). Follow-up measures were obtained 3 and 6 months after the study concluded. Results showed that patients who received ACT interventions scored significantly lower on BDI and BAI when compared to standard treatment on both follow-up tests as well as on the first follow-up for OCDS. The authors concluded that the intervention based on ACT was effective in lowering both drinking and anxiety-depression states.

Final Considerations

The present chapter aimed to outline some clinical challenges in interventions for licit substance dependence – especially alcohol and tobacco. Both substances are highly consumed worldwide and present multiple deleterious health effects to users. Behavior analysis and the clinical practice based on its principles help us to functionally understand psychoactive drug consumption behaviors and – especially regarding alcohol and tobacco – allow us to analyze and raise hypotheses on the variables involved in their consumption.

Social acceptance of both substances allows us to infer that their consumption is less intensely punished when compared to illicit substances. Low response costs involved in obtaining alcohol and tobacco as well as the scientific findings on response cost allow us to understand why consumption happens in multiple contexts and functionally relates to multiple events. Control exerted by both positive and negative reinforcers in various contexts is presented as an additional challenge that requires a thorough functional analysis prior to defining intervention procedures. Lastly, both experiments described here point to an effectiveness of interventions based on behavioral principles as a safe therapeutic pathway focused on lowering alcohol and tobacco consumption.

References

Alling, K., & Poling, A. (1995). The effects of differing response-force requirements on fixed-ratio responding of rats. *Journal of the Experimental Analysis of Behavior, 63*(3), 331–346. https://doi.org/10.1901/jeab.1995.63-331

Brasil. (1996). *Lei n° 9.294, de 15 de julho de 1996*. Dispõe sobre as restrições ao uso e à propaganda de produtos fumígeros, bebidas alcoólicas, medicamentos, terapias e defensivos agrícolas, nos termos do § 4° do art. 220 da Constituição Federal.

Cole, M. L., & Bonem, M. K. (2000). The A-B-C's of smoking cessation: Using behavioral strategies to help undergraduates stop smoking. *The Behavior Analyst Today, 1*(4), 89–101. https://doi.org/10.1037/h0099893

Exame.(2019,August2).*ETCO:57%doscigarrosvendidosnoBrasilsãoilegais*.Retrievedfromhttps://exame.abril.com.br/negocios/releases/etco-57-dos-cigarros-vendidos-no-brasil-sao-ilegais/

Forbes (2018, September 4). *Quanto custa um maço de cigarro ao redor do mundo*. Retrieved from https://forbes.com.br/listas/2018/09/quanto-custa-um-maco-de-cigarros-ao-redor-do-mundo/

Hayes, S., Pistorello, J., & Biglan, A. (2008). Terapia de Aceitação e Compromisso: modelo, dados e extensão para a prevenção do suicídio. *Revista Brasileira De Terapia Comportamental E Cognitiva, 10*(1), 81–104. https://doi.org/10.31505/rbtcc.v10i1.234

Higgins, S. T., Delaney, D. D., Budney, A. J., Bickel, W. K., Hughes, J. R., & Foerg, F. (1991). A behavioral approach to achieving initial cocaine abstinence. *The American Journal of Psychiatry., 148*, 1218–1224.

Luce, S. C., Christian, W. P., Lipsker, L. E., & Hall, R. V. (1981). Response cost: A case for specificity. *The Behavior Analyst, 4*, 75–80.

Matos, M. A. (2001). Comportamento governado por regras. *Revista Brasileira De Terapia Comportamental E Cognitiva, 3*(2), 51–66. https://doi.org/10.31505/rbtcc.v3i2.135

McLellan, A. T., Lewis, D. C., O'Brien, C. P., & Kleber, H. D. (2000). Drug dependence, a chronic medical illness: Implications for treatment, insurance, and outcome evaluation. *Journal of the American Medical Association, 284*, 1689–1695.

Ministério da Saúde. Instituto Nacional de Câncer (INCA). (2019a). *Convenção Quadro para o Controle do Tabaco*. Retrieved from http//www.inca.gov.br/tabagismo/frameset.asp?Item=cquadro3&link=historico.hm

Ministério da Saúde. Instituto Nacional de Câncer (INCA). (2019b). *Tabagismo no Brasil*. Retrieved from http://www.inca.gov.br/tabagismo/frameset.asp?item=dadosnum&link=brasil.htm.

O Globo. (2019, May 13). *Ministério da Justiça estuda reduzir o imposto do cigarro para conter o contrabando; comunidade médica critica*. Retrieved from https://g1.globo.com/ciencia-e-saude/noticia/2019/05/13/ministerio-da-justica-estuda-reduzir-o-imposto-do-cigarro-para-conter-o-contrabando-comunidade-medica-critica.ghtml

Pietras, C. J., & Hackenberg, T. D. (2005). Response-cost punishment via token loss with pigeons. *Behavioural Processes, 69*(3), 343–356. https://doi.org/10.1016/j.beproc.2005.02.026

Rachlin, H. (2000). *The science of self-control*. Harvard University Press.

Robbins, T. W., & Everitt, B. J. (1996). Neurobehavioural mechanisms of reward and motivation. *Current Opinion in Neurobiology, 6*, 228–236.

Sidman, M. (1995). *Coerção e suas implicações*. Editorial Psy.

Skinner, B. F. (1953). *Science and human behavior*. MacMillan.

Thekiso, T. B., Murphy, P., Milnes, J., Lambe, K., Curtin, A., & Farren, C. K. (2015). Acceptance and commitment therapy in the treatment of alcohol use disorder and comorbid affective disorder: A pilot matched control trial. *Behavior Therapy, 46*(6), 717–728.

Venturi, G. (2017). Consumo de drogas, opinião pública e moralidade: motivações e argumentos baseados em uso. *Tempo Social, 29*(2), 159–185.

Weiner, H. (1962). Some effects of response cost upon human operant behavior. *Journal of the Experimental Analysis of Behavior, 5*(2), 201–208. https://doi.org/10.1901/jeab.1962.5-201

World Health Organization. (2018, September 21). Retrieved from https://www.who.int/news-room/detail/21-09-2018-harmful-use-of-alcohol-kills-morethan-3-million-people-each-year-most-of-them-men

Index

S. M. Oliani et al. (eds.), *Behavior Analysis and Substance Dependence*,
https://doi.org/10.1007/978-3-030-75961-2

D

T